Acute Myocardial Infarction

Books Available in Cardiovascular Clinics Series

Brest	1/1	Hypertensive Cardiovascular Disease
Brest	1/2	Coronary Heart Disease
Downing	2/1	Congenital Heart Disease
Gifford	3/1	Peripheral Vascular Disease
Fowler	6/3	Diagnostic Methods in Cardiology
Vidt	7/1	Cleveland Clinic Cardiovascular Consultations
Brest et al.	7/2	Innovations in the Diagnosis and Management of Acute Myocardial Infarction
Spodick	7/3	Pericardial Diseases
Rahimtoola	8/2	Coronary Bypass Surgery
Rios	8/3	Clinical Electrocardiographic Correlations
Onesti, Brest	9/1	Hypertension
Kotler, Segal	9/2	Clinical Echocardiography
Brandenburg	10/3	Office Cardiology
Castellanos	11/1	Cardiac Arrhythmias: Mechanisms and Management
Engle	11/2	Pediatric Cardiovascular Disease
Rackley	11/3	Critical Care Cardiology
Noble, Rothbaum	12/1	Geriatric Cardiology
Rahimtoola	13/1	Controversies in Coronary Artery Disease
Spittell	13/2	Clinical Vascular Disease
Fowler	13/3	Noninvasive Diagnostic Methods in Cardiology
Goldberg	14/1	Coronary Artery Spasm and Thrombosis
Dreifus	14/2	Pacemaker Therapy
Conti	14/3	Cardiac Drug Therapy
Schroeder	15/1	Invasive Cardiology
Wenger	15/2	Exercise and the Heart, ed. 2
Josephson	15/3	Sudden Cardiac Death
Dreifus	16/1	Cardiac Arrhythmias: Electrophysiologic Techniques and Management
Frankl, Brest	16/2	Valvular Heart Disease: Comprehensive Evaluation and Management
Rackley	16/3	Advances in Critical Care Cardiology
Kotler, Steiner	17/1	Cardiac Imaging: New Technologies and Clinical Applications
Fisk	17/2	The Right Heart
McGoon	17/3	Cardiac Surgery, ed. 2
Mehta	18/1	Thrombosis and Platelets in Myocardial Ischemia
Waller	18/2	Contemporary Issues in Cardiovascular Pathology
David	18/3	Ambulatory Monitoring of the Cardiac Patient
Shaver	19/1	Cardiomyopathies: Clinical Presentation, Differential Diagnosis, and Management
Goldberg	19/2	Coronary Angioplasty
Douglas	19/3	Heart Disease in Women

Acute Myocardial Infarction

Carl J. Pepine, M.D. / Editor

Professor of Medicine
Associate Director, Division of Cardiology
University of Florida
Chief, Cardiology Section
Gainesville Veterans Administration Medical Center
Gainesville, Florida

CARDIOVASCULAR CLINICS

Albert N. Brest, M.D. / Editor-in-Chief

James C. Wilson Professor of Medicine
Director, Division of Cardiology
Jefferson Medical College
Philadelphia, Pennsylvania

F. A. DAVIS COMPANY • Philadelphia

Printed in the United States of America

Last digit indicates print number: 10 9 8 7 6 5 4 3 2 1

NOTE: As new scientific information becomes available through basic and clinical research, recommended treatments and drug therapies undergo changes. The author(s) and publisher have done everything possible to make this book accurate, up-to-date, and in accord with accepted standards at the time of publication. However, the reader is advised always to check product information (package inserts) for changes and new information regarding dose and contraindications before administering any drug. Caution is especially urged when using new or infrequently ordered drugs.

Library of Congress Cataloging in Publication Data

Cardiovascular clinics. 20/1

Philadelphia, F. A. Davis, 1969–
v. ill. 27 cm.
Editor: v. 1- A. N. Brest.
Key title: Cardiovascular clinics, ISSN 0069-0384.
1. Cardiovascular system—Diseases—Collected works. I. Brest, Albert N., ed.
[DNLM: W1 CA77N]
RC681.A1C27 616.1 70-6558
ISBN 0-8036-6858-9 MARC-S

Preface

Few areas in clinical medicine have been associated with as much excitement and undergone as much change over the past several years as acute myocardial infarction. The changes have resulted from important advances in our understanding of the pathophysiology of acute myocardial ischemia and infarction in addition to the development and application of extremely aggressive new approaches to management of these patients. The purpose of this book is to synthesize these advances and place them into perspective for the clinician.

We begin by examining the pathophysiology of acute ischemia, infarction, and postischemic injury. This introductory chapter is followed by chapters that review our new thinking about various clinical aspects of acute myocardial infarction. Many of these topics would have been mentioned scarcely, if at all, in a text written a decade ago on this subject.

The authors have emphasized our new understanding of ischemic injury, infarction, and management while integrating this new information with the prevailing views. Thus, Part 2 includes chapters that discuss three etiologies of acute myocardial infarction: atherosclerotic and nonatherosclerotic coronary artery factors, thrombosis/platelets and other blood factors, and coronary artery spasm.

In the third part, our authors approach diagnosis of acute myocardial infarction from several angles, including discussion of early biochemical markers of myocardial necrosis, radionuclide assessment, silent myocardial infarction, and differences between Q-wave and non-Q-wave infarcts. Following a chapter devoted solely to myocardial infarction in young people and in women, the final section looks at the latest management approaches, including both intracoronary and intravenous thrombolysis as well as other pharmacologic and mechanical interventions, use of beta-adrenergic blockers and conventional drug therapy, and management of arrhythmias. The final chapter examines the process of risk stratification after myocardial infarction, including fundamental aspects of cardiac function as well as comorbid factors as they are determined prior to hospital discharge.

Because of the latest data as well as the different perspectives presented in this volume, *Acute Myocardial Infarction* will provide both the experienced cardiologist and the clinician who has not been concentrating in this area with valuable information.

Finally, I wish to thank all of my colleagues who provided important contributions to this book. Their breadth of experience allows this book to stand alone as a reference source for all of those who are involved in the care of patients with myocardial infarction.

Carl J. Pepine

Editor's Commentary

The last issue of CARDIOVASCULAR CLINICS that was devoted to myocardial infarction was published in 1975. The many evolutions since then include enhanced understanding of pathophysiology (e.g., roles of spasm and thrombosis), new therapeutic interventions (e.g., thrombolytic therapy and angioplasty), and advances in risk profiling (e.g., early exercise testing). The current issue puts into perspective both ongoing advances and conventional approaches to clinical recognition and management of acute myocardial infarction. I am extremely grateful to Carl Pepine for his guidance in the formulation of this issue, and both of us are indebted to the individual authors for their exemplary contributions.

Albert N. Brest, M.D.
Editor-in-Chief

Contributors

Juan Jose Badimon, Ph.D.
Assistant Professor of Medicine
Mount Sinai School of Medicine
New York, New York

Lina Badimon, Ph.D.
Associate Professor of Medicine
Mount Sinai School of Medicine
New York, New York

Barry D. Bertolet, M.D.
University of Florida
College of Medicine
Gainesville, Florida

Albert N. Brest, M.D.
James C. Wilson Professor of Medicine
Director, Division of Cardiology
Jefferson Medical College
Philadelphia, Pennsylvania

L. Maximilian Buja, M.D.
Gill Professor of Pathology
University of Texas
Southwestern Medical Center
Dallas, Texas

Robert P. Byington, Ph.D.
Assistant Professor of Epidemiology
Wake Forest University
Bowman Gray School of Medicine
Center for Prevention Research and Biometry
Winston-Salem, North Carolina

C. Richard Conti, M.D.
Professor of Medicine
Chief, Division of Cardiology
University of Florida
College of Medicine
Gainesville, Florida

Anne B. Curtis, M.D.
Assistant Professor of Medicine
Director, Clinical Electrophysiology
Department of Medicine
Division of Cardiology
University of Florida
Gainesville, Florida

Curt D. Furberg, M.D., Ph.D.
Professor of Medicine
Director, Center for Prevention Research and Biometry
Bowman Gray School of Medicine
Winston-Salem, North Carolina

Valentin Fuster, M.D., Ph.D.
Arthur M. and Hilda A. Master Professor of Medicine
Chief, Division of Cardiology
Department of Medicine
Mount Sinai Medical Center
New York, New York

Robert S. Gibson, M.D.
Professor of Medicine
Co-Director, Cardiovascular Noninvasive Imaging
Director of Stress Testing and
Doppler Echocardiography Laboratories
University of Virginia Medical Center
Charlottesville, Virginia

Sheldon Goldberg, M.D.
Professor of Medicine
Associate Director, Division of Cardiology
Jefferson Medical College
Director, Cardiac Catheterization Laboratory
Thomas Jefferson University Hospital
Philadelphia, Pennsylvania

Scott E. Hessen, M.D.
Division of Cardiology
Jefferson Medical College
Philadelphia, Pennsylvania

James A. Hill, M.D.
Associate Professor of Medicine
Division of Cardiology
University of Florida
College of Medicine
Director, Cardiac Catheterization Laboratory
Shands Hospital at the University of Florida
Gainesville, Florida

Douglas H. Israel, M.D.
Division of Cardiology
Mount Sinai School of Medicine
New York, New York

Deborah A. Jalowiec, M.D.
Instructor of Medicine
Division of Cardiology
University of Florida
College of Medicine
Gainesville, Florida

Charles R. Lambert Jr., M.D., Ph.D.
Assistant Professor of Medicine
Division of Cardiology
University of Florida
Director, Cardiac Catheterization Laboratories
Gainesville Veterans Administration Medical Center
Gainesville, Florida

Michael Mansour, M.D.
Division of Cardiology
University of Florida
Gainesville, Florida

Carl J. Pepine, M.D.
Professor of Medicine
Associate Director, Division of Cardiology
University of Florida
Chief, Cardiology Section
Gainesville Veterans Administration Medical Center
Gainesville, Florida

Peter Puleo, M.D.
Assistant Professor of Medicine
Bugher Foundation Center for Molecular Biology
Baylor College of Medicine
Director of the Coronary Care Unit
Ben Taub General Hospital
Houston, Texas

Charles E. Rackley, M.D.
Anton and Margaret Fuisz Professor of Medicine
Division of Cardiology
Georgetown University Medical Center
Washington, D.C.

Robert Roberts, M.D.
Professor of Medicine
Chief, Cardiology
Director, Bugher Foundation Center for Molecular Biology
Baylor College of Medicine
Houston, Texas

Allan M. Ross, M.D.
Professor of Medicine
Director, Division of Cardiology
George Washington University Medical Center
Washington, D.C.

Lowell F. Satler, M.D.
Clinical Assistant Professor of Medicine
Division of Cardiology
Georgetown University Medical Center
Washington, D.C.

Bernardo Stein, M.D.
Division of Cardiology
Mount Sinai School of Medicine
New York, New York

Bruce F. Waller, M.D.
Professor of Pathology and Medicine
Director, Section of Cardiovascular Pathology
Research Associate, Krannert Institute of Cardiology
Indiana University School of Medicine
Indianapolis, Indiana

James T. Willerson, M.D.
Rogers Professor of Medicine
Director, Cardiology Division
University of Texas Southwestern Medical Center
Parkland Memorial Hospital
Dallas, Texas

Andrew Zalewski, M.D.
Assistant Professor of Medicine
Division of Cardiology
Jefferson Medical College
Cardiac Catheterization Laboratory
Thomas Jefferson University Hospital
Philadelphia, Pennsylvania

Contents

PART 1

Introduction

CHAPTER 1

New Concepts in the Pathophysiology of Acute Myocardial Ischemia and Infarction and Their Relevance to Contemporary Management

Carl J. Pepine, M.D.

Important advances have occurred over the past decade in our understanding of the pathophysiology of acute myocardial ischemia and infarction. These advances have resulted in application of very aggressive new approaches to the management of this condition. The purpose of this chapter is to review these advances and discuss their importance in the care of patients with acute myocardial infarction.

PATHOPHYSIOLOGY OF ACUTE MYOCARDIAL ISCHEMIA, INFARCTION AND POSTISCHEMIC INJURY

The basic process by which coronary artery disease produces morbidity and mortality and alters quality of life is *acute myocardial ischemia.* A period of myocardial ischemia precedes and encompasses all acute myocardial infarctions, and a thorough understanding of ischemia is essential to the recognition and management of the patient with suspected infarction. Traditionally, it has been accepted that ischemia results when the myocardial oxygen supply–demand relationship decreases to a critical level in a region of the left ventricle.

Myocardial Oxygen Supply

Myocardial oxygen supply is determined largely by oxygen delivered via coronary blood flow. Myocardial oxygen delivery is controlled by processes that regulate coronary flow, which are determined by hydraulic, rheologic, and anatomic factors. The hydraulic factors include: coronary perfusion pressure, which is related to systemic blood pressure, left ventricular diastolic pressure, and the time

Table 1–1. Coronary Anatomic Factors Involved in the Pathophysiology of Acute Myocardial Infarcation

Coronary atherosclerosis	Thrombus
Coronary artery spasm	Platelet aggregation
Endothelial dysfunction	Leukocytes
Plaque rupture/hemorrhage/disruption	Eicosanoids

available for diastolic coronary flow (i.e., diastolic filling period); the latter is inversely related to heart rate. The rheologic factors center on blood viscosity, which relates closely to the concentration of large molecules in the blood, such as fibrinogen.

The coronary anatomic factors are determined by the caliber of both the arteriolar bed and the larger coronary arteries (Table 1–1). Coronary vessel caliber is controlled by a number of processes, some of which influence vascular smooth muscle activation. These processes may act via medial receptors or recently demonstrated endothelial mechanisms. Some vasoconstrictors (e.g., alpha-adrenergic agonists) and vasodilators (e.g., $beta_2$-adrenergic agonists) act via medial receptors to reduce or increase blood flow, respectively. Increases in blood flow may be induced also by acetylcholine, histamine, 5-HT, ADP (from aggregating platelets), thrombin, and other agents that activate specific endothelial receptors to induce formation of endothelium-derived relaxation factor (EDRF) or factors. These factors in turn cause dilatation of coronary arteries.[1–3] In addition, one EDRF also has platelet antiaggregation activity.[4] One of these EDRFs appears to be nitric oxide, which, in turn, mediates local coronary smooth muscle relaxation via activation of guanylate cyclase to generate cyclic guanosine monophosphate (cGMP).[5,6] This local *endogenous* mechanism for coronary dilation appears to act in a manner analogous to *exogenously* administered organic nitrates. This common mechanism to generate nitric oxide and coronary dilation suggests possibilities for replacement of defective EDRF by nitrates.

Atherosclerosis (thickened intima and plaque) and probably other processes such as coronary artery spasm and inflammation appear to be associated with various degrees of endothelial cell dysfunction and reduced production of EDRF. In animal studies, 15 minutes of smooth muscle activation, which did produce narrowing severe enough to reduce blood flow, and noncritical external constriction have resulted in marked morphologic changes in endothelial cells and platelet deposition.[7–9] EDRF is also released by increases in shear stress at the endothelial surface, which occurs when coronary blood flow rate increases.[1,2] The resultant "flow-dependent dilation" of the large capacitance arteries that occurs probably serves to optimize their impedance characteristics in the setting of arteriolar dilation.[10] When a stenosis becomes flow-limiting, an important stimulus for EDRF release from less diseased adjacent endothelium is lost. Reduction in EDRF release will favor further reduction of artery size, and loss of platelet antiaggregant activity will favor platelet aggregation and deposition as well as vasoconstriction.[11] This development is particularly important in eccentric stenoses where a segment of relatively normal endothelium is in series with the atherosclerotic plaque. Thus, the aforementioned circumstances set the stage for defective coronary dilation, constriction, and thrombotic occlusion, which may lead to acute myocardial infarction.

Coronary artery constriction (i.e., coronary artery spasm) is well documented as a cause of acute ischemia leading to myocardial infarction in patients with variant angina.[12–14] Coronary artery constriction probably plays an important role in the development of myocardial infarction in some other patients with unstable angina pectoris.[15] Coronary constriction is probably operative also in a larger number of patients who have signs and symptoms of ischemic injury that wax and wane in the early stage of myocardial infarction.[16] Intermittent coronary occlusion has been documented during continuous intracoronary infusion of streptokinase given in the early stages of acute myocardial infarction. In such patients, nitrate administration during reocclusion may re-establish patency of the infarct-related artery in many cases. Thus, defective coronary artery dilation, constriction, and thrombosis, in various combinations, all probably operate in the peri-infarction period in many patients.

Inflammatory and immunologically-mediated injury, and white blood cells in particular, seem also to play a role in acute myocardial infarction in many animal models and are likely to be invoked in human myocardial ischemic injury and infarction as well.[17] Increased subendothelial infiltration of the proximal coronary artery segments with monocytes and macrophages has been found in patients dying within 1 month of presentation with unstable angina.[49] In patients with coronary arteritis and even coronary atherosclerosis, a role for macrophages and neutrophils has been suggested. White cells, via the release of leukotrienes, may constrict coronary arteries and also activate platelets.[18] Neutrophils are also a rich source of oxygen-derived free radicals, and this mechanism may contribute to membrane damage during reoxygenation in both coronary vessels and myocardium.[19] In addition, leukocyte plugging of small capillaries has been found in animal infarction models.[20] Structurally-damaged endothelium (e.g., plaque rupture, fissuring, and disruption) also enhances platelet adherence and aggregation, fibrin deposition, leukocytes, and nonocclusive thrombus formation. Lack of normal endogenous relaxation–dilatation mechanisms, thrombotic elements, and local release of vasoactive substances (such as thromboxane, serotonin, and leukotrienes) set the stage for reduction of regional blood flow to limit myocardial oxygen delivery in a variable fashion.

Some noncoronary factors, such as arterial blood oxygen content, hemoglobin concentration, and blood viscosity, also play important roles in reducing myocardial oxygen supply in selected patients.

Myocardial Oxygen Demand

Myocardial oxygen demand is determined largely by heart rate, contractility, and left ventricular systolic wall stress. The latter is related directly to peak left ventricular pressure (i.e., systolic blood pressure in the absence of outflow obstruction) and chamber size, and inversely to left ventricular wall thickness.

Duration

The duration as well as the amount of myocardium involved in the supply–demand imbalance are of central importance in determining the clinical outcome of a given acute ischemic episode. Brief periods (i.e., several minutes) of temporary decrease in the myocardial oxygen supply–demand ratio promptly result in *transient ischemia.* Transient ischemia involving myocardium of a critical size is usually associated with reversible changes of the electrocardiogram (ST segment shifts), myocardial blood flow distribution (thallium 201 perfusion defects), contractile function (dyskinesis), and occasionally a subjective sensation perceived as chest discomfort (angina pectoris and its equivalents). This form of ischemic injury is usually reversible without detectable consequences. More prolonged (i.e., 30 to 40 min) disruptions in the myocardial supply–demand balance, such as those resulting from occlusive coronary thrombus and perhaps very frequent but brief episodes, such as those resulting from coronary spasm and/or nonocclusive thrombus, have the potential to result in myocardial injury that has both reversible and permanent components (i.e., necrosis or dysrhythmias like ventricular tachycardia), which may lead to death. When evidence for myocardial necrosis can be detected, acute myocardial infarction is said to have evolved. However, with newer and more sensitive laboratory methods, the demarcation between severe reversible ischemic injury and permanent injury or infarction has become less distinct.

Terms like "acute coronary insufficiency" and "threatened myocardial infarction" have been used to describe patients with prolonged severe ischemic injury without evidence for infarction. Under some conditions, severe ischemic injury may produce severe myocardial dysfunction without evidence for necrosis, which persists for a long period after the supply–demand imbalance has been corrected. Functional, ultrastructural, and biochemical abnormalities in the myocardium may persist for some time despite restoration of perfusion. It may be days or even weeks before function is restored to normal. This phenomenon has been called *"myocardial stunning."*[21] Stunning occurs in situations in which there is acute occlusion of a vessel, which then opens to reperfuse that myocardial region. Myocardial stunning is probably closely related to *"postischemic"* or *"reperfusion-related injury"* encountered in animal models of acute infarction undergoing early reperfusion. The term *"hibernating myocardium"* refers to a more chronic reduction in blood flow or increase in oxygen demand to cause ischemia. The myocardium then down-regulates or depresses its function to match its oxygen supply.[22] This new concept of "down-regulation" of myocardial function is an attractive contrast to the prevailing view that the myocardium always "commits suicide" when its blood flow is reduced to a critical level for a long period. With this new concept, a new equilibrium between myocardial oxygen supply and demand is established at a level that does not result in myocardial necrosis. However, any additional impairment in oxygen supply or increase in oxygen demand may disturb this new equilibrium and prompt progression to necrosis. Positron emission tomography (PET) can identify hibernating myocardial segments by quantification of blood flow and regional metabolic activity.[23,24] Thus, hypokinetic areas that have reduced blood flow but are metabolically active have been shown to lose their dysfunction after successful reperfusion by bypass surgery.

This revision of classic concepts has important implications relative to coronary bypass surgery, silent ischemia, ischemic cardiomyopathy, and the prolonged period of depressed regional myocardial function encountered after successful reperfusion of patients with acute myocardial infarction using thrombolytic drugs or percutaneous transluminal coronary angioplasty (PTCA). Induction, detection, and control over this down-regulation of myocardial function should offer many attractive avenues for management of myocardial infarction patients prior to or after reperfusion.

ISCHEMIA AND INFARCTION DURING DAILY LIFE: THE ROLE OF SILENT ISCHEMIA AND INFARCTION

Silent myocardial ischemia and infarction have been subjects of considerable study recently because of their high frequency in out-of-hospital studies. Myocardial ischemia occurring in ambulatory patients has been characterized during normal daily life using the electrocardiogram as an objective marker for ischemia. Findings from these studies have led to modification of traditional views of the pathophysiology of ischemia and infarction. Previously, characterization of transient ischemic episodes was based upon reports of angina and studies done in the exercise laboratory. The prevailing view suggested that ischemic episodes were painful and evoked by increasing myocardial oxygen demands that exceed a fixed ceiling of myocardial oxygen supply reserve, which could be utilized by the coronary circulation to meet the increasing demands (Fig. 1–1). Conversely, absence of pain, despite physical effort to increase myocardial oxygen demands, implied a sense of security in that ischemia and infarction were not present even in the setting of severe coronary artery disease. This view with respect to effort was then modified, except for the rare patient with variant angina.

Recent studies in ambulatory patients, however, have now documented many more silent than painful ischemic episodes in symptomatic individuals without exercise stress.[25] There is considerable overlap in the duration and severity of abnormalities related to the extent and magnitude of ischemic myocardial dysfunction. Because silent ischemic episodes go unrecognized, many episodes are prolonged (>20 min) and may even be associated with signs of more severe ischemic dysfunction when compared with ischemic episodes accompanied by pain. Silent myocardial infarction is also recognized to occur frequently, but the precise relationship between silent transient ischemia and infarction is not yet known.[26]

Studies from several groups of patients indicate that ischemia (silent plus painful) occurs during the day in a characteristic *circadian pattern*. Ischemic

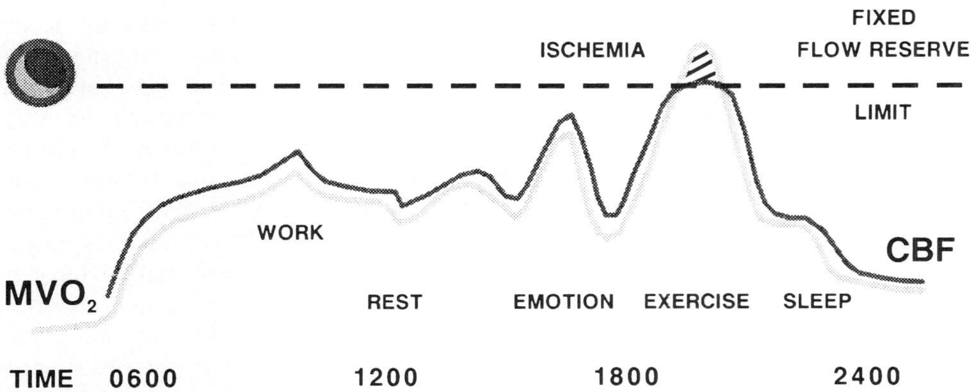

Figure 1–1. Traditional concept of transient myocardial ischemia held that coronary atherosclerosis produces a fixed limit to coronary flow reserve. Accordingly, patients can increase myocardial oxygen demands (MVO_2) over a wide range of cardiac work, including emotional and exercise activities. These demands are met by appropriate increases in coronary blood flow (CBF) until MVO_2 increases exceed the fixed flow reserve and ischemia occurs.

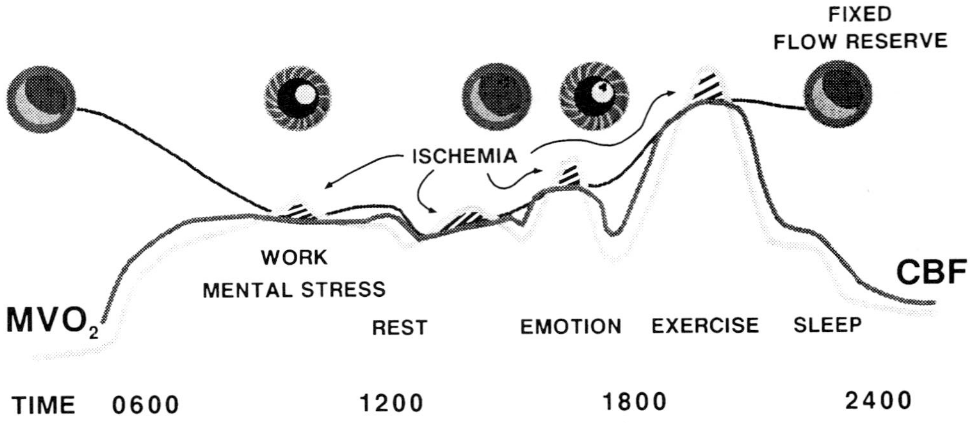

Figure 1–2. Revised concept of myocardial ischemia suggests that the coronary artery stenosis must be considered as a dynamic rather than a fixed obstruction. Changes in smooth muscle tone, in platelet aggregability, and other factors alter lumen size so that flow reserve is variable. When sympathetic nervous system activation takes place in the early morning, increases in myocardial oxygen demand may or may not be met by appropriate increases in coronary flow. Cognitive and emotional activities seem to increase myocardial oxygen demand above the level that can be met by coronary flow. Hence, this revised concept explains how ischemia may occur many times throughout the day and tends to be most frequent in the hours after waking and is infrequent in the late evening and early morning hours. Here, ischemia is most often silent.

activity tends to cluster in a time period that begins shortly after waking, peaks at about noon, and decreases in frequency throughout the afternoon and evening (Fig. 1–2). In the period between midnight and waking, ischemic episodes are very infrequent. This pattern relates temporally to the period of heightened sympathetic activation, and $beta_1$-adrenergic blockade prevents most of this morning increase in ischemia.[27] The aforementioned diurnal pattern is the same as that observed for acute myocardial infarction, sudden cardiac death, and ventricular ectopic activity in the postinfarction patient.[28] These latter events are also modified by beta blockade, supporting the concept of a common pathogenesis.

The majority of silent ischemic episodes detected out-of-the-hospital occur at heart rates lower than those reached by these same patients at the onset of ischemia during an exercise test.[29] This finding, coupled with data indicating that heart rate and blood pressure are not significantly changed just *before the onset* of ischemia, suggests that myocardial oxygen delivery is reduced at times when most ischemic episodes occur in a free-living environment. Analysis of activities at the onset of acute myocardial ischemia, as well as infarction, reveals that relatively low-level activities are often associated with these episodes. This finding supports the heart rate and blood pressure data suggesting a lower myocardial oxygen demand at the onset of silent episodes in the ambulatory environment compared with ischemia induced in the exercise laboratory. These results imply that myocardial oxygen supply, or the functional reserve of the coronary arteries, is not fixed but varies throughout the day, depending on previously unrecognized "stressors." Stressors present in the daily life of these patients that have been identified as important triggers of ischemia include mental activity associated with cognitive tasks (e.g., mental arithmetic), cold exposure, and cigarette smoking (see Fig. 1–2).

In addition, continuous electrocardiographic monitoring studies, in either the coronary care unit or ambulatory setting, indicate that heart rate increases during the actual ischemic episode regardless of the presence or absence of pain. This rise in heart rate appears, in part, mediated by $beta_1$-adrenergic activity and increases myocardial oxygen demands while limiting the time available for diastolic coronary blood flow. Therefore, this heart rate increase would be expected to increase the magnitude and duration of an ischemic episode. The foregoing findings suggest that dynamic changes in coronary artery size, in addition to changes in oxygen demand, may play an important role in the pathogenesis of ischemia and infarction.

Strong evidence has emerged to indicate that characteristics of these ischemic episodes are important determinants of prognosis. Frequent and prolonged episodes of silent ischemia at low heart rates, as encountered in unstable angina and postinfarction patients, identify a subset of patients at high risk for acute myocardial infarction and sudden death.[30–32] Recent data in apparently stable patients with angina show a similar association between outcome and ischemic activity detected during daily life.[33] There is new evidence to suggest that this transient ischemic activity may be a clinical marker for coronary artery endothelial dysfunction and that it identifies a patient subset with an unstable ischemic syndrome that may not be manifested by pain. In contrast, ischemia occurring only at high heart rates, such as those reached during high-level exercise tests, appears to identify a patient subset at relatively low risk for myocardial infarction and death. This type of ischemic response may serve as a marker for the patient subset with relatively normal coronary endothelial function, which is indicative of a more stable ischemic syndrome and better outcome.

Silent myocardial infarction is an important problem that occurs in many patients and must have been preceded by a silent ischemic episode. Recently, silent infarction has been shown to have prognostic implications, in terms of subsequent death and reinfarction, that are the same as painful myocardial infarction.

CONTEMPORARY MANAGEMENT OF MYOCARDIAL INFARCTION

This improved understanding of the pathophysiology of myocardial ischemic injury has led to many advances in the management of myocardial infarction. Management of the patient with known or suspected acute myocardial infarction, however, still begins with *confirmation of the diagnosis.* The diagnosis of acute myocardial infarction has been enhanced by development and application of more sensitive and specific techniques to evaluate myocardial injury and necrosis. The diagnosis is still most often suspected based upon a clinical presentation characterized by prolonged, severe chest pain. It is now well accepted, however, that at least 25 percent to 30 percent of all myocardial infarctions may be *silent or unrecognized* and detected only from interval electrocardiograms that reveal residual Q wave evidence of infarction. The true frequency of silent infarction probably is underestimated inasmuch as a proportion of those patients with painful infarctions who develop Q waves are known to have these Q waves disappear over time. In addition, patients who die suddenly or in the early hours after infarction are often classified as sudden deaths rather than acute myocardial infarction. Finally, there are an unknown number of patients who have both clinically and electrocardiographically silent or unrecognized myocardial infarctions. Many with non-Q-wave myocardial infarction may fit this category.

Based on the foregoing, a high index of suspicion is clearly needed for the diagnosis of myocardial infarction. The practitioner, however, needs to know that clinical findings may be neither present nor typical in many cases. So in all cases the diagnosis of acute myocardial infarction must be documented by laboratory tests. These tests routinely include electrocardiographic and serum enzyme evidence for myocardial necrosis.

Over the past decade, *serum enzyme* and *isoenzyme levels* have become the final arbiters by which acute myocardial necrosis is documented and the diagnosis of myocardial infarction is confirmed or excluded. Because of the poor sensitivity of single measurements of cardiac enzyme levels, these assays should not be used alone in the emergency room to exclude myocardial infarction. If myocardial infarction is suspected, creatine kinase (CK) and its MB fraction should be measured at admission and again approximately 12 to 24 hours later. If reperfusion is suspected, sampling should be at approximately 8 hours. If myocardial infarction may have occurred more than 20 hours before the initial evaluation, then levels of lactic dehydrogenase isoenzyme may increase the diagnostic accuracy and should be measured. Properly used, these assays are remarkably sensitive, but as with all tests, optimal interpretation requires insight into technical pitfalls and other causes of misleading results.

Avid infarction imaging with 99m-technetium-labeled pyrophosphate provides a window for detection of ischemic myocardial damage, which extends to approximately 7 days. This test may be useful in selected cases both to confirm the diagnosis and to localize the extent. Nonreversible thallium 201 or rubidium 82 perfusion defects, using single photon or positron emission tomographic (i.e., SPECT or PET) imaging during and after stress, may assist in diagnosis of myocardial infarction in selected cases. Advances in PET imaging using other labels allows accurate separation of perfused but *non-viable* regions from *viable* myocardial regions, as noted earlier in discussion of hibernating myocardium. This technology is now available in many centers and will soon be much more widely available. The information obtained has very important application relative to reperfusion and *reperfusion-related injury* and may even help in answering the clinical question of who should receive reperfusion therapy.

There are now considerable data supporting the importance of classifying patients with acute myocardial infarction by those who develop Q waves on the electrocardiogram and those who do not. The term *"Q wave infarction"* has replaced the term "transmural infarction" because morphologic studies have shown a lack of specificity of Q waves as a marker for infarction involving all layers of myocardium. The term *"non-Q-wave infarction"* has replaced "subendocardial infarction" also because of lack of morphological limitations to this region. Patients with non-Q-wave infarction, however, represent an increasing proportion of myocardial infarctions identified. This increase may be due to improved sensitivity and wider application of CK-MB assay and possibly because some current treatments (e.g., calcium antagonists, beta blockers, nitrates) of patients with chronic recurrent or acute ischemia actually limit injury and prevent development of Q wave infarction. Patients with *non-Q-wave infarction* appear to behave as though they have had partial reperfusion. They have smaller infarctions and reduced early mortality compared with those who have Q wave infarctions. They, however, also appear to be a higher risk for early reinfarction, angina, and perhaps death compared with patients who have Q wave infarctions. Patients with non-Q-wave infarction also have a relatively low likelihood of totally occlusive coronary artery thrombus at early angiography compared with those who have Q wave infarction. Thus, the patient with non-Q-wave infarction has a greater likelihood of having a patent but highly stenosed infarct-related coronary artery and limited initial myocardial damage to the region served by that artery. But this non-Q-wave infarction patient has a high likelihood of residual or recurrent ischemia with its attendant risks (i.e., recurrent ischemia, myocardial infarction, and death).

Treatment of Acute Myocardial Infarction

Treatment of acute myocardial infarction has undergone remarkable evolution over the past several years as a result of many important developments. The pathophysiology of acute myocardial infarction has been clarified. It has been shown that coronary artery thrombus is present in most patients presenting with Q wave myocardial infarction.[34] Early administration of thrombolytic agents in the form of direct (urokinase), indirect (streptokinase), and tissue type (rtPA) plasminogen activators, results in lysis of coronary thrombus in a high frequency of patients.[35–38] Reperfusion associated with early thrombolysis or PTCA is associated with improved left ventricular function. Additionally, a large data base derived from several well-controlled trials indicates that a substantial proportion of patients who receive early thrombolytic therapy alone or in combination with PTCA have significant prolongation of life.[36,39,40] Male patients $\leq$65 years old receiving thrombolytic agents intravenously *within 4 hours* of the onset of symptoms associated with acute anterior myocardial infarction comprise the group most likely to have improved survival. Data concerning recurrent ischemia and/or reinfarction or infarct extension after apparently successful thrombolysis and the role for more definitive revascularization procedures such as early PTCA or coronary artery bypass grafting (CABG) are evolving. These revascularization strategies may be used alone or in combination with thrombolysis.

Although there is still dispute concerning the precise role of these treatments and their timing in management of evolving myocardial infarction, there is general agreement in several important areas. One is that the mortality in patients after acute myocardial infarction, both early and late, is directly influenced by the degree of ensuing left ventricular dysfunction, which in turn is dependent upon the size of the infarcted myocardial region. Accordingly, limiting the extent of damage would be expected to lessen the impact of myocardial infarction in terms of left ventricular dysfunction and should, therefore, improve subsequent survival and function. It is also agreed that the time interval between the onset of abrupt coronary occlusion and institution of any intervention to limit ischemic injury and infarction-related damage should be relatively brief. This time interval probably should not exceed 6 hours and should be shorter when possible. Treatments that may extend this interval are needed, and it is rational to attempt to reduce myocardial oxygen requirements and improve collateral blood flow during this period. Finally, severe residual stenosis persisting after successful reperfusion limits the potential for reperfusion-related salvage of tissue and impairs recovery of ventricular function. Therefore, some definitive procedure to deal with important residual stenosis, when present, is an essential part of the followup management of patients undergoing thrombolytic therapy. More prolonged infusion of thrombolytic agents followed by PTCA and CABG at some point after thrombolysis (either early or later) needs to be considered when important residual stenoses are detected. Although the timing of these revascularization procedures is not yet resolved, they are likely to be effective adjuncts to the use of thrombolysis alone in order to provide maximal salvage of injured myocardium, preserve ventricular function, and extend survival.

Recently, considerable evidence has been presented to suggest that reperfusion is associated with some degree of *postreperfusion* or *postischemic injury* that extends and amplifies the myocardial damage.[41,42] The precise contribution of this postreperfusion injury process to the outcome of human myocardial infarction is unknown at present. Data from animal models, however, suggest that postreperfusion injury may be both important and extensive in terms of the recovery of function of the left ventricle. *"Free-radical-induced injury," calcium overload* or gain, and microvascular and membrane disruption all appear to be involved. Animal models suggest that pretreatment with calcium antagonists and beta blockers may be important to help limit injury. Use of free-radical scavengers (super-oxide dismutase) or prevention of more reactive hydroxy- free-radical formation (e.g., deferoxamine) at the time of reperfusion appears to be effective in animal models. Whether or not these agents are effective in human infarction has not yet been determined, but clinical trials are underway.

The process of *remodeling of the left ventricle* during acute myocardial infarction is much more complex than previously thought. At least two general processes appear to be involved in the regional shape distortion of the left ventricle that occurs after myocardial infarction. *"Infarct expansion"* is a term used to describe the increase in ventricular size that occurs as a result of acute stretching, thinning, and dilation of the injured myocardial segment.[43,44] An expansion index derived from the echocardiogram may be determined as the relationship between the infarct- and non-infarct-containing segment. Infarct expansion plays an important role in the pathogenesis of persistent cardiac dilation, aneurysm formation, ventricular septal defect, and free-wall rupture.[45] Infarct expansion and rupture are more common in Q wave infarction and first infarctions. Recently, use of indomethacin or ibuprofen for postinfarction pericarditis has been suggested as a risk factor for infarct expansion.[46,47] "Extension" and "reinfarction" are used interchangeably to signify additional new damage due to repeat myocardial injury that may occur after the initial injury. Extension is usually documented by new CK-MB rise and is associated with a hospital mortality many times higher than that encountered in those without extension. Recurrent ischemia, ST segment depression, and history of previous infarction are risk factors for extension.[48] "Thinning" relates to the thickness of the infarcted segment. A thinning index may be determined from the echocardiogram as the relationship between infarct and normal wall thickness. An understanding of these processes will help to determine which patients develop ventricular septal rupture and/or aneurysm.

IMPLICATIONS FOR MANAGEMENT OF PATIENTS WITH ACUTE MYOCARDIAL INFARCTION

The foregoing concepts suggest a need for classification of patients with acute myocardial infarction according to the timing of the process of infarction in order to provide optimal management. Patients presenting in the *initial hours* of infarction, for perhaps up to 6 hours after onset of symptoms, should be considered to be in the *evolving infarction phase* between reversible and nonreversible ischemic injury. The period from approximately 6 hours after the onset of symptoms until hospital discharge represents a period when little or no reversible injury is present. This interval may be thought of as the *completed infarction phase.* The time period from discharge until approximately 8 to 12 weeks represents further healing until the infarcted segment reaches maximal strength, and risk of events begins to plateau. During this period the patient slowly attempts to return to this previous level of activities. This may be thought of as the *convalescent* phase.

EVOLVING MYOCARDIAL INFARCTION

Management of the patient in the evolving phase should focus on several important initial steps: (1) attempting to confirm the diagnosis, (2) assessing possible risks and benefits of early reperfusion therapy, and (3) choosing the type(s) of therapy (e.g., restore coronary blood flow, reduce myocardial oxygen demand, or both) (Table 1–2). The latter decision is very important as an attempt to reduce the rate at which myocardial tissue is irreversibly damaged and to restore function to irreversibly damaged tissue. Inasmuch as no form of reperfusion therapy is immediately effective in restoring blood flow, this treatment may extend the time interval for reperfusion to be effective and permit more optimal myocardial salvage. These three initial steps in the approach to management must be completed rapidly and usually at the bedside to avoid delays and are in addition to conventional management.

The clinical diagnosis is usually rapidly confirmed by the presence of ECG changes (acute ST segment elevation, loss of R wave amplitude, Q waves, or

Table 1–2. Objectives in Management of Acute Myocardial Infarction

A. Evolving Infarction Phase (onset to 6 hr)
   1. Admit to CCU
   2. Confirm diagnosis
   3. Assess risks and benefits of thrombolytic therapy
   4. Attempt to preserve ischemic myocardium
B. Completed Infarction Phase (>6 hr to just before discharge)
   1. Prevent complications
   2. Identify patients who are at early high risk
   3. Initiate secondary prevention
C. Convalescent Infarction Phase (predischarge evaluation to 8 weeks)
   1. Risk assessment
   2. Begin rehabilitation
   3. Continue secondary prevention

pathological T wave changes) and, on occasion, elevated CK levels. The serious risks of thrombolytic therapy are largely limited to bleeding and allergic reactions. Candidates must not have a history of recent bleeding (6 weeks), peptic ulcer disease, stroke or surgical procedures. Previous exposure to streptokinase is also a contraindication to its reuse because it is highly antigenic; shortly after its use, high titers of antibodies to it are found. Other risk factors that may limit benefits include severe hypertension, recent central vascular invasive procedures, and comorbid conditions (e.g., advanced age, cancer) which are likely to reduce life expectancy to a greater extent than acute myocardial infarction.

Conventional management of the patient with known or suspected evolving myocardial infarction should consist of admission to the coronary care unit, with electrocardiographic and frequent blood pressure monitoring. Low-risk patients can probably be admitted directly to intermediate-type care units. Oxygen and intravenous analgesic agents are still recommended but without convincing documentation of their benefit. Intravenous anticoagulation with heparin should be strongly considered in patients without contraindications for anticoagulation. In particular, those with large anterior infarctions, heart failure, large hearts, or atrial fibrillation should be anticoagulated unless contraindications are present. In patients receiving thrombolytic agents that produce a "systemic lytic state" (e.g., rtPA, streptokinase), heparin use should be delayed. In this phase, arrhythmias must be recognized and treated promptly to prevent a deleterious rise in myocardial oxygen demand (tachyarrhythmia) or decrease in myocardial oxygen supply (bradyarrhythmia). Fever also must be treated promptly to prevent a rise in myocardial oxygen demand. Other drug therapies include *intravenous nitroglycerin* in an attempt to improve coronary collateral flow, dilate coronary arteries, reverse coronary spasm, and reduce myocardial oxygen demands. Intravenous administration of *beta-adrenergic blockers* followed by oral use to reduce myocardial oxygen consumption and preserve ischemic myocardium should be considered also. These latter drugs have been shown to be very beneficial and should be employed unless there are contraindications.

Decisions relative to *thrombolytic therapy* center around rtPA and may also include use of streptokinase or urokinase in some cases. A number of newer, more clot-specific second- and third-generation (acylated streptokinase, pro-urokinases, FAB-urokinase, FAB-streptokinase, and PEG-coated streptokinase) fibrinolytic agents may be capable of inducing thrombolysis with relatively little associated fibrinogen degradation and, therefore, may cause less bleeding. They are undergoing clinical investigation in the United States and abroad. These agents were developed on the theory that they will activate only plasminogen that is bound to fibrin in preformed thrombus. Also, the use of various combinations of thrombolytic agents may provide possible synergy and more rapid and efficient thrombolysis.

In this phase, coronary angiography should be reserved for those patients who are at risk of losing a substantial mass of myocardium, judged from clinical features such as pulmonary congestion or cardiogenic shock owing to left ventricular dysfunction and perhaps those with extensive electrocardiographic changes indicative of anterior-septal or anterior-lateral myocardial infarction. In selected patients with severe hemodynamic impairment, use of the intra-aortic balloon pump and coronary angiography followed by PTCA or CABG should also be considered.

Completed Myocardial Infarction

This phase includes the period from approximately 6 hours after onset to the predischarge evaluation. Decisions made relative to management in this phase should be contingent upon an estimate of short-term prognosis. If prognosis is judged to be poor on the basis of clinical findings and noninvasive estimates of left ventricular function or signs and/or symptoms of continued ischemia are present, and if it is thought that the outcome may be improved by urgent revascularization, then coronary angiography is indicated. Although cardiac catheterization can be done safely, the risks and complications of CABG appear to be greater in the patient with recent infarction than in those who have depressed left ventricular function without recent infarction. Therefore, it is preferable, when possible, to allow healing and compensatory changes to occur over 2 to 3 weeks before proceeding to bypass surgery. Hence, when possible, such patients should have invasive studies postponed until the convalescent phase. There is general agreement, however, that patients experiencing hemodynamic compromise, congestive heart failure with associated findings to suggest rupture of the intraventricular septum, acute mitral regurgitation, or pseudoaneurysm at any time in the postinfarction period should undergo emergency cardiac catheterization with appropriate angiographic studies. Most such events occur within the first week following infarction. Over the past several years, reports suggest that *early* surgical intervention for ventricular septal rupture results in substantially improved survival compared with later intervention. In such patients undergoing catheterization and surgery, use of the intra-aortic balloon pump and intravenous nitroprusside often improves hemodynamic dysfunction and may reduce risks associated with these procedures. The information needed from catheterization studies in this phase is a precise estimate of residual left ventricular function, evaluation of associated mitral insufficiency, and determination of the extent and severity of coronary artery disease.

Approximately 10 percent to 15 percent of acute myocardial infarction patients will develop signs and/or symptoms of acute unstable ischemia within the first week after onset of infarction. When *unstable postinfarction angina* develops within the first week and remains refractory to medical therapy, there is a high risk of recurrent myocardial infarction or death occurring during hospitalization. In addition, such patients have very high mortality within 6 months. Early coronary angiography is clearly indicated, with a consideration of prompt revascularization if warranted.

Convalescent Infarction Phase

This phase begins just before hospital discharge and continues to approximately 8 weeks. During this phase, pre- and post-discharge *risk assessment* is initiated and *rehabilitation* takes place also. Risk assessment is made from clinical (e.g., age, previous myocardial infarction, heart failure, ventricular arrhythmias) and noninvasive findings.

The average mortality rate for the first year after discharge for acute infarction ranges from approximately 6 percent to 10 percent. The obligation of the physician in this phase is to identify those patients who may be at higher risk. Prognosis, in my opinion, is best judged on the basis of extent of left ventricular dysfunction, history of ischemic heart disease before infarction, and presence of inducible myocardial ischemia. This judgment can be made in most patients without cardiac catheterization. Risk is clearly increased in patients with postinfarction angina or exercise tests identifying ischemia, reduced ejection fraction, signs and symptoms of heart failure, and frequent or complex ventricular arrhythmias as well as those with non-Q-wave myocardial infarction. The physician's obligation is to identify such patients and recommend coronary angiography and revascularization options if appropriate, in an attempt to modify this risk.

The single most important factor related to subsequent risk is residual left ventricular function, and I believe that a noninvasive assessment of left ventricular ejection fraction should be done in all postinfarction patients. I use radionuclide imaging or quantitative two-dimensional echocardiography just prior to discharge. Patients with an ejection fraction ≥50 percent have an exceedingly low event rate over the next 5 years. Patients with ejection fractions <20 percent have an exceedingly high event rate but also they have a very high surgical mortality. Therefore, unless findings indicative of ventricular aneurysm are present, the evaluation should probably stop in those with poor left ventricular function (ejection fractions <20 percent). An exception to this recommendation would be the patient who has signs and symptoms of severe heart failure and who is a candidate for cardiac transplantation. Patients with ejection fractions >20 percent should undergo predischarge, symptom- or heart-rate-limited exercise testing to attempt to identify ischemia, using the electrocardiographic, tomographic thallium 201 perfusion or radionuclide ventriculographic responses. In patients with angina or laboratory findings suggesting ischemia (ST segment depression ≥1 mm, reversible thallium perfusion defect, or reduction in ejection fraction or regional wall motion) during relatively low-level exercise and those who have signs or symptoms of left ventricular failure or those with non-Q-wave myocardial infarction, coronary angiography is indicated. In addition, those with moderate to severe left ventricular dysfunction (ejection fraction ≤40 percent) associated with significant ventricular arrhythmias also should be considered for coronary angiography.

Treatment in this phase should consist of beta blockers, if they have not been initiated previously, provided contraindications are not present, and aspirin. Both of these agents have the potential to reduce events in patients following myocardial infarction and should be continued for at least 2 years or longer. Intense risk factor modification directed at secondary prevention is also in order.

SUMMARY

Acute myocardial infarction is one of the most challenging and changing areas in clinical medicine. This introduction should provide both an overview and necessary background for the clinician to make full use of the remaining chapters in this monograph.

REFERENCES

1. Rubanyi, GM, Romeo, CJ, and Vanhoutte, PM: Flow induced release of endothelium-derived relaxing factor. Am J Physiol 250:H1145, 1986.
2. Pohl, U, Holtz, J, Busse, R, et al: Crucial role of endothelium in the vasodilator response to increased flow in vivo. Hypertension 8:37, 1986.

3. Vanhoutte, PM: Vascular physiology: The end of the quest? Nature 327:459, 1987.
4. Azuma, H, Ishikawa, M, Sekizaki, S, et al: Endothelium-dependent inhibition of platelet aggregation. Br J Pharmacol 88:411, 1986.
5. Palmer, RMJ, Ferrige, AG, and Moncada S: Nitric oxide release accounts for the biological activity of endothelium-derived relaxing factor. Nature 327:524, 1987.
6. Murad, F: Cyclic guanosine monophosphate as a mediator of vasodilation. J Clin Invest 78:1, 1987.
7. Joris, I and Majno, G: Endothelial changes induced by arterial spasm. Am J Pathol 102:346, 1981.
8. Kurgan, A, Gertz, SD, and Wajnberg, RS: Intimal changes associated with arterial spasm induced by periarterial application of calcium chloride. Exp Mol Pathol 39:176, 1983.
9. Gertz, DS, Uretsky, G, Rebecka, S, et al: Endothelial cell damage and thrombus formation after partial arterial constriction: Relevance to the role of coronary artery spasm in the pathogenesis of myocardial infarction. Circulation 63:476, 1981.
10. Bassenge, E and Stewart, DJ: Differential effects of isosorbide-5-mononitrate on epicardial coronary arteries and relevant hemodynamic parameters: Special aspects of nitrate action. In Julian, DG, Rittinghausen, R, and Uberbacher, HJ (eds): Mononitrates II. Springer-Verlag, New York, 1987, pp 13–19.
11. Folts, JD, Gallaggher, K, and Rowe, FF: Blood flow reductions in stenosed canine coronary arteries: Vasospasm or platelet aggregation. Circulation 65:248, 1982.
12. Roberts, WC, Curry, RC, Isner, JM, et al: Sudden death in Prinzmetal's angina with coronary spasm documented by angiography. Analysis of three necropsy patients. Am J Cardiol 50:203, 1982.
13. Walling, A, Waters, DD, Miller, D, et al: Long-term prognosis of patients with variant angina. Circulation 76:990, 1987.
14. Nakamura, M, Takeshita, A, and Nose, Y: Clinical characteristics associated with myocardial infarction, arrhythmias, and sudden death in patients with vasospastic angina. Circulation 75:1110, 1987.
15. Biagini, A, Mazzei, MG, Carpeggiani, C, et al: Vasospastic ischemic mechanism of frequent asymptomatic transient ST-T changes during continuous electrocardiographic monitoring in selected unstable angina patients. Am Heart J 103:13, 1982.
16. Hackett, D, Davies, G, Chierchia, S, et al: Intermittent coronary occlusion in acute myocardial infarction. N Engl J Med 317:1055, 1987.
17. Engler, R: Consequences of activation and adenosine-mediated inhibition of granulocytes during myocardial ischemia. Fed Proc 46:2407, 1987.
18. Mullane, KM, Salmon, JA, and Kraemer, R: Leukocyte-derived metabolites of arachidonic acid in ischemia-induced myocardial injury. Fed Proc 46:2422, 1987.
19. Simpson, PJ, Mickelson, JK, and Lucchesi, BR: Free radical scavengers in myocardial ischemia. Fed Proc 46:2413, 1987.
20. Schnid-Schoenbein, GW: Capillary plugging by granulocytes and the no-reflow phenomenon in the microcirculation. Fed Proc 46:2397, 1987.
21. Braunwald, E and Kloner, RA: The stunned myocardium: Prolonged, postischemic ventricular dysfunction. Circulation 66:1146, 1982.
22. Braunwald, E and Rutherford, JD: Reversible ischemic left ventricular dysfunction: Evidence for the "hibernating myocardium." J Am Coll Cardiol 8:1467, 1986.
23. Marshall, RC, Tillisch, JH, Phelps, ME, et al: Identification and differentiation of resting myocardial ischemia and infarction in man with positron computed tomography[18], F-labeled fluorodeoxyglucose and N-13 ammonia. Circulation 67:766, 1983.
24. Tillisch, J, Brunken, R, Marshall, R, et al: Reversibility of cardiac wall-motion abnormalities predicted by positron tomography. N Engl J Med 314:884, 1986.
25. Pepine, CJ: Clinical aspects of silent myocardial ischemia in patients with angina and other forms of coronary heart disease. Am J Med 80:25, 1986.
26. Kannel, WB and Abbott, RD: Incidence and prognosis of unrecognized myocardial infarction: An update on the Framingham Study. N Engl J Med 311:1144, 1984.
27. Imperi, GA, Lambert, CR, Coy, K, et al: Effects of titrated metoprolol on silent myocardial ischemia in ambulatory patients with coronary artery disease. Am J Cardiol 60:519, 1987.
28. Tofler, GH, Brezinski, D, Schafer, AI, et al: Concurrent morning increase in platelet aggregability and the risk of myocardial infarction and sudden cardiac death. N Engl J Med 316:1514, 1987.
29. Muller, JE, Ludmer, PL, Willich, SN, et al: Circadian variation in the frequency of sudden cardiac death. Circulation 75:131, 1987.

30. Gottlieb, SO, Weisfeldt, ML, Ouyang, P, et al: Silent ischemia predicts infarction and death during 2 year follow-up of unstable angina. J Am Coll Cardiol 10:756, 1987.
31. Nademannee, K, Intarachot, V, Josephson, MA, et al: Prognostic significance of silent myocardial ischemia in patients with unstable angina. J Am Coll Cardiol 10:1, 1987.
32. Johnson, SM, Mauritson, DR, Winniford, MD, et al: Continuous electrocardiographic monitoring in patients with unstable angina pectoris: Identification of high-risk subgroup with severe coronary disease, variant angina, and/or impaired early prognosis. Am Heart J 103:4, 1982.
33. Rocco, MB, Barry, J, Campbell, S, et al: Circadian variation of transient myocardial ischemia. J Am Coll Cardiol 7:191A, 1986.
34. DeWood, MA, Spore, J, Notske, R, et al: Prevalence of total coronary occlusion during the early hours of transmural myocardial infarction. N Engl J Med 303:897, 1980.
35. Kennedy, JW, Ritchie, JK, Davis, KB, et al: Western Washington randomized trial of intracoronary streptokinase in acute myocardial infarction. N Engl J Med 309:1477, 1983.
36. Gruppo Italiano per lo Studio della Streptochinasi nell'Infarto Miocardico (GISSI): Effectiveness of intravenous thrombolytic treatment in acute myocardial infarction. Lancet 1:397, 1986.
37. The ISAM Study Group: A prospective trial of intravenous streptokinase in acute myocardial infarction (ISAM): Mortality, morbidity, and infarct size at 21 days. N Engl J Med 314:1465, 1986.
38. Guerci, AD, Gerstenblith, G, Brinker, JA, et al: A randomized trial of intravenous tissue plasminogen activator for acute myocardial infarction with subsequent randomization to elective coronary angioplasty. N Engl J Med 317:1613, 1987.
39. White, HD, Norris, RM, Brown, MA, et al: Effect of intravenous streptokinase on left ventricular function and early survival after acute myocardial infarction. N Engl J Med 317:850, 1987.
40. ISIS Steering Committee: Intravenous streptokinase given within 0–4 hours of onset of myocardial infarction reduced mortality in ISIS-2. Lancet 1:502, 1987.
41. Weisfeldt, ML: Reperfusion and reperfusion injury. Clin Res 35:13, 1987.
42. Bolli, R, Zhu, W, Hartley, CJ, et al: Attenuation of dysfunction in the postischemic 'stunned' myocardium by dimethylthiourea. Circulation 76:458, 1987.
43. Hutchins, GM and Bulkley, BH: Infarct expansion versus extension: Two different complications of acute myocardial infarction. Am J Cardiol 41:1127, 1978.
44. Schuster, EM and Bulkley, BM: Expansion of transmural myocardial infarction: A pathophysiologic factor in cardiac rupture. Circulation 60:1532, 1979.
45. Eaton, LH and Bulkley, BH: Expansion of acute myocardial infarction: Its relationship to infarct morphology in a canine model. Circ Res 49:80, 1981.
46. Rostami, A, Basualdo, CA, and Jugdutt, BI: Does indomethacin or ibuprofen therapy for postinfarction pericarditis cause myocardial infarct expansion? (abstract). Clin Res 33:222A, 1985.
47. Boden, WE and Sadaniantz, A: Ventricular septal rupture during ibuprofen therapy for pericarditis after acute myocardial infarction. Am J Cardiol 55:1631, 1985.
48. Muller, JE, Rude, RE, Braunwald, E, et al: Myocardial infarct extension: Occurrence, outcome and risk factors in the multicenter investigation of limitation of infarct size. Ann Intern Med 108:1, 1988.
49. Sato, T, Takebayashi, S, and Kohchi, K: Increased subendothelial infiltration of the coronary arteries with monocytes/macrophages in patients with unstable angina: Histological data on 14 autopsied patients. Atherosclerosis 68: 191, 1987.

CHAPTER 2

Changing Outcome in Acute Myocardial Infarction

Lowell F. Satler, M.D.
Charles E. Rackley, M.D.

In 1968, a surprising epidemiologic phenomenon emerged: after decades of increase, mortality rates from ischemic heart disease in the United States began to decline. Between the years 1968 and 1976, the rates declined by 21 percent,[1-3] and additional data suggest that the decline continued in the years 1976 to 1980.[1-3] Although the single most important contributing factor in this reduction remains unclear, one of the possible components is a reduction in mortality due to acute myocardial infarction. The purpose of this chapter is to examine the role of pharmacologic, mechanical, and other supportive interventions designed to limit infarct size and to decrease mortality.

DEVELOPMENT OF THE CORONARY CARE UNIT

The earlier coronary care units were designed specifically to detect fatal arrhythmias so that prompt resuscitation could be provided. It is estimated currently that the incidence of primary ventricular fibrillation after hospital arrival is 4.5 percent among these patients.[4] Pooled data suggest that 94 percent are resuscitated successfully originally and about 88 percent survive to leave the hospital.[4] If coronary care units significantly reduce the mortality associated with malignant ventricular ectopy in about 5 percent of patients, one would expect that it would be simple to demonstrate their effectiveness in reducing mortality in acute infarction. Randomized trials, however, have challenged the efficiency of the coronary care unit. Mather and coworkers[5] evaluated 1895 patients and then randomized 24 percent of them to home versus hospital care. At followup 330 days later, survival was actually better among patients randomized to home care. Hill and associates[6] evaluated 500 patients treated by a hospital-based medical team that was sent to the patient's home as soon as possible after the onset of potential myocardial infarction (MI) symptoms. After 2 hours of observation at home, 70 percent of patients were randomized to home versus hospital care. At followup 6 weeks later, mortality was 11 percent for the hospital group and 13 percent among the home group. Despite these negative results, the coronary care unit goals have expanded beyond arrhythmia prophylaxis and treatment to become the center of all efforts to control ischemia and limit infarct size.

THE IMPORTANCE OF ARRHYTHMIA PROPHYLAXIS

Prophylactic anti-arrhythmic therapy[7,8] has been used to reduce mortality. The use of lidocaine was supported by studies suggesting a reduction in the incidence of ventricular fibrillation (VF) associated with acute MI. Lie and colleagues[7] documented a significant reduction in the incidence of VF; however, mortality was similar between the groups. More recently, Dunn and coworkers[8] failed to demonstrate any reduction in the incidence of VF; and because the toxicity of lidocaine may outweigh its benefit, prophylactic use has been challenged. The use of prophylactic lidocaine may be most valuable in facilities with poor monitoring capabilities.[9]

HEMODYNAMIC MONITORING

The prognosis and the clinical status are related to both the cardiac output and wedge pressure[10,11] (Table 2–1). Although the use of the pulmonary artery catheter often results in significant changes in therapy, there has been no clinical evidence that its application alters mortality.[12] Its major benefit may be the reduction of iatrogenic errors by providing immediate hemodynamic evidence for or against a pharmacologic intervention.

NITRATES

Nitrates have been shown in both clinical and experimental infarction to improve left ventricular function, thus increasing cardiac output and reducing filling pressure.[13,14] In addition, by reducing blood pressure and relieving coronary spasm, they reduce oxygen demand and increase coronary flow.[14,15] Vasodilators, however, may also have adverse effects. Reflex tachycardia may increase cardiac work and reduced arterial pressure may decrease coronary artery blood flow to ischemic myocardium.[16]

To determine the net effects of these treatments, several trials of intravenous nitrates in acute MI have been conducted[17–26] (Table 2–2). Owing to the small size of the studies, none of them likely would have been able to detect a moderate

Table 2–1. Relationship of Clinical Status to Cardiac Output and Wedge Pressure

Subset	PCW >18	CI <2.2 liters/min/m^2	Mortality (%)
I	−	−	3
II	+	−	9
III	−	+	23
IV	+	+	51

PCW = pulmonary capillary wedge; CI = cardiac index.

Table 2–2. Mortality in Randomized Nitrate Trials in AMI[39]

Trial	Nitrate	Deaths: Allocated Nitrate	Deaths: Allocated Control	Two Sided p Value
Hockings[17]	NP	7/25 (28%)	9/25 (36%)	NS
Durrer[18]	NP	9/163 (6%)	20/165 (12%)	<0.05
Cohn[19]	NP	69/407 (17%)	77/405 (19%)	NS
Chiche[20]	NTG	3/50 (6%)	8/45 (18%)	NS
Bussman[21]	NTG	4/31 (13%)	12/29 (41%)	<0.02
Flaherty[22]	NTG	11/56 (20%)	11/48 (23%)	NS
Nelson[23]	NTG	0/14 (0%)	0/14 (0%)	NS
Jaffe[24]	NTG	4/57 (7%)	2/57 (4%)	NS
Lis[25]	NTG	5/64 (8%)	10/76 (13%)	NS
Jugdutt[26]	NTG	24/154 (16%)	44/156 (28%)	<0.01
TOTAL		136/1021 (13.3%)	193/1020 (18.9%)	<0.001

NP = nitroprusside; NTG = nitroglycerin.

reduction in mortality. Yusuf and associates[27] recently combined data from 10 trials of patients randomized to intravenous nitrates in acute MI, and they found a striking 35 percent reduction in mortality. Although these promising results represent an overview of trials that were not separately persuasive, the evidence appears significant enough to justify routine nitrate use.

GLUCOSE–INSULIN–POTASSIUM

Agents that could provide metabolic support for the ischemic myocardium and, in addition, might prevent damage caused by ischemia have not been fully explored to date. The only promising therapeutic intervention is the intravenous administration of a glucose–insulin–potassium solution, which has demonstrated a reduction of infarct size, both by itself[28] and in combination with reperfusion interventions,[29] as well as a reduction in mortality[30] (Fig. 2–1). Its mechanism of

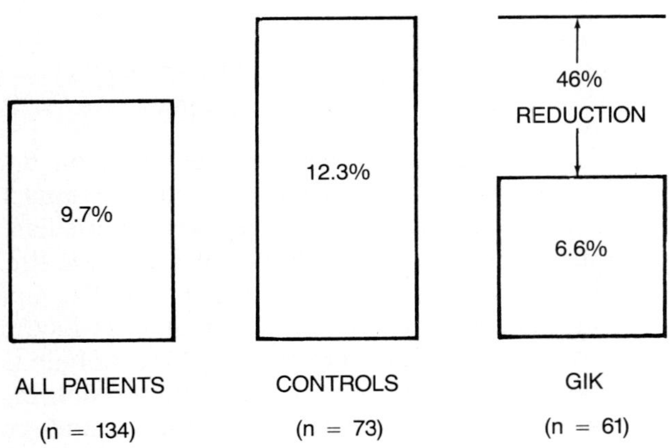

Figure 2–1. Hospital mortality in infarct patients.

action has remained unclear, although it has been postulated that it provides the metabolic substrate required at the time of active ischemia when the anaerobic myocardium switches over from free fatty acids to glucose.[31] Glucose–insulin–potassium metabolically antagonizes catecholamines by decreasing fatty acid production.[32]

BETA BLOCKERS

Profound reductions in long-term mortality following MI have been documented using timolol,[33] metoprolol,[34] and propranolol[35] when these drugs were started within weeks after infarction and continued for years. Most studies involving early (within 4 hour) use of beta blockers have suggested a reduction in infarct size,[36,37] whereas the use of beta blockers administered late has shown no such benefit. Two large scale mortality base studies, ISIS[38] (atenolol) and MIAMI[39] (metoprolol), have demonstrated clear salutary effects of beta blocker in at least some subgroups, which may be related to a decreased incidence of myocardial rupture.[40]

CALCIUM CHANNEL BLOCKERS

The rationale for using calcium channel blockers to reduce mortality includes: (1) reduced incidence of coronary spasm[41]; (2) improved coronary blood flow to the ischemic zone[42]; (3) reduced oxygen demand; and (4) protection of ischemic cells by inhibition of intracellular calcium accumulation.[43] Despite these theoretical advantages, clinical trials have been disappointing. In the Nifedipine Angina Myocardial Infarction Study,[44] patients were randomized to nifedipine or placebo at an interval of 4.6 hours from the onset of symptoms. Infarct size was identical in both groups but 2-week mortality was significantly higher in the nifedipine group. In the Norwegian Nifedipine Study,[45] 227 patients were treated within 12 hours of onset of infarction. No difference in infarct size or mortality was noted. The Danish Multicenter Group[46,47] that studied verapamil in acute myocardial infarction reported the results of a randomized trial in 1436 patients. Mortality at 6 months was 12.8 percent in the verapamil group, compared with 13.9 percent in the placebo group ($p = NS$).

PHARMACOLOGIC AND MECHANICAL REVASCULARIZATION

The rationale for reperfusion interventions is based on definitive angiographic and operative studies of DeWood and colleagues,[48] who documented that acute thrombotic occlusion of the coronary artery is the immediate event leading to myocardial infarction. Early and rapid thrombolysis should limit the range of ischemic injury and the extent of subsequent infarction. This approach should allow for better preservation of myocardial function and a reduction in mortality.

It has now become apparent that intravenous thrombolytic therapy administered very early is best, as shown in large studies using 1.5 million units of streptokinase given over a period of 60 minutes. These studies include completed trials in Italy (GISSI),[49] the Netherlands,[50] West Germany (Intravenous Streptokinase

Table 2–3. Trials of IV STK in the Treatment of Myocardial Infarction

	Mortality			
Trial	**SK Group (%)**	**Control Group (%)**	**Reduction (%)**	**p Value**
GISSI (Italy)[49]	10.7	13.0	18	<0.0002
Netherlands[50]	8.6	15.9	46	0.01
ISAM (West Germany)[51]	5.2	6.5	20	NS
Western Washington[52]	6.3	9.7	35	NS
New Zealand[53]	2.5	12.9	81	0.012
ISIS-2 (Great Britain)[54]	8.0	12.0	33	

in Acute Myocardial Infarction—ISAM),[51] the United States (Western Washington Study),[52] and New Zealand,[53] as well as the ongoing ISIS Study in Great Britain (International Studies of Infarct Survival—ISIS-2)[54] (Table 2–3). Even in the studies that showed no overall difference in mortality,[51,52] the data indicated important effects of therapy (i.e., higher global and regional ejection fractions 3 to 4 weeks after the administration of streptokinase,[51] and a significant 2-year difference in survival in treated patients with anterior wall infarctions[52]). Impressive data were provided by the GISSI trial,[49] in which 11,806 patients had a reduction in overall mortality of 18 percent at 3 weeks, with more advantages observed the earlier treatment was begun, and a maximum reduction of 47 percent in 1277 patients treated within 1 hour. In addition to its impressive effect on mortality, intravenous streptokinase has been shown in randomized placebo-controlled trials to improve myocardial function,[51–53] presumably by limiting the area of ischemia and infarction. Similarly, the beneficial effect on pre-discharge ejection fraction of the infusion of single-chain tissue plasminogen activator[55] also could reasonably be expected to translate into a survival benefit. Recent data also suggest that anisoylated plasminogen streptokinase activator complex (APSAC) may provide survival expectations that exceed those achieved with streptokinase. Administration of APSAC in high doses by means of short infusions given over a period of 2 to 5 minutes has produced reperfusion rates of 50 percent or more[56]; a recent study comparing APSAC with placebo[57] found an overall reduction in mortality of 48 percent in patients treated up to 6 hours after the onset of pain.

The relatively safe and effective use of streptokinase in coronary care units, as well as community hospitals, suggests that all thrombolytic agents will find broad application in the management of acute myocardial infarction. The best candidates for such therapy are patients in the earliest phase, especially within 4 hours after the onset of pain. The many patients who will be cared for in hospitals without facilities for performing invasive coronary procedures should benefit from thrombolytic therapy to the same degree reported in the GISSI studies.[49] Alternatively, patients who are transported to centers with coronary catheterization facilities and facilities for invasive procedures[58–60] are more likely to be managed by thrombolytic therapy, followed by angiography, and perhaps angioplasty or surgery. Thrombolytic therapy will therefore be used either alone or in combination with other techniques for vascular reperfusion, depending on the hospital setting and the prevailing attitudes about rational, long-range management.

SUMMARY

Beta blockers, glucose–insulin–potassium, nitrates, and thrombolytic interventions have been demonstrated to reduce the mortality of acute MI. Because of the number of interventions available, it will become progressively more difficult to isolate their additional benefits. The next challenge will be to determine the ideal combination of interventions to limit infarct size maximally in the context of early reperfusion, thereby limiting reperfusion injury and further improving salvage.

REFERENCES

1. Cooper, R, Stamler, J, Dyer, A, et al: The decline in mortality from coronary heart disease, U.S.A., 1968–1975. J Chronic Dis 31:709, 1978.
2. Kannel, WB and Thom, TJ: Implications of the recent decline in cardiovascular mortality. J Cardiovasc Med 4:983, 1979.
3. Stern, MP: The recent decline in ischemic heart disease mortality. Ann Intern Med 91:630, 1979.
4. Goldman, L and Batsford, WP: Risk–benefit stratification as a guide to lidocaine prophylaxis of primary ventricular fibrillation in acute myocardial infarction: An analytic review. Yale J Biol Med 52:455, 1979.
5. Mather, HG, Morgan, DC, Pearson, NG, et al: Myocardial infarction: A comparison between home and hospital care for patients. Br Med J 1:925, 1976.
6. Hill, JD, Hampton, JR, and Mitchell, JRA: A randomised trial of home-versus-hospital management for patients with suspected myocardial infarction. Lancet 1:837, 1978.
7. Lie, KI, Wellens, HJ, van Capelle, FJ, et al: Lidocaine in the prevention of primary ventricular fibrillation: A double-blind, randomized study of 212 consecutive patients. N Engl J Med 291:1324, 1974.
8. Dunn, HM, McComb, JM, Kinney, CD, et al: Prophylactic lidocaine in the early phase of suspected myocardial infarction. Am Heart J 110:353, 1985.
9. Wyman, MG and Hammersmith, L: Comprehensive treatment plan for the prevention of primary ventricular fibrillation in acute myocardial infarction. Am J Cardiol 33:661, 1974.
10. Forrester, JS, Diamond, G, Chatterjee, MB, et al: Medical therapy of acute myocardial infarction by application of hemodynamic subsets (first of two parts). N Engl J Med 295:1356, 1976.
11. Forrester, JS, Diamond, G, Chatterjee, MB, et al: Medical therapy of acute myocardial infarction by application of hemodynamic subsets (second of two parts). N Engl J Med 295:1404, 1976.
12. Robin, ED: The cult of the Swan-Ganz catheter. Ann Intern Med 103:445, 1985.
13. Franciosa, JA, Gulha, NH, Limas, CJ, et al: Improved left ventricular function during nitroprusside infusion in acute myocardial infarction. Lancet 1:650, 1972.
14. Shell, WE and Sobel, BE: Protection of jeopardized ischemic myocardium by reduction of ventricular afterload. N Engl J Med 291:481, 1974.
15. Conti, CR: Nitrate therapy for ischaemic heart disease. Eur Heart 6(SupplA):3, 1986.
16. Jugdutt, B: Myocardial salvage by intravenous nitroglycerin in conscious dogs: Loss of beneficial effect with marked nitroglycerin-induced hypotension. Circulation 68:673, 1983.
17. Hockings, BEF, Cope, GD, Clarke, GM, et al: Randomized controlled trial of vasodilator therapy after myocardial infarction. Am J Cardiol 48:345, 1981.
18. Durrer, JD, Lie, KI, van Capelle, FJL, et al: Effect of sodium nitroprusside on mortality in acute myocardial infarction. N Engl J Med 306:1121, 1982.
19. Cohn, JN, Franciosa, JA, Francis, GS, et al: Effect of short-term infusion of sodium nitroprusside on mortality rate in acute myocardial infarction complicated by left ventricular failure. Results of a VA Cooperative Study. N Engl J Med 306:1129, 1982.
20. Chiche, P, Baligadoo, SJ, and Derrida, JP: A randomized trial of prolonged nitroglycerin infusion in acute myocardial infarction. Circulation 59& 60:II-165, 1979.
21. Bussmann, WD, Passek, D, Seidel, W, et al: Reduction of CK and CK-MB indexes of infarct size by intravenous nitroglycerin. Circulation 63:615, 1981.
22. Flaherty, JT, Becker, LC, Bulkley, BH, et al: A randomized prospective trial of intravenous nitroglycerin in patients with acute myocardial infarction. Circulation 68:576, 1983.

23. Nelson, GIC, Silke, B, Ahuja, RC, et al: Haemodynamic advantages of isosorbide dinitrate over furosemide in acute heart-failure following myocardial infarction. Lancet 1:730, 1983.
24. Jaffe, AS, Geltman, EM, Tiefenbrunn, AJ, et al: Reduction of infarct size in patients with inferior infarction with intravenous glyceryl trinitrate. A randomized study. Br Heart J 49:452, 1983.
25. Lis, Y, Bennett, D, Lambert, G, et al: A preliminary double-blind study of intravenous nitroglycerin in acute myocardial infarction. Intensive Care Med 10:179, 1984.
26. Jugdutt, BI, Wortman, C, and Warnica, WJ: Does nitroglycerin therapy in acute myocardial infarction reduce the incidence of infarct expansion? J Am Coll Cardiol 5:477, 1985.
27. Yusuf, S, Collins, R, MacMahon, S, et al: Effect of intravenous nitrates on mortality in acute myocardial infarction: An overview of the randomised trials. Lancet 1:1088, 1988.
28. Mantle, JA, Rogers, WJ, Smith, LR, et al: Clinical effects of glucose–insulin–potassium on left ventricular function in acute myocardial infarction: Results from a randomized clinical trial. Am Heart J 102:313, 1981.
29. Satler, LF, Green, CE, Kent, KM, et al: Metabolic support during coronary reperfusion. Am Heart J 114:54, 1987.
30. Rogers, WJ, Stanley, AW, Breinig, JB, et al: Reduction of hospital mortality rate of acute myocardial infarction with glucose–insulin–potassium infusion. Am Heart J 92:441, 1976.
31. Schelbert, HR, Henze, E, Schon, HR, et al: C-11 palmitate for the noninvasive evaluation of regional myocardial fatty acid metabolism with positron computed tomography. III. In vivo demonstration of the effects of substrate availability of myocardial metabolism. Am Heart J 105:492, 1983.
32. McDaniel, HG, Papapietro, SE, Rogers, WJ, et al: Glucose–insulin–potassium induced alterations in individual plasma free fatty acids in patients with suspected acute myocardial infarction. Am Heart J 102:10, 1981.
33. Norwegian Multicenter Study Group: Timolol-induced reduction in mortality and reinfarction in patients surviving acute myocardial infarction. N Engl J Med 304:801, 1981.
34. Hjalmarson, A, Herlity, J, Malek, I, et al: Effect on mortality of metoprolol in acute myocardial infarction: A double-blind randomized trial. Lancet 2:823, 1981.
35. Beta-Blocker Heart Attack Trial Research Group: A randomized trial of propranolol in patients with acute myocardial infarction: 1. Mortality results. JAMA 247:1707, 1982.
36. Yusuf, S, Peto, R, Lewis, J, et al: Beta blockade during and after myocardial infarction: An overview of the randomized trials. Prog Cardiovasc Dis 27:335, 1985.
37. Yusuf, S, Sleight, P, Rossi, P, et al: Reduction in infarct size, arrhythmias and chest pain by early intravenous beta blockade in suspected acute myocardial infarction. Circulation 67 (Suppl I):I-32, 1983.
38. ISIS-1 (First International Study of Infarct Survival) Collaborative Group: Randomised trial of intravenous atenolol among 16,027 cases of suspected acute myocardial infarction: ISIS-1. Lancet 2:57, 1986.
39. The MIAMI Trial Research Group: Metoprolol in acute myocardial infarction (MIAMI): A randomized placebo-controlled international trial. Eur Heart J 6:199, 1985.
40. ISIS-1 (First International Study of Infarct Survival) Collaborative Group: Mechanisms for the early mortality reduction produced by beta-blockade started early in acute myocardial infarction: ISIS-1. Lancet 1:921, 1988.
41. Maseri, A, L'Abbate, A, Baroldi, G, et al: Coronary vasospasm as possible cause of myocardial infarction: A conclusion derived from the study of "preinfarction" angina. N Engl J Med 299:1271, 1978.
42. Henry, PD, Shuchleib, R, Borda, LJ, et al: Effects of nifedipine on myocardial perfusion and ischemic injury in dogs. Circ Res 43:372, 1978.
43. Antman, EM, Stone, PH, Muller, JE, et al: Calcium channel blocking agents in the treatment of cardiovascular disorders. Part I: Basic and clinical electrophysiologic effects. Ann Intern Med 93:875, 1980.
44. Muller, JE, Morrison, J, Stone, PH, et al: Nifedipine therapy for patients with threatened and acute myocardial infarction: A randomized, double-blind, placebo-controlled comparison. Circulation 69:740, 1984.
45. Sirnes, PA, Uverskeid, MD, Pedersen, TR, et al: Evolution of infarct size during the early use of nifedipine in patients with acute myocardial infarction: The Norwegian Nifedipine Multicenter Trial. Circulation 70:638, 1984.
46. The Danish Study Group on Verapamil in Myocardial Infarction: Verapamil in acute myocardial infarction. Eur Heart J 5:516, 1984.

47. Danish Multicenter Study Group on Verapamil in Myocardial Infarction: Verapamil in acute myocardial infarction. Am J Cardiol 54:24E, 1984.
48. DeWood, MA, Spores, J, Notske, R, et al: Prevalence of total coronary occlusion during the early hours of transmural myocardial infarction. N Engl J Med 303:897, 1980.
49. GISSI: Effectiveness of intravenous thrombolytic treatment in acute myocardial infarction. Lancet 1:397, 1986.
50. Simoons, ML, Serruys, PW, van den Brand, M, et al: Early thrombolysis in acute myocardial infarction: Limitation of infarct size and improved survival. J Am Coll Cardiol 7:717, 1986.
51. The ISAM Study Group: A prospective trial of intravenous streptokinase in acute myocardial infarction (ISAM): Mortality, morbidity, and infarct size at 21 days. N Engl J Med 314:1465, 1986.
52. Kennedy, JW, Martin, GV, Davis, KB, et al: The Western Washington intravenous streptokinase in acute myocardial infarction randomized trial. Circulation 77:345, 1988.
53. White, HD, Norris, RM, Brown, MA, et al: Effect of intravenous streptokinase on left ventricular function and early survival after acute myocardial infarction. N Engl J Med 317:850, 1987.
54. ISIS-2 (Second International Study of Infarct Survival) Steering Committee: Intravenous streptokinase given within 0–4 hours of onset of myocardial infarction reduced mortality in ISIS-2. Lancet 1:502, 1987.
55. Guerci, AD, Gerstenblith, G, Brinker, JA, et al: A randomized trial of intravenous tissue plasminogen activator for acute myocardial infarction with subsequent randomization to elective coronary angioplasty. N Engl J Med 317:1613, 1987.
56. Anderson, JL, Rothbard, RL, Hackworthy, RA, et al: Multicenter reperfusion trial of intravenous anisoylated plasminogen streptokinase activator complex (APSAC) in acute myocardial infarction: Controlled comparison with intracoronary streptokinase. J Am Coll Cardiol 11:1153, 1988.
57. AIMS Trial Study Group: Effect of intravenous APSAC on mortality after acute myocardial infarction: Preliminary report of a placebo-controlled clinical trial. Lancet 1:545, 1988.
58. Topol, EF, Fung, AY, Kline, E, et al: Safety of helicopter transport and out-of-hosptial intravenous fibrinolytic therapy in patients with evolving myocardial infarction. Cathet Cardiovasc Diagn 12:151, 1986.
59. Topol, EJ, Califf, RM, George, BS, et al: A randomized trial of immediate versus delayed elective angioplasty after intravenous tissue plasminogen activator in acute myocardial infarction. N Engl J Med 317:581, 1987.
60. European Cooperative Study Group for Recombinant Tissue-Type Plasminogen Activator (rTPA): Thrombolysis with tissue plasminogen activator in acute myocardial infarction: No additional benefit from immediate percutaneous coronary angioplasty. Lancet 1:197, 1988.

PART 2

Etiology

CHAPTER 3

Atherosclerotic and Nonatherosclerotic Coronary Artery Factors in Acute Myocardial Infarction

Bruce F. Waller, M.D.

Acute myocardial infarction (AMI) is the endpoint of a series of events surrounding the reduction and, in general, the interruption of coronary arterial supply to the myocardium. Various diseases of the coronary arteries are responsible for altered coronary blood flow and, collectively, may be referred to as "coronary artery disease." *Atherosclerosis* is the most common cause of coronary artery disease, but many other *nonatherosclerotic* disease processes involve the coronary arteries and reduce blood flow (Table 3–1). Unfortunately, "coronary artery disease" is frequently used synonymously with "coronary artery atherosclerosis." Coronary artery diseases can reduce or interrupt coronary blood flow by fixed luminal obstructions *(internal narrowing),* encroachment on the lumen by disease of the arterial wall *(external narrowing)*, or both. Reduction in coronary arterial blood flow also may result from dynamic changes in the walls of an otherwise normal artery *(spasm)* or from myocardial oxygen demand–supply disproportion *(left ventricular outflow obstruction).*

In view of current trends at rapid coronary artery reperfusion to salvage jeopardized myocardium during evolving acute myocardial infarction, the various etiologies of coronary artery disease must be kept in mind. The purpose of this chapter is to review atherosclerotic and nonatherosclerotic coronary artery factors in the genesis of acute myocardial infarction.

STATUS OF THE CORONARY ARTERIES AT NECROPSY IN PATIENTS WITH FATAL ACUTE MYOCARDIAL INFARCTION

Approximately 4 to 7 percent of all patients with acute myocardial infarction (and nearly four times this percentage for patients aged <35 years) do not have atherosclerotic coronary artery disease as demonstrated by coronary arteriogra-

Table 3–1. Nonatherosclerotic Causes of Coronary Artery Disease (Myocardial Infarction Without Coronary Atherosclerosis)

1. Congenital Anomalies
   A. Anomalous origin from the aorta
      1. Right from left sinus of Valsalva
      2. Left from right sinus of Valsalva
      3. Single coronary artery
      4. Atresia of coronary ostium
      5. High-takeoff coronary ostium
      6. Ostial ridges
   B. Anomalous origin from the pulmonary trunk
   C. Fistula
   D. Myocardial bridges ("tunneled" epicardial coronary artery)
2. Embolus
   A. Natural
      1. Thrombus
      2. Tumor
      3. Calcium
      4. Vegetation (infective, noninfective)
   B. Iatrogenic
      1. Cardiac surgery
      2. Cardiac catheterization
      3. Coronary angioplasty
      4. Prosthetic valves
   C. Paradoxical
3. Dissection
   A. Coronary artery
   B. Aortic
4. Spasm
5. Trauma
   A. Nonpenetrating
   B. Penetrating
   C. Surgery
   D. Catheterization
6. Arteritis
   A. Takayasu disease
   B. Polyarteritis nodosa
   C. Systemic lupus erythematosus
   D. Kawasaki syndrome (mucocutaneous lymph node syndrome)
   E. Syphilis
   F. Other infections (infective endocarditis, salmonella, parasites)
   G. Burger's disease
   H. Giant cell
7. Metabolic Disorders
   A. Mucopolysaccharidoses (Hurler, Hunter)
   B. Homocystinuria
   C. Fabry disease
   D. Amyloid
8. Intimal Proliferation
   A. Irradiation therapy
   B. Cardiac transplantation
   C. Fibromuscular hyperplasia (methylsergide therapy)
   D. Ostial cannulation
   E. Transluminal balloon angioplasty
   F. Idiopathic infantile arterial calcification (juvenile internal sclerosis)
9. External Compression
   A. Aortic aneurysm
   B. Tumor metastases
   C. Muscle bridges

Table 3–1 *Continued*

10. Thrombosis Without Underlying Atherosclerotic Plaque
    A. Polycythemia
    B. Thrombocytosis
    C. Hypercoagulability
11. Myocardial Oxygen Demand–Supply Disproportion
    A. Aortic stenosis
    B. Systemic hypotension
    C. Carbon monoxide poisoning
    D. Increased myocardial function (thyrotoxicosis)
12. Intramural coronary artery disease (small vessel disease)
    A. Hypertrophic cardiomyopathy
    B. Amyloid
    C. Cardiac transplantation
    D. Neuromuscular
    E. Diabetes mellitus
13. Normal coronary arteries

(Adapted from Cheitlin, et al,[143] Baim and Harrison,[144] and Alpert and Braunwald.[1])

phy, at necropsy, or both.[1–4] In view of the fact that coronary angiography simply represents a "lumenogram," the specificity for etiology of the coronary luminal narrowing is extremely low. Review of necropsy studies[2–4] suggests that approximately 95 percent of patients with fatal acute myocardial infarction have at least one major epicardial coronary artery (left anterior descending, left circumflex, right, left main) with severe luminal narrowing or total occlusion (Fig. 3–1). The remaining 5 percent of patients have normal major epicardial coronary arteries. Of the 95 percent of patients with severe coronary luminal narrowing, 95 percent of these patients have typical atherosclerotic plaque with (85 percent) or without (15 percent) superimposed thrombus. The remaining 5 percent of the patients with severe coronary luminal narrowing have a host of etiologies (see Table 3–1) including coronary arteritis, trauma, systemic metabolic disorders, intimal fibrous proliferation, and coronary emboli. (Certain medical centers with large populations of cardiac transplant patients will exceed the 5 percent nonatherosclerotic approximation owing to the high frequency of intimal fibrous proliferation in the coronary arteries late after transplantation.) Of the 5 percent necropsy patients with fatal acute myocardial infarction with normal or nearly normal epicardial coronary arteries, perhaps 50 percent to 60 percent of these patients represent clinical coronary spasm, but the remaining 40 percent to 50 percent represent a combination of congenital coronary artery anomalies, spontaneous recanalization, and coronary supply–myocardial demand mismatches.

ATHEROSCLEROTIC CORONARY ARTERY DISEASE

Atherosclerosis is *a disease of the intima* and can be defined as a "variable combination of changes in the intima of the arteries consisting of an accumulation of lipids, complex carbohydrates, blood and its products, fibrous tissue and calcific deposits, and associated (secondarily) with medial changes."[3] Our understanding of the evolution of the atherosclerotic plaque (Fig. 3–2) from the fatty streak, to the fibrous-atheromatous plaque, to the complicated plaque interacting with various biophysical and biochemical factors has changed over the last 10

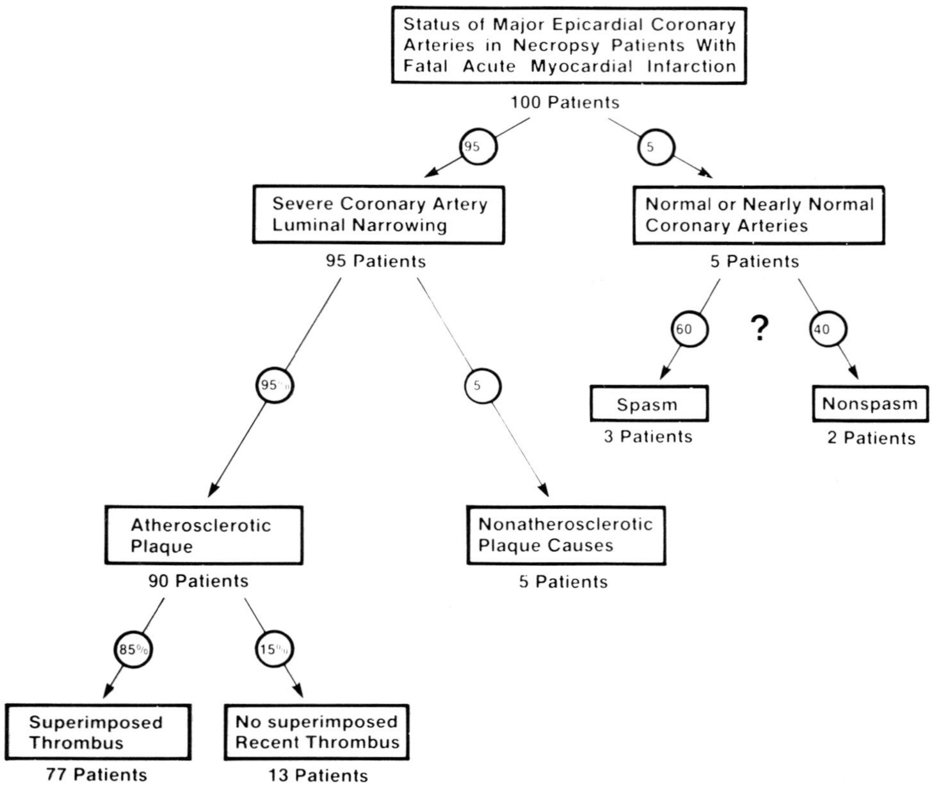

Figure 3–1. Diagram displaying the approximate breakdown of the status of major epicardial coronary arteries in necropsy patients with fatal acute myocardial infarction.

years. In the past, two major hypotheses for the pathogenesis of atherosclerotic plaque included the "incrustation"[5] theory of Rokitansky[6] (intimal fibrous thickening results from fibrin-platelet deposition with secondary accumulation of lipids) and the "imbibition"[5] hypothesis of Virchow[7] (a transudation of blood lipids into the vessel wall). Today these theories have been integrated into a hypothesis that includes the interaction of blood elements and lipids with the arterial wall, and these events are modified by various risk factors (Figs. 3–2 and 3–3).[5] The major critical events in the development of the atherosclerotic plaque appear to be: *endothelial injury* (fissures, cracks); *arterial wall platelet–fibrin interaction* and subsequent *smooth muscle cell proliferation; lipid entry* and accumulation; *fibrosis;* development of *thrombi* (repeat of injury–repair process); and finally, *ulceration* and *calcification.*[5] This current "response-to-injury" hypothesis suggests that repeated or continuous injury is necessary for the development of the fibrofatty plaque (see Fig. 3–3). In the face of chronic injury, smooth muscle cells derived from coronary media and/or intima form a matrix for the fibrofatty plaque. A new thickened intima, developed in stages in response to repeated injuries, consists of layers of smooth muscle cells, collagen, and elastic fibers. Fibrin-platelet thrombi also form on the neointimal surface and contribute to the plaque formation and plaque growth.

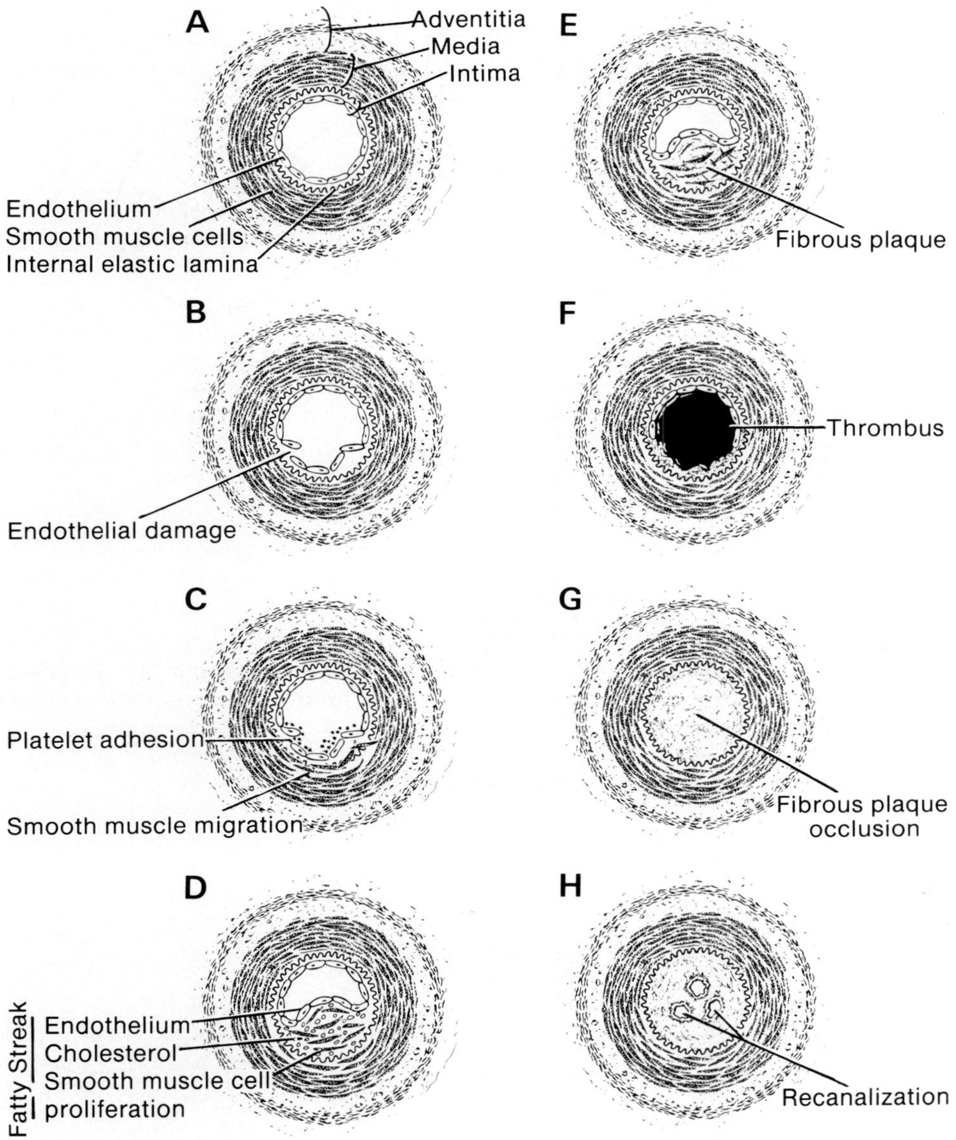

Figure 3–2. Evolution of atherosclerotic plaque showing the concept of endothelial injury with smooth muscle migration, incorporation of lipid, and the formation of a fibrous plaque. Coronary thrombosis may result with subsequent organization. (Modified from Fuster and Kottke.[5])

MYOCARDIAL INFARCTION AND CORONARY ARTERIAL OBSTRUCTION—THE "INFARCT ARTERY"

Myocardial infarction with or without complications of aneurysm formation or dilated cardiomyopathy occurs in hearts with generally two or three of the major epicardial coronary arteries severely diseased by atherosclerotic plaque. Most transmural infarcts occur distal to a totally occluded coronary artery. Col-

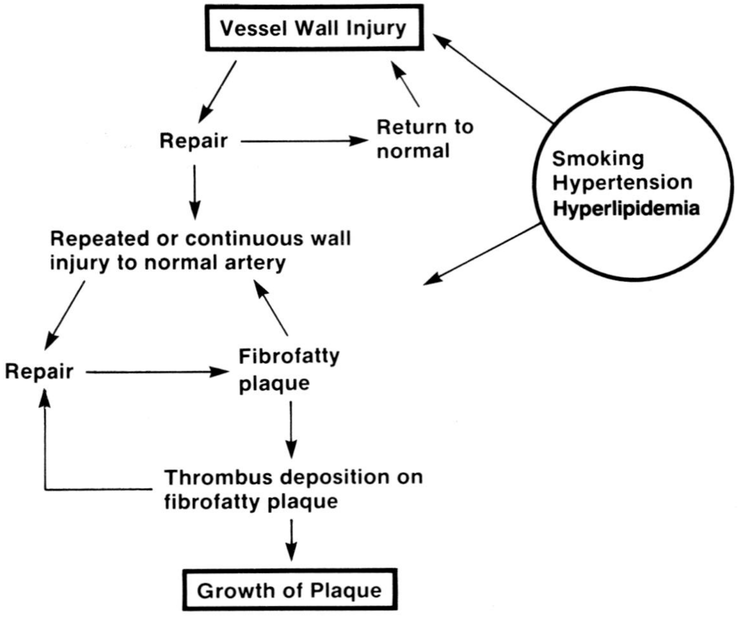

Figure 3–3. Diagram showing the evolution of atherosclerotic plaque based on the "vessel-wall injury" hypothesis. External factors ("risk factors"—smoking, hypertension, hyperlipidemia) influence and promote vessel wall injury.

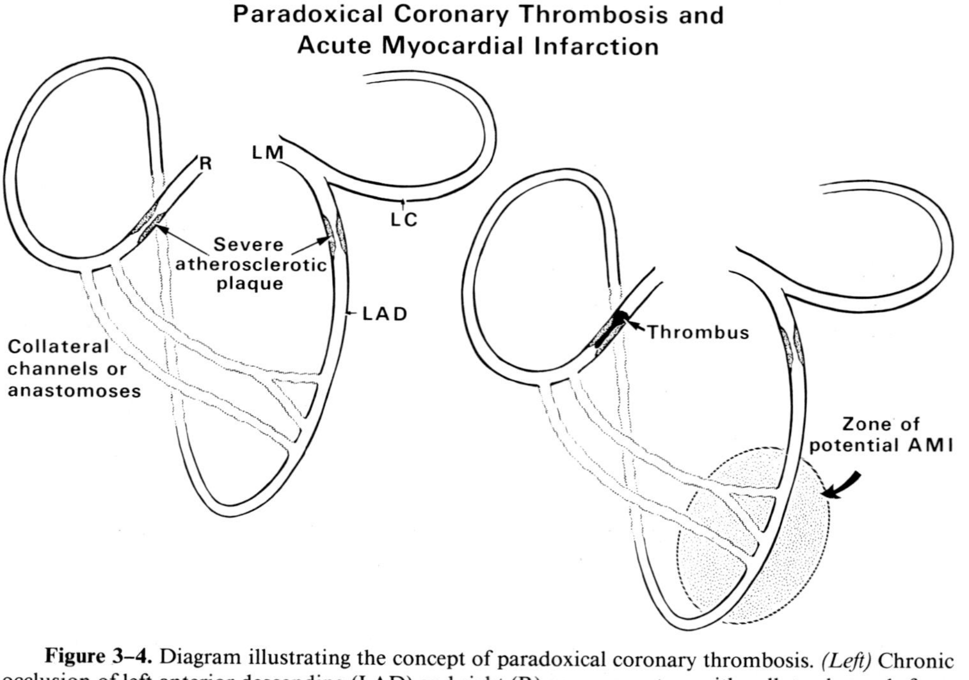

Figure 3–4. Diagram illustrating the concept of paradoxical coronary thrombosis. *(Left)* Chronic occlusion of left anterior descending (LAD) and right (R) coronary artery with collateral vessels from the R supplying the distal LAD. *(Right)* Sudden thrombotic occlusion of R coronary artery produces acute myocardial infarction (AMI) in distribution of LAD. LC = left circumflex; LM = left main.

lateral blood flow, level of metabolism, presence and location of stenoses in other arteries, rate of development of the coronary obstruction, and the amount of muscle supplied by the obstructed vessel are factors affecting the viability of the myocardium distal to the occlusion.[2]

Obstruction of the left anterior descending coronary artery usually is associated with infarction of the anterior (anteroseptal) left ventricle but also may be associated with infarction of apical regions of the left ventricle, basal to mid portions of the left ventricle. Obstruction of the left circumflex artery can cause infarction of the lateral or inferoposterior wall of the left ventricle, whereas occlusion of the right coronary artery usually results in infarction of the posterior wall of the left ventricle, apical portions of the ventricular septum, and posteromedial papillary muscle. The "infarct artery" has been the subject of intense interest with recent efforts at acute reperfusion therapy during evolving AMI. *In approximately 90 percent of acute myocardial infarcts, the infarct artery corresponds to the distribution just described. In the remaining 10 percent, infarcts occur at a location different from the recently occluded coronary artery* (Fig. 3–4). This form of infarction has been termed "ectopic infarction",[7A] infarction at a distance,[7B] and "paradoxical coronary thrombosis".[7C] For example, following the gradual occlusion of the left anterior descending coronary artery, the anteroseptal wall of the left ventricle may be maintained by collateral vessels arising from the right coronary artery. In this situation, sudden occlusion of the *right* coronary artery may cause infarction of the *anteroseptal* left ventricular wall (see Fig. 3–4).

Plaque Fissure

In addition to the importance of "plaque fissure" in the genesis and continued evolution of atherosclerotic plaque described above, recent pathologic studies,[8–11] in which coronary thrombi found in fatal cases of acute myocardial infarction were reconstructed from serial histologic sections, have shown that nearly all were related to rupture or fissuring of underlying atherosclerotic plaques.[8,9] As described above, rupture of a plaque leads to communication between the lipid content of the plaque and luminal blood products; thrombus develops over the rupture site and then propagates (Figs. 3–5 and 3–6). The head of the thrombus (related to the underlying plaque) is different in composition from the thrombus propagating distally[10]; the former is rich in platelets, whereas the latter contains a higher proportion of fibrin. Increasing angiographic information suggests that *coronary thrombosis and plaque fissures are the "connecting link" between patients with unstable angina pectoris and acute myocardial infarction* (Fig. 3–7).[10A,12–15] Eccentric coronary stenosis with a narrow neck or irregular borders or both is the most common morphologic feature on angiography in both acute myocardial infarction and unstable angina pectoris (Fig. 3–8).[15] This angiographic pattern probably represents either a disrupted atherosclerotic plaque, partially occlusive or lysed thrombus, or both. The predominance of this coronary luminal morphology in both unstable angina pectoris and acute myocardial infarction suggests a link between the two conditions such that unstable angina and acute myocardial infarction may form a *continuous spectrum* with the clinical outcome dependent on the amount of platelet deposition, degree of underlying stenosis, associated coronary artery spasm, and the presence or absence of collateral circulation. Levin and Fallon[16] published a valuable study in which postmortem angiography and subsequent histologic sections *correlated the irregular luminal borders seen*

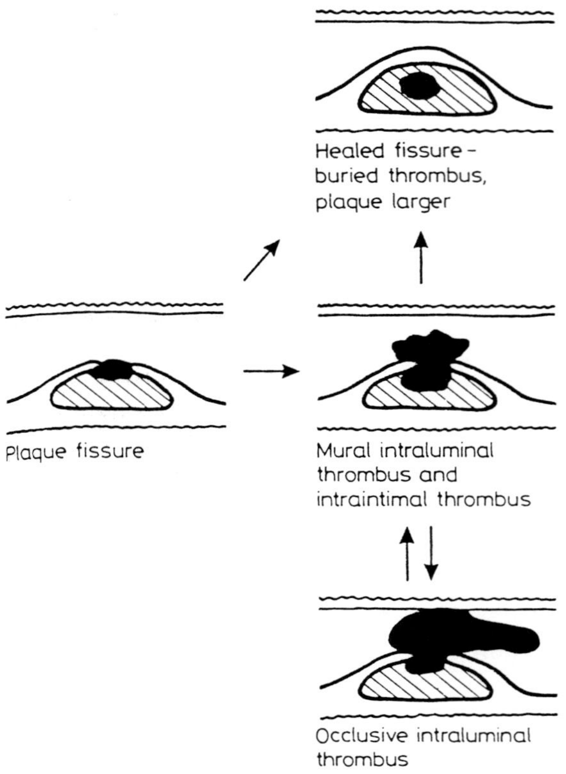

Figure 3–5. Diagram showing the relation between clinical expressions of ischemic heart disease and the histopathologic stages of plaque fissuring. (Modified from Davies and Thomas.[10A])

angiographically with histologically "complicated plaques" (plaque rupture, hemorrhage, and superimposed partially occluding thrombus). In contrast, the angiographic stenosis with smooth borders without intraluminal lucencies were associated with histologically "uncomplicated" plaques (intact intimal surfaces with no superimposed thrombus). These angiographic and histologic findings have potentially major therapeutic importance in support of antithrombotic and possibly thrombolytic therapy in patients with unstable angina pectoris.[17]

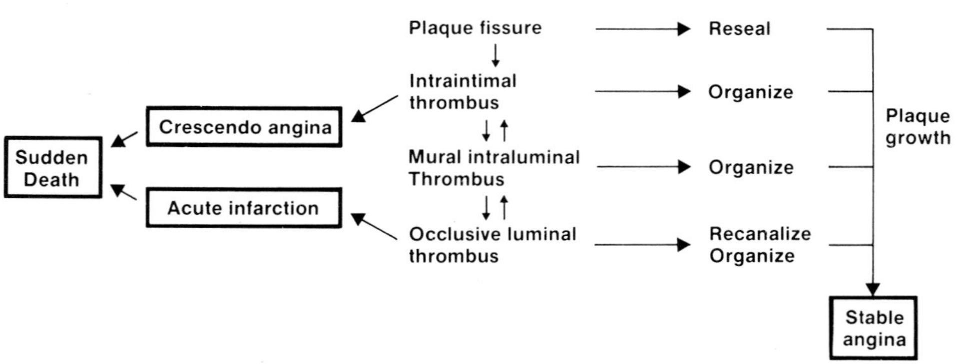

Figure 3–6. Diagram illustrating the evolution of a plaque fissure to reseal and stabilize or to progress to thrombotic occlusion. (From Davies and Thomas,[10A] with permission.)

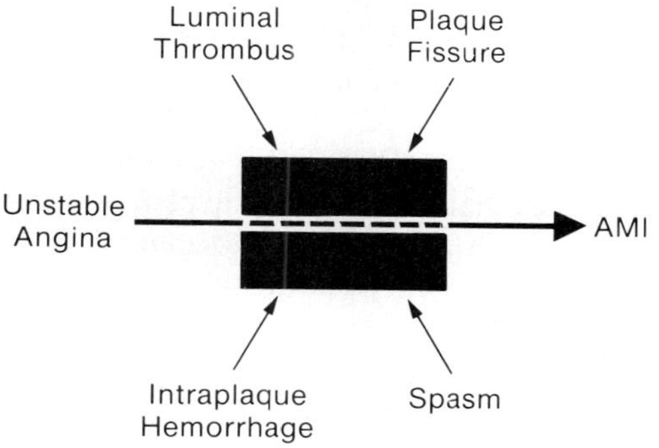

Figure 3–7. Diagram showing the various "missing links" in the spectrum of unstable angina pectoris and evolving acute myocardial infarction. The development of plaque hemorrhage and luminal thrombus formation are common denominator factors in both clinical events.

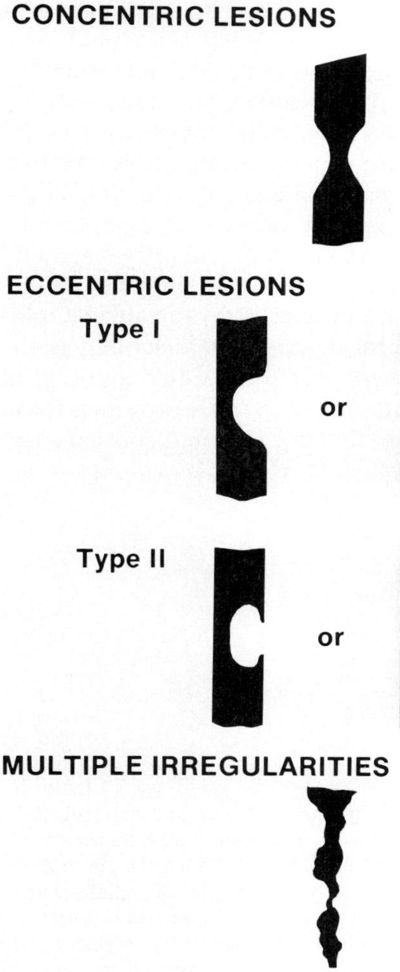

Figure 3–8. Diagram of coronary artery angiographic patterns associated with the pathogenesis of unstable angina pectoris and acute myocardial infarction. Type II eccentric lesions are associated with a high frequency of plaque fissures, disruption, and fibrin-platelet thrombus formation. (From Ambrose, et al,[15] with permission.)

Diffuse versus Focal Nature of Atherosclerotic Plaque

Discussion continues as to whether coronary atherosclerotic plaque is a *diffuse* or *focal* process (Fig. 3–9). One group of investigators believes that the atherosclerotic process in patients with clinical evidence of coronary heart disease is diffuse involving, for practical purposes, all segments of all four major coronary arteries[18] (see Fig. 3–9). On the other hand, another group of investigators believes that atherosclerotic plaque occurs focally along the length of the involved artery with segments of normal artery often present between diseased segments (see Fig. 3–9).[19] In addition, the focal nature is exemplified also by histology of each coronary artery segment—one arc of artery is commonly involved and not the other.[19] If one defines diffuse as "widely scattered or widely spread," then coronary atherosclerotic disease appears to be diffuse in nature. If, on the other hand, one defines diffuse as "involving every segment of the entire tree," then atherosclerotic disease is not a diffuse process but rather it is a focal (localized or concentrated) process. Coronary atherosclerosis can also be considered as "extensive" in that there are usually several coronary vessels involved as well as a multiplicity of lesions with the involved artery.

The importance of this issue arises in the discussion of differences found in coronary narrowing observed angiographically during life versus that observed histologically at necropsy. Generally, the coronary angiogram underestimates the amount of atherosclerotic plaque present.[19A] The coronary angiogram is a picture of the coronary lumen, and, as such, one measures diameter reduction based upon a "peak-and-valley" effect of a diseased coronary artery. Angiographically, one compares a site of maximal narrowing with an adjacent site of "presumed" normal coronary artery to determine the percentage of coronary diameter deduction. If coronary artery atherosclerosis is a diffuse process, then the angiographically presumed normal coronary segment used for comparison is actually a diseased coronary segment and the angiogram *underestimates* the amount of coronary atherosclerosis. If, on the other hand, the atherosclerotic process is focal, then a presumed normal coronary artery may, in fact, be a normal coronary seg-

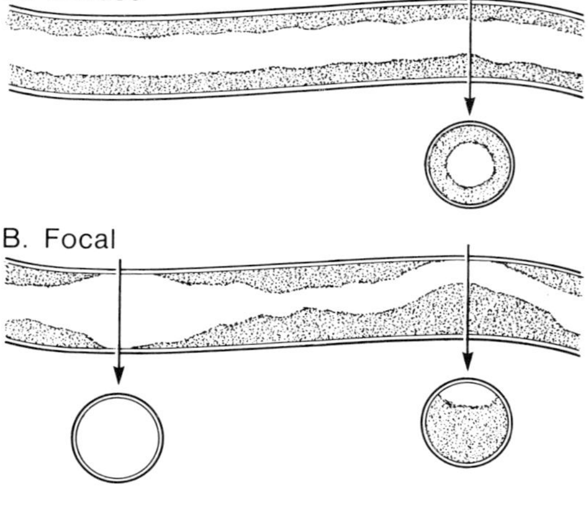

Figure 3–9. Diagram showing the 2 patterns of coronary atherosclerosis. (*A*) Diffuse pattern in which the entire artery has varying degrees of atherosclerotic plaque. (*B*) Focal or extensive pattern in which normal coronary segments are interposed between diseased segments, or there is one portion of the coronary artery wall free of disease (eccentric plaque).

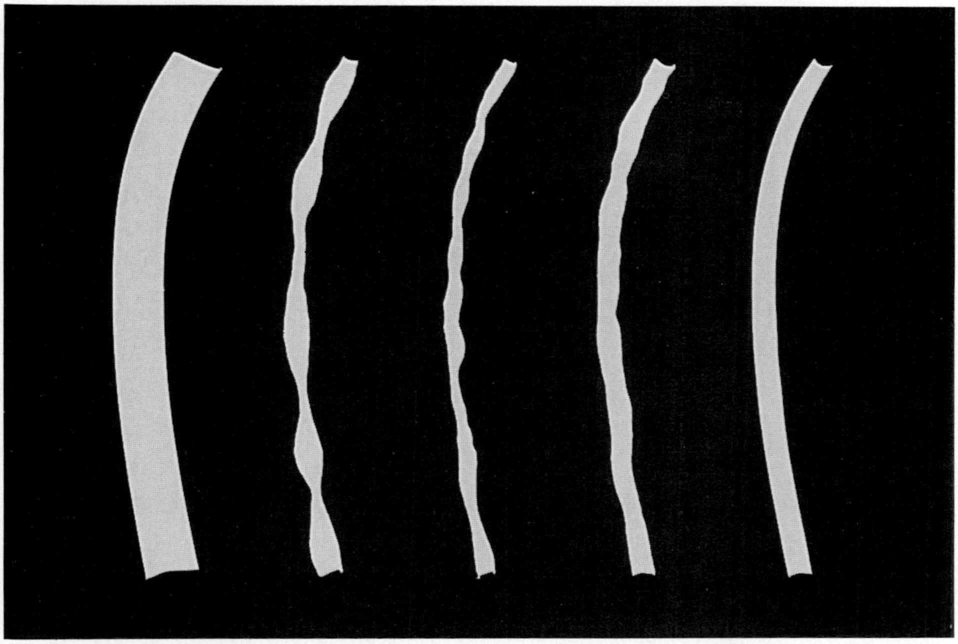

Figure 3–10. Five diagrams portraying different coronary angiograms of the left anterior descending coronary artery. The first *(far left)* is probably interpreted as a "normal" vessel, the next as "multiple coronary aneurysms," the third as "severe coronary disease," the next as "minor luminal irregularities," and the last as "normal," or "normal small vessel." However, the coronary angiogram represents a "lumenogram," and the respective coronary arteries are shown in Figure 3–11.

ment, and the postmortem examination may *overestimate* the amount of coronary atherosclerosis (Figs. 3–10 and 3–11).

Coronary Artery Lumen

The residual lumen in nonoccluded atherosclerotic coronary arteries cross-sections varies in its *shape,* and the lumen shape changes throughout its *course* along the length of a given artery (Figs. 3–12 through 3–15). The coronary artery lumen becomes a tortuous and irregular tube. The residual, nonoccluded coronary artery lumen has been described as *concentric, eccentric, semilunar, polymorphous eccentric, eccentric slit-like,* and *central.* Basically, the variation in the distribution of atherosclerotic plaque along the circumference of coronary arteries results in two major types of cross-sectional luminal shapes: *concentric* and *eccentric* (see Fig. 3–12).[20] If the atherosclerotic plaque is distributed along the entire vessel circumference, the cross-sectional coronary lumen is located centrally and is called a central or concentric type lumen (see Figs. 3–12 and 3–13).[20] If, however, the plaque fails to involve the entire coronary artery circumference, leaving a variable arc of normal wall, the residual cross-sectional lumen is called eccentric (see Figs. 3–12 and 3–14).[20] The eccentric lumen has been further subdivided into "slit-like," "polymorphous," or "semilunar types."[20,21] Although the polymorphous type of eccentric lumen may be observed with variable degrees of obstruction, the slit-like eccentric lumen is always associated with severe (>75 percent) cross-sectional area narrowing.

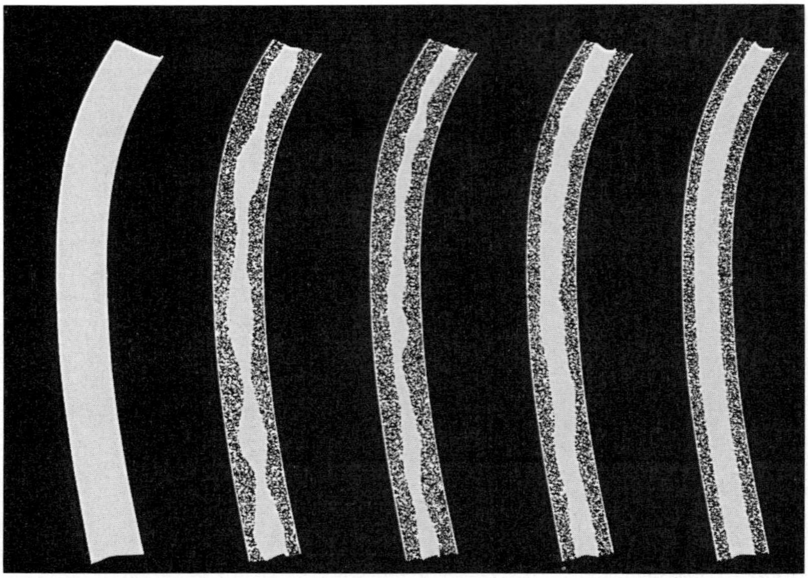

Figure 3–11. Corresponding five coronary arteries illustrated in Figure 3–10. The first coronary artery is "normal." The second coronary artery has diffuse coronary atherosclerosis *(stippled area)*, giving a "peak-and-valley effect that could be misinterpreted as coronary aneurysms. The third vessel had diffuse and severe coronary atherosclerosis. The next coronary artery also has diffuse and moderately severe disease, but because the "peak-and-valley" effect of atherosclerosis is minimal, the coronary angiogram may be interpreted as "minor luminal irregularities." The last vessel has the same external diameter as the first normal vessel but has diffuse and concentric atherosclerotic plaque mimicking a small normal coronary artery.

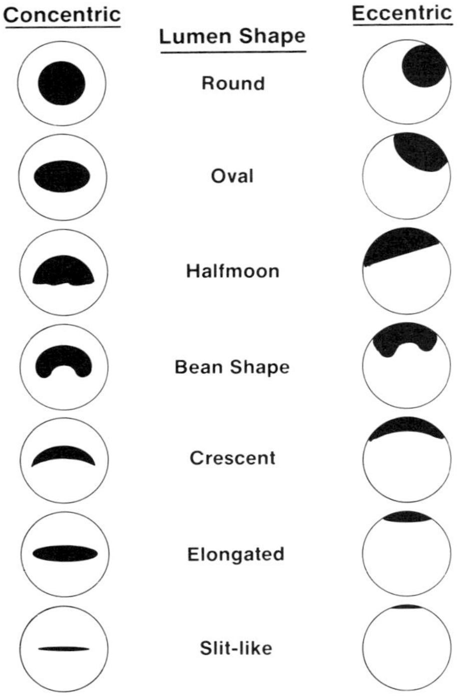

Figure 3–12. Diagram showing the various luminal shapes observed in coronary arteries with *concentric* and *eccentric* lumens.

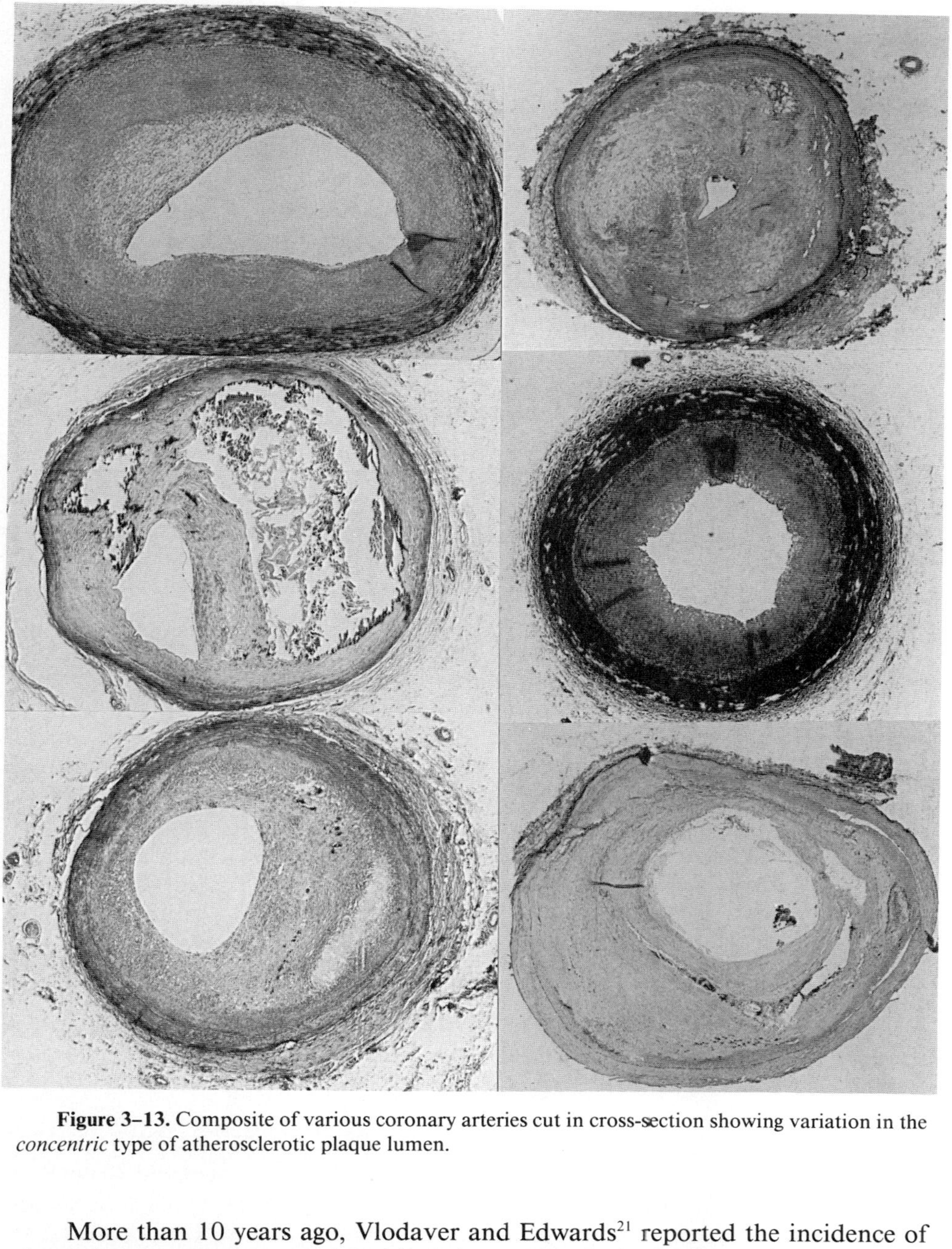

Figure 3–13. Composite of various coronary arteries cut in cross-section showing variation in the *concentric* type of atherosclerotic plaque lumen.

More than 10 years ago, Vlodaver and Edwards[21] reported the incidence of the various types of coronary luminal shapes. On the basis of examination of 200 atherosclerotic coronary artery sections, the frequency of three types of coronary lumen was: 30 percent concentric, 41 percent eccentric polymorphous, and 29 percent eccentric slit-like. Thus, in 70 percent of the cross-sections studied the residual lumen was *eccentric,* and in only 30 percent was the lumen *concentric.* Baroldi[22] examined 1069 sites of severe (>70 percent) diameter reduction and found that 46 percent of the coronary luminal shapes were concentric, 24 percent

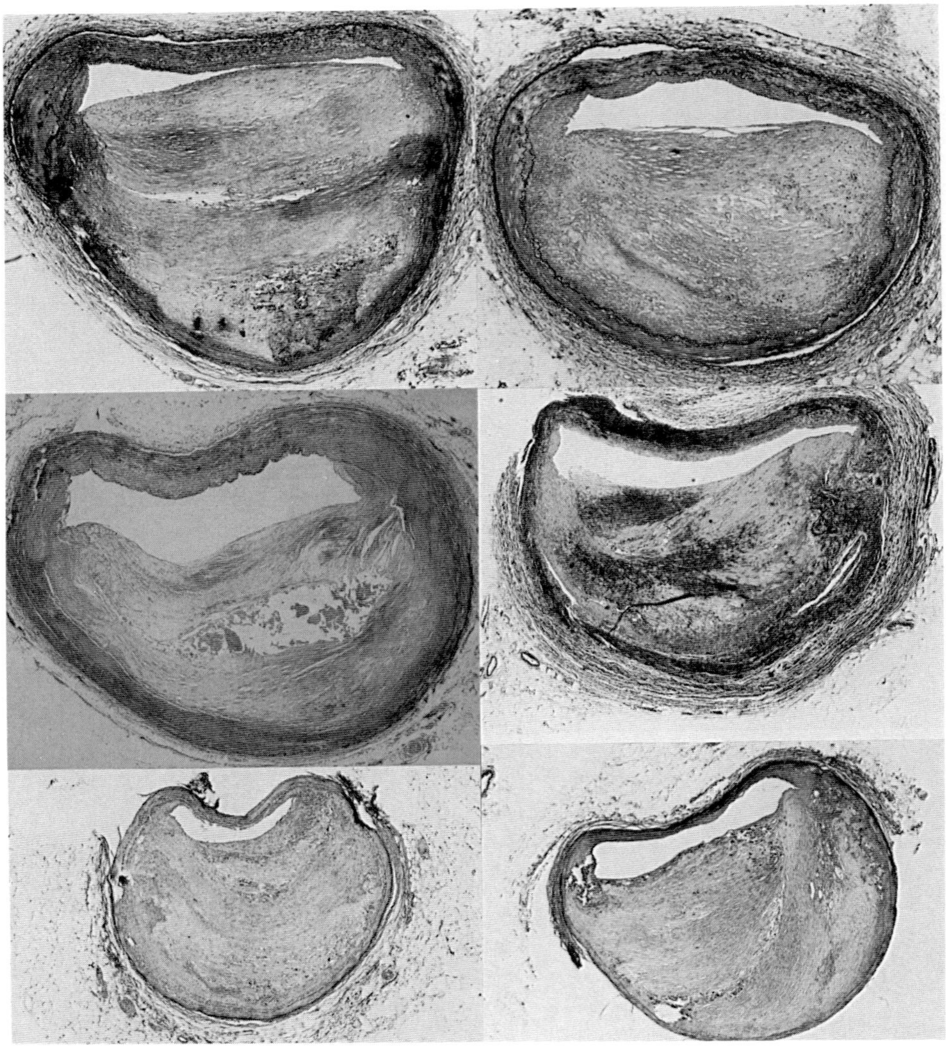

Figure 3–14. Composite of various coronary arteries cut in cross-section showing variation in the *eccentric* type of atherosclerotic plaque lumen. Various names such as "polymorphous" or "slit-like" have been applied to some of these shapes.

were eccentric (lateral lumen position but still encircled by plaque) and 30 percent were "semilunar" (a variable arc of free wall). I recently reviewed 500 atherosclerotic sections from major epicardial coronary arteries (each section narrowed at least 75 percent in cross-sectional area) and found luminal patterns were *concentric* in 26 percent and *eccentric* in 74 percent.[23] Thus, of over 1750 atherosclerotic coronary sections in three studies, the luminal shape was *concentric* in 34 percent and various forms of *eccentric* in 66 percent of sections (see Figs. 3–13 through 3–15).

Recently, Saner and colleagues[24] provided a timely and clinically relevant morphometric analysis of the arc of disease-free wall in the eccentric type of cor-

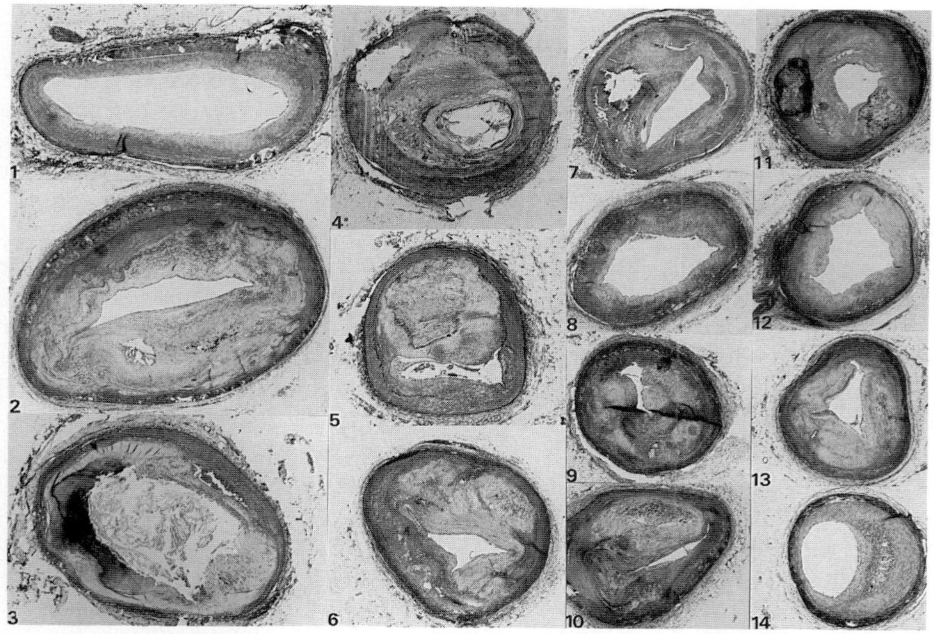

Figure 3–15. Consecutive serial 5-mm long cross-sections of the left anterior descending coronary artery showing the variations in luminal shapes throughout the course of the artery (#1 = proximal; #14 = distal). The arteries have been oriented with the top of each picture indicating the artery wall closest to the visceral pericardium and the bottom part of each picture closest to the myocardium. Note the arterial lumen shifts back and forth between upper and lower and right and left sides of the cross-section. Elastic stain, each at 12.

onary lumen. In an analysis of 100 coronary segments narrowed 50 percent to 90 percent in cross-sectional area by atherosclerotic plaque, 17 percent to 23 percent (mean 20 percent) of the vessel circumference was disease-free. The percent of disease-free wall arc length did not differ significantly with increasing severity of luminal obstruction, with location of the lesion within the same or different arteries, or among coronary segments with different diameters. The presence of the disease-free wall segment has clinical importance in at least three areas: (1) the accuracy with which angiography reflects the morphologic features of the diseased artery, (2) coronary spasm, and (3) mechanism of coronary angioplasty and subsequent "restenosis" of previously dilated arteries.

Variability in coronary luminal shape represents one of the explanations for the angiographic underestimation of vessel narrowing. Both eccentric and concentric luminal shapes present difficulties in accurately grading the amount of diameter reduction with respect to a normal coronary lumen. A "normal" coronary angiogram does not necessarily mean a normal coronary artery wall and may actually correspond histologically to a severely narrowed coronary segment composed of serial polymorphous or semilunar type lumens. Moreover, a long regular concentric stenosis may produce an angiographically "small normal vessel" (see Figs. 3–10 and 3–11). Of the two types of coronary lumen, the eccentric, and, in particular, the slit-like lumen, appears more likely to pose a problem for angiographic underestimation because the length of the luminal slit frequently approaches the full dimension of the diameter of the original lumen. Spears and colleagues[25] indicated that the maximal potential in estimating angiographic luminal narrowing is proportional to the degree of ellipticity (eccentricity). When the ratio of major to minor axis of the eccentric lumen increases, the potential angiographic error increases considerably. With the advent of triaxial motion capability, the use of multiple angulated angiographic views will improve the angiographic–morphologic correlation by minimizing the effects of the disease-free wall.[19A]

Saner and colleagues[24] speculate that the normal or nearly normal arc of the coronary wall may be capable of "reacting" to humoral or neurogenic stimuli resulting in an increased or decreased luminal diameter. The extent to which dynamic augmentation or contraction of the coronary lumen is possible appears to be a function of the extent and location of smooth muscle in the coronary wall (Figs. 3–16 and 3–17). Isner and associates[26] reported smooth muscle cell depletion (medial attenuation) accompanying advanced degrees of luminal narrowing by atherosclerotic plaque. These observations support the concepts of Saner and colleagues[24] that dynamic alterations of coronary lumen are unlikely to occur along the circumference of coronary artery containing atherosclerotic plaque, but rather along the disease-free circumference of the coronary artery. Although only approximately 20 percent of the vessel circumference is disease-free, the effects of humoral or neurogenic stimuli on this small segment may be quite influential on the overall degree of luminal narrowing. It is known that atherosclerotic lesions do not produce clinical symptoms of ischemia until approximately 75 percent cross-sectional area luminal reduction has occurred. Thus, given an eccentric lesion with 70 percent cross-sectional area reduction, contraction (spasm) of the plaque-free wall of only 5 percent to 10 percent could convert a clinically silent stenosis into a clinically symptomatic and possibly fatal lesion (see Fig. 3–16).

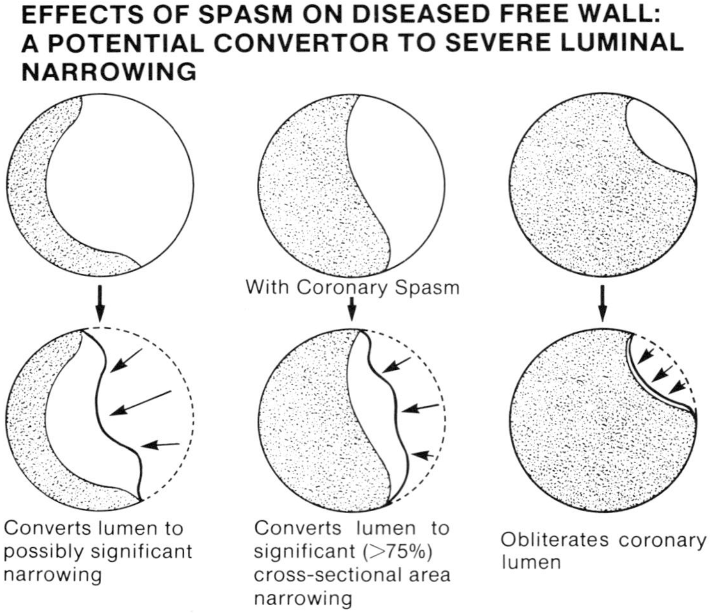

Figure 3–16. Diagram showing the adverse effects of spasm on arc of disease-free wall. Spasm can convert an asymptomatic lesion into a symptomatic lesion.

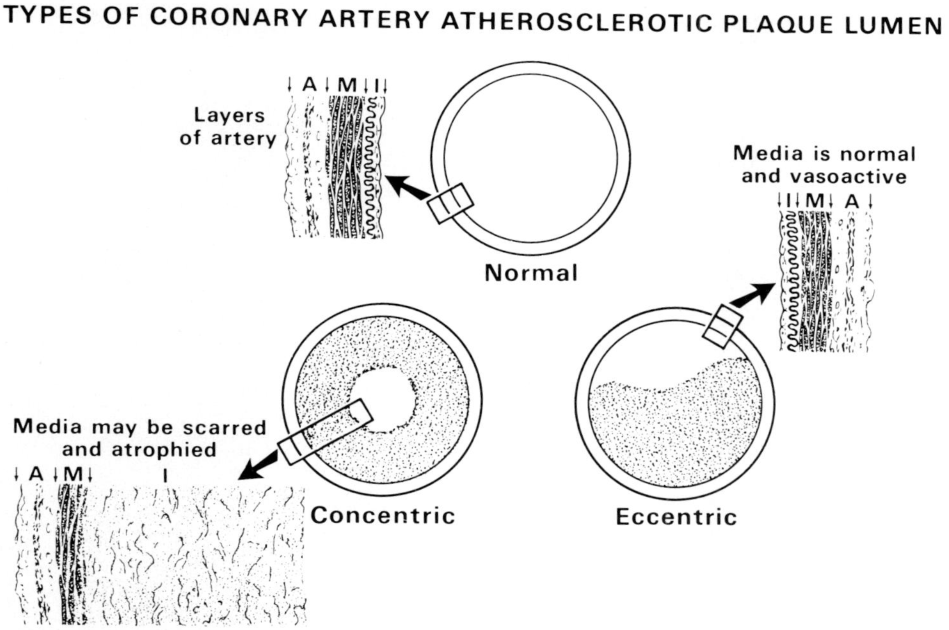

Figure 3–17. Diagram showing variation in coronary media in relation to concentric and eccentric atherosclerotic plaque. Nonatrophied media may be vasoactive and convert insignificant luminal narrowing to significant narrowing.

The distribution of atherosclerotic plaque and the resulting luminal configuration are linked directly to currently understood mechanisms of balloon angioplasty. To date, at least five possible mechanisms exist for successful balloon angioplasty: (1) plaque compression, (2) focal plaque "fracture" or "splitting," (3) stretching of the plaque-free wall in eccentric lesions, (4) stretching of coronary segments without plaque damage, and (5) focal plaque rupture with localized dissection.[26A] Of these possibilities, the second, fourth, and third mechanisms (in the order of decreasing importance) appear most likely. Morphometric data provided by Saner and colleagues[24] and the high frequency of eccentric type coronary lumen in severely diseased vessels[21–23] suggest that *stretching of the plaque-free wall may be a more frequent mechanism of clinically successful coronary angioplasty than previously thought.* In addition, dilation of the disease-free arc without damage to plaque on the remaining portions of the wall may provide a partial explanation for early "restenosis" after an angiographically successful dilation. Stretching of the plaque-free wall segment may result initially in coronary luminal increase but several weeks later in gradual "relaxation" of this overstretched segment ("restitution of tone") ("restenosis"). In addition to stretching, the plaque-free segment may be susceptible to spasm (see above), resulting in acute luminal closure during or shortly after the dilation procedure.

Quantitation of Luminal Stenosis and Length of Stenosis

Atherosclerotic plaque encroaches to various degrees upon the coronary artery lumen. In experimental studies, a 75 percent luminal cross-sectional area reduction is required to decrease flow (i.e., produce clinically significant [symptomatic] coronary artery disease). Thus, in general, greater than 75 percent

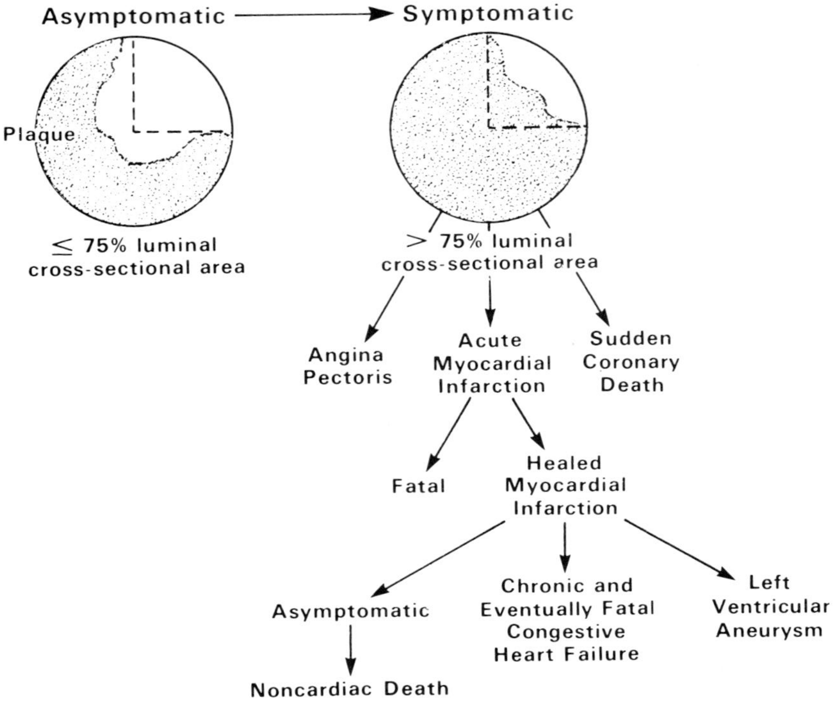

Figure 3–18. Various clinical presentations of atherosclerotic coronary heart disease based on the degree of luminal cross-sectional area reduction.

cross-sectional area luminal reduction at necropsy is considered *significant* coronary artery atherosclerosis (Fig. 3–18). In addition to *stenosis of the lumen,* the *length of stenoses* is also a factor in the reduction of blood flow: "the effectiveness of a given localized constriction in reducing flow may be large or small and will vary in inverse relation to the peripheral resistance of the vascular bed and the lumen area of the constricted segment and in direct relation to the axial length of the constricted area, flow velocity, and blood viscosity."[27] In this regard, Baroldi[29] examined the length of 565 severe (≥70 percent cross-sectional area reduction) stenoses and found the coronary artery lesion length was less than 5 mm in 13 percent, between 5 mm and 20 mm in 38 percent, and greater than 20 mm in 49 percent. Thus, nearly half of the segments severely narrowed in cross-sectional area were narrowed a considerable length. Included in this study were 100 severe stenoses from the infarct artery of necropsy patients with fatal acute myocardial infarction.

Topography of Atherosclerotic Coronary Artery Disease

Many necropsy studies have evaluated the major epicardial coronary arteries in patients with fatal atherosclerotic coronary heart disease.[28–98] Efforts have been made to assess the degree of coronary atherosclerosis and to compare various subsets of patients as to the *location* of severe stenoses (*which* major arteries, *how many* major arteries, *where in* the major coronary arteries [proximal versus distal]) and the *amount or extent* of atherosclerotic disease (*how many segments*

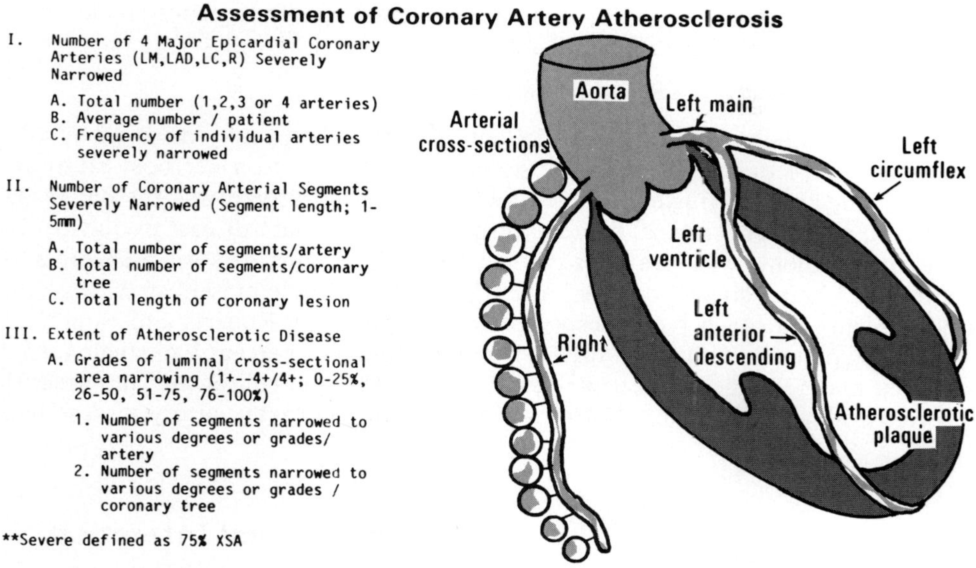

Figure 3–19. Diagram showing various ways of assessing the amount and degree of coronary atherosclerosis. One may simply *count* the number of four major vessels severely narrowed; one can *serially section* the arteries in cross-sectional fashion and *determine the number of segments* severely diseased; and one can determine the *extent* of atherosclerosis by *grading* luminal cross-sectional area (see Table 3–2).

per artery or *what degree of narrowing* per segment, average degree luminal narrowing per artery, per heart) (Fig. 3–19). Different methods of examination (gross inspection, postmortem angiography or casts, histological cross-sections, longitudinal dissections) and different methods of quantifying plaque (cross-sectional

Table 3–2. Quantitative Analysis of Amounts of Coronary Atherosclerotic Plaques

Author (Year of Study)	Interval (mm) of Consecutive Serial Coronary Segments
Osborn (1963)	4
Fulton (1965)	2
Baroldi (1967)	3
Friedman (1973)	5
Liberthson (1974)	1
Perper (1975)	2
Pomerance (1975)	3–4*
Crawford (1977)	5†
Roberts (1979)	5†

*Grading system of luminal XSA narrowing: 0–25%, 26–50%, 51–75%, 76–100%, total occlusion.

†Grading system of luminal narrowing: 0–33%, 33–67%, 67–75%, 76–100%; stenosis scoring system (0–9).

‡Grading system of luminal narrowing: 0–25%, 26–50%, 51–75%, 76–100% (96–100); stenosis scoring system (0–4).

area [various degrees or grades], diameter reduction, gross inspection) make comparison of these studies difficult (Table 3–2).

How Many Vessels Are Severely Narrowed?

The number of major epicardial coronary vessels severely diseased by atherosclerotic plaque varies with the necropsy study.[78–98] In a necropsy study by Berger and Stary,[62] single-, double-, and triple-vessel disease was present in 38 percent, 33 percent, and 20 percent, respectively (left main disease excluded). In necropsy patients with previous clinical history of angina pectoris, Lenegre and Himbert[74] found single-, double-, and triple-vessel disease present in 22 percent, 30 percent, and 48 percent, respectively. In a study by Roberts and Buja[46A] of necropsy patients with acute myocardial infarction, 14 percent had single artery disease and 53 percent had triple-vessel disease. Pitt and colleagues[64] reported 31 percent of cases without a history of symptomatic coronary artery disease had

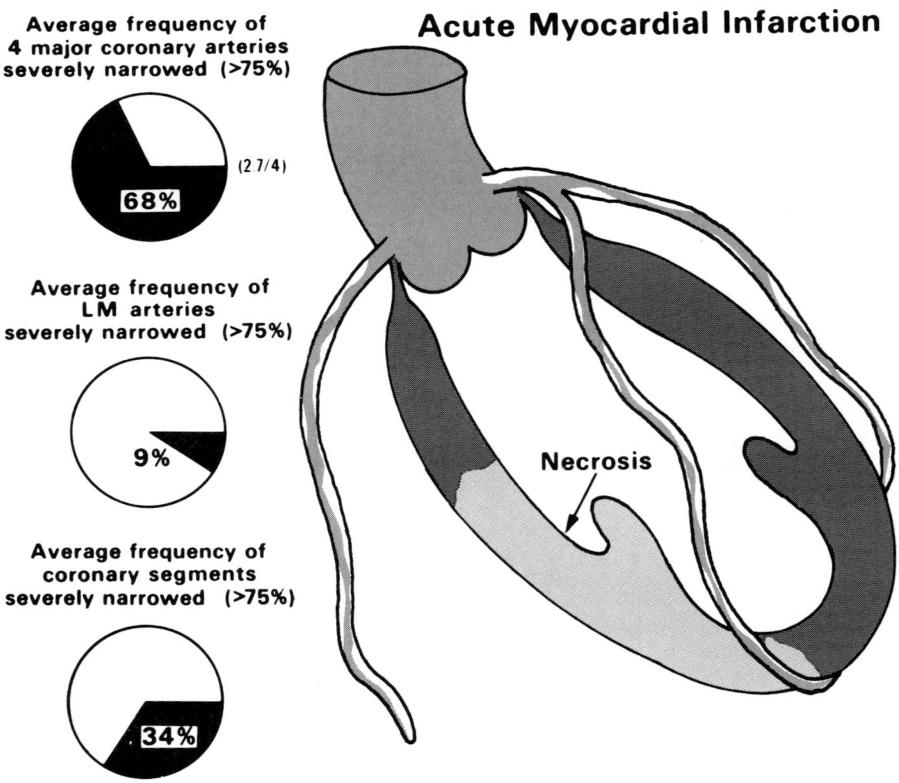

Figure 3–20. Extent and degree of coronary atherosclerosis in patients with fatal *acute myocardial infarction.* The top left pie diagram represents the average number of four major epicardial coronary arteries (left main [LM]; left anterior descending; left circumflex; right) narrowed >75 percent in cross-sectional area by plaque. The middle pie diagram represents the average frequency of LM coronary arteries narrowed >75 percent in cross-sectional area. The bottom pie diagram represents the average frequency of serial cross-sectional segments of the entire coronary tree narrowed >75 percent in cross-sectional area in studies in which consecutive serial coronary sectioning was performed (see Table 3–2).

double- or triple-vessel disease, compared with 61 percent of patients with such a history. Pathologic studies generally agree that in patients with symptomatic coronary heart disease, at least one major vessel is severely narrowed by plaque and usually two or three major vessels are severely narrowed.

If patients with fatal coronary events are subgrouped according to clinical manifestation (Figs. 3–20 through 3–29), *the average number (frequency) of four major coronary arteries* (left main, left anterior descending, left circumflex, right) *narrowed >75 percent in cross-sectional area is similar: angina pectoris*—3.0/4 (stable angina), 3.2/4 (unstable angina); *acute myocardial infarction*—2.7/4; *healed myocardial infarction*—2.2/4 (small infarct), 2.2/4 (large infarct); *left ventricular aneurysm*—2.5/4; *ischemic cardiomyopathy*—2.5/4; *angina pectoris and aortocoronary bypass grafting*—2.8/4; *angina pectoris and balloon angioplasty*—2.0/4; angina pectoris and *death in the cardiac catheterization laboratory*—3.6/4; *sudden coronary death*—2.4/4 (with previous clinical ischemia), 2.7/4 (without previous clinical ischemia). Combining all subsets, *the average number of arteries severely narrowed is 2.7/4 (68 percent).*

Comparison of the number of major coronary arteries severely narrowed at necropsy with the age at death discloses that single-vessel disease is more common in patients under age 41 years and in patients over age 89 years (Figs. 3–30

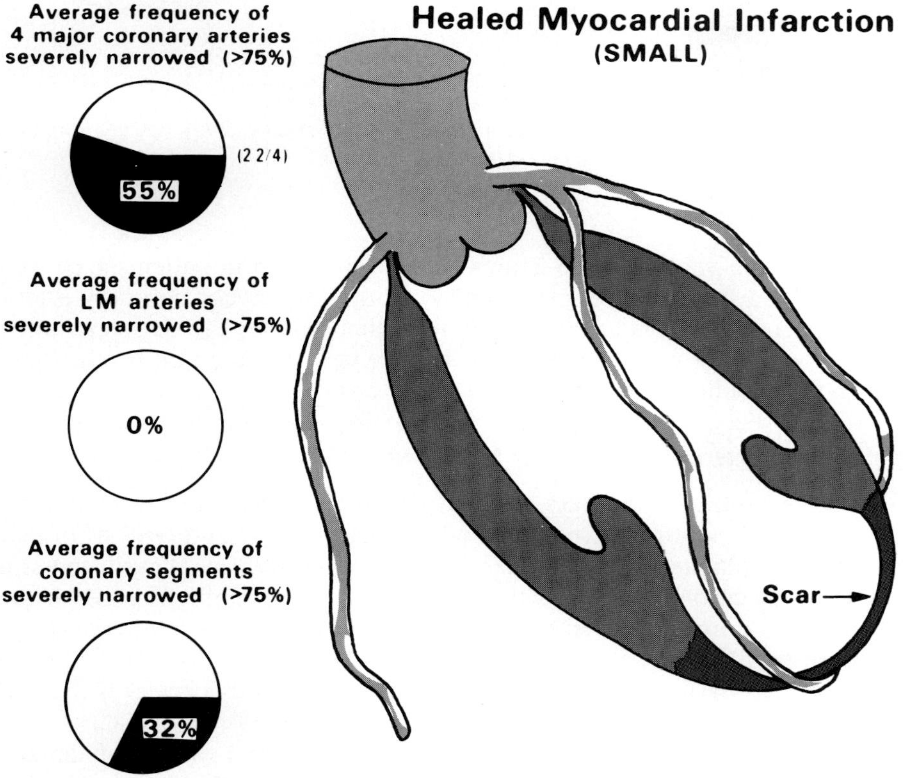

Figure 3–21. Extent and degree of coronary atherosclerosis at necropsy in patients with *small healed myocardial infarction.* Pie diagrams as described in Figure 3–20.

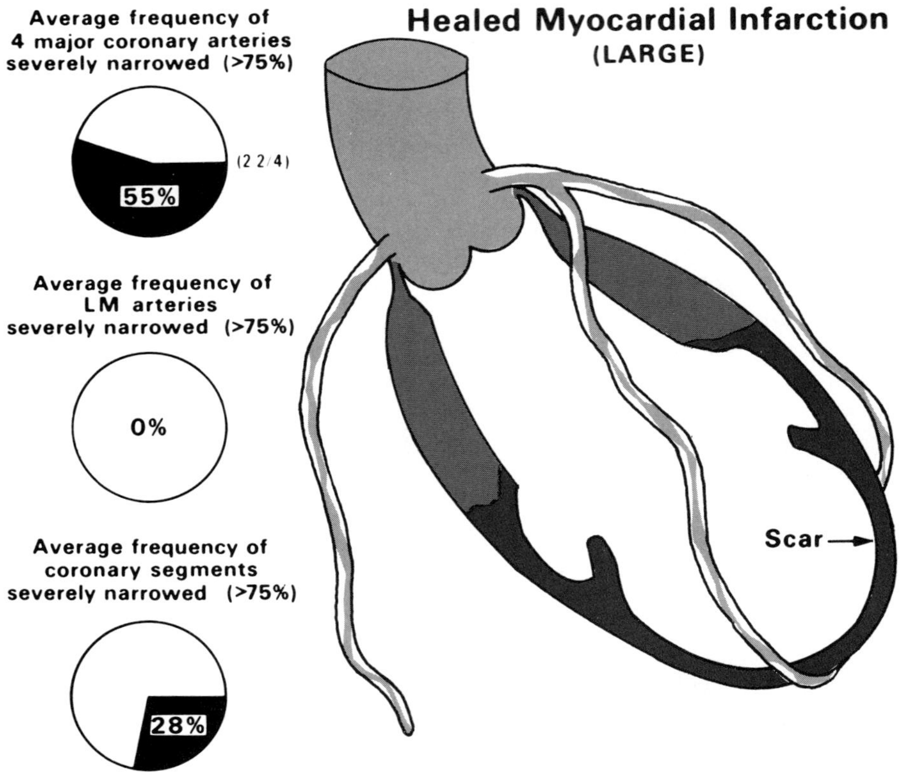

Figure 3–22. Extent and degree of coronary atherosclerosis at necropsy in patients with *large, healed myocardial infarction.* Pie diagrams as described in Figure 3–20.

and 3–31). Triple-vessel disease is most frequently found in patients aged 41 to 89 years. The average number (frequency) of the four major coronary arteries severely narrowed by plaque is similar in patients under age 41 years and in patients over age 89 years: 2.4/4, 2.2/4, respectively; but the number is slightly higher in the middle age group 41 to 89 years: 2.7/4.

Which Major Arteries Are Severely Narrowed?

Multiple studies[28–98] address the topic of which of the major epicardial coronary arteries are severely narrowed and how factors of age and type of coronary event influence plaque location. Four necropsy studies indicate that the left anterior descending coronary artery is the most frequently severely diseased (58 percent) coronary artery (Fig. 3–32). The left anterior descending coronary artery is followed in frequency by the right coronary artery (33 percent) and the left circumflex coronary artery (26 percent). The left main coronary artery is least frequently involved (16 percent) (see Figs. 3–20 through 3–29).

In view of the high frequency of severe involvement of the left anterior descending coronary artery by atherosclerotic plaque, this artery has gone by several aliases: "the artery of occlusion," "the artery of sudden death," "the widow-

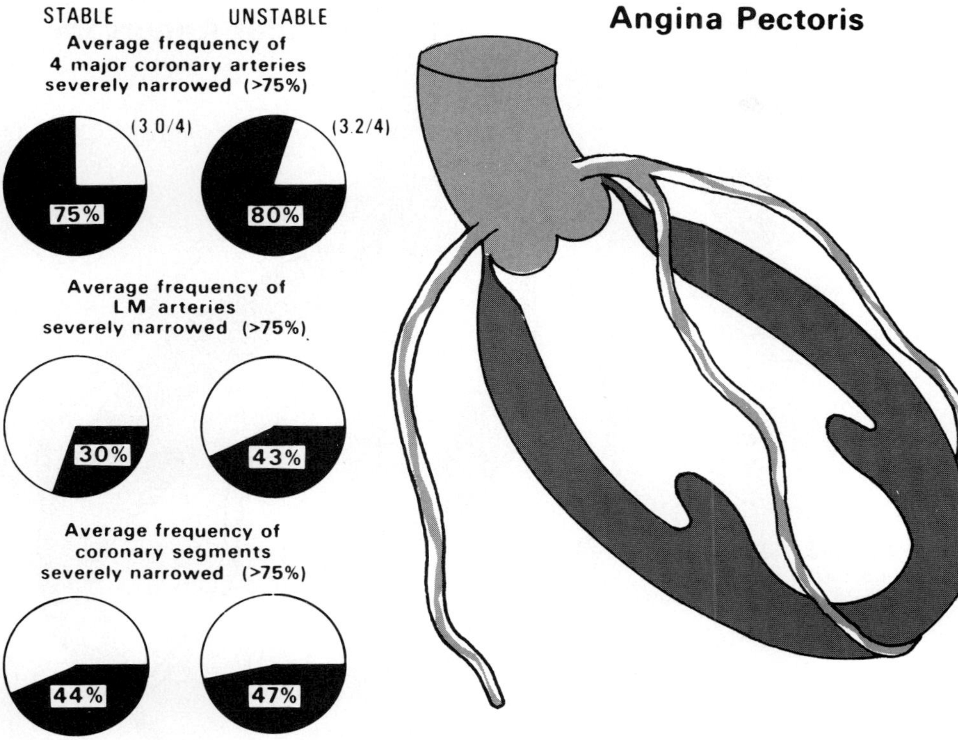

Figure 3–23. Extent and degree of coronary atherosclerosis at necropsy in patients with *stable and unstable angina pectoris.* Pie diagrams as described in Figure 3–20.

maker," "the artery of coronary thrombosis," "the artery of PTCA," and "the artery of acute reperfusion."

The dominance of the left anterior descending coronary artery with respect to patient age is shown in Figure 3–33. The left anterior descending coronary artery remains the most frequently diseased vessel in the young, middle-aged, and elderly necropsy patient. The left main coronary artery is commonly severely narrowed in patients aged under 41 years (see Fig. 3–30) and in patients aged 41 to 89 years, but this is rarely, if ever, found in patients over 89 years.

How Much of the Coronary Tree Is Diseased?

Several authors[78–98] have attempted to quantify how much of each artery or how much of the entire coronary tree is severely narrowed by atherosclerotic plaque. The epicardial coronary tree has been cut in consecutive serial coronary cross-sections measuring 1 mm to 5 mm in length, and each segment has been graded as to the amount of luminal narrowing (see Table 3–2). Various scoring or grading systems have been devised[80,92,98] in order to make comparative studies of various subsets of patients with fatal or nonfatal coronary events. These coronary score systems are a convenient way of expressing the overall status of the

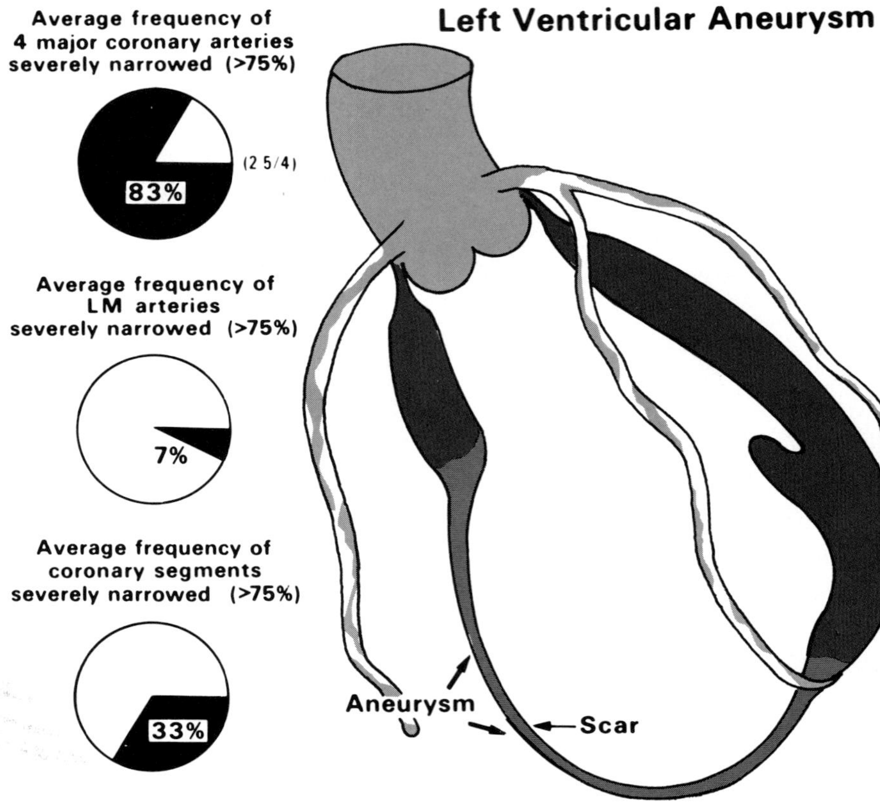

Figure 3–24. Extent and degree of coronary atherosclerosis at necropsy in patients with *left ventricular aneurysm* following acute myocardial infarction. Pie diagrams as described in Figure 3–20.

degree of coronary artery stenosis. If patients with fatal coronary events are grouped according to various clinical manifestations (see Figs. 3–20 through 3–29), *the average frequency of various coronary segments narrowed >75 percent is similar: angina pectoris*—44 percent (stable angina), 47 percent (unstable angina); *acute myocardial infarction*—34 percent; *healed myocardial infarction*—32 percent (small infarct), 29 percent (large infarct); *left ventricular aneurysm*—33 percent; *ischemic cardiomyopathy*—29 percent; *angina pectoris and balloon angioplasty*—9 percent; angina pectoris and *death in the cardiac catheterization laboratory*—58 percent; *sudden coronary death*—25 percent (with previous clinical ischemia), 30 percent (without previous clinical ischemia). Combining all subgroups, *the average frequency of coronary segments severely narrowed is 35 percent.*

Left Main Coronary Artery Stenosis

Severe luminal narrowing of the left main coronary artery has been associated with several clinical "risk" factors. Left main coronary disease is seen more frequently in necropsy patients with a history of *angina pectoris, type 2 hyper-*

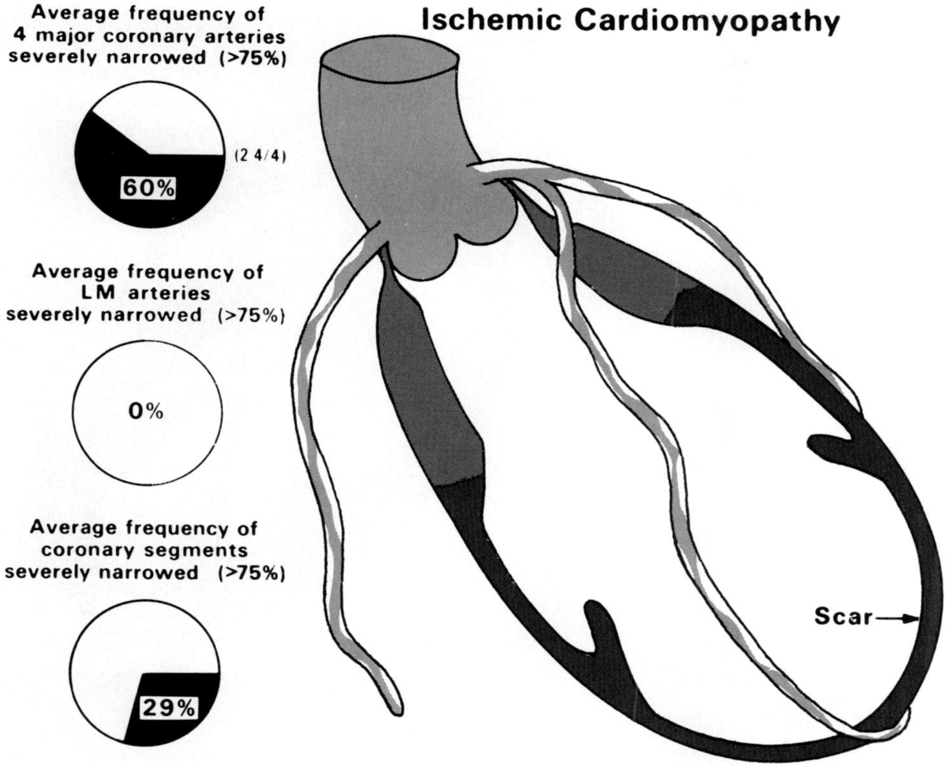

Figure 3–25. Extent and degree of atherosclerosis at necropsy in patients with *ischemic cardiomyopathy* (coronary dilated cardiomyopathy). Pie diagrams as described in Figure 3–20.

lipoproteinemia,[99] *diabetes mellitus,*[100,101] and *triple-vessel coronary artery disease. Isolated* severe left main disease is a rare necropsy finding.

Coronary Ostial Stenosis

Narrowing at the aortic origin of a coronary artery (ostial stenosis) may result from atherosclerotic or nonatherosclerotic conditions affecting either the aorta, coronary artery, or both.[102] Atherosclerotic conditions such as syphilis[103] and homozygous Type II hyperlipoproteinemia may cause severe ostial stenosis secondary to severe plaquing in the ascending aorta. Ostial stenosis may be associated with acute myocardial infarction. In a study by Heggtveit,[104] "paraostial" obstructive atherosclerosis was present in 73 percent of patients with fatal acute myocardial infarction. In 5 percent of patients, the ostial stenosis was considered responsible for the infarction. Ostial stenosis of the right coronary artery was more frequent than the left. In a study of 213 coronary casts by Baroldi and Scomazzoni,[90] the frequency of severe ostial stenosis (including the first 2 mm of the left main artery) was as follows: 3 patients (1 percent) with left ostial stenosis (2 isolated), all without acute myocardial infarction; 11 patients (5 percent) with right ostial stenosis (3 isolated), 7 of whom had acute or healed myocardial infarction.

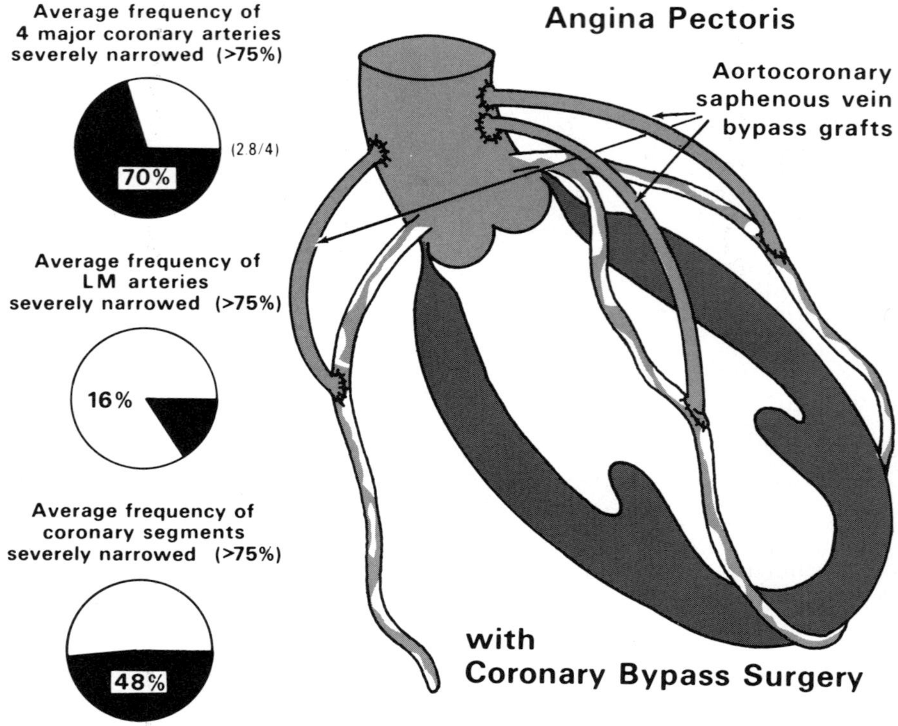

Figure 3–26. Extent and degree of coronary atherosclerosis at necropsy in patients with *angina pectoris who underwent aortocoronary saphenous vein bypass graft surgery.* Pie diagrams as described in Figure 3–20.

CORONARY ARTERY THROMBOSIS AND ACUTE MYOCARDIAL INFARCTION

The role of coronary thrombosis in the genesis of AMI remains controversial.[105–109] Herrick's article in 1912[110] attracted widespread interest in the concept of acute coronary artery occlusion producing acute myocardial infarction. The terms "coronary thrombosis" and "coronary occlusion" became virtually synonymous with AMI.[109,110] This view was held for many years until Blumgart and associates[111,112] demonstrated pathologic specimens in which coronary occlusion was found in the absence of AMI.

Since Virchow's triad of factors predisposing to thrombogenesis (alterations of arterial wall, patterns and/or rates of blood flow, blood components[108]), much has been learned about the pathogenesis of coronary thrombosis. Focal endothelial injury or disruption exposing subendothelial connective tissues to circulating platelets and fibrin is currently held as the initial stimulus to coronary artery thrombosis (Figs. 3–5, 3–6, and 3–34 through 3–37). Mechanisms that may be responsible for the arterial wall disruption involve hemodynamic stresses, intraplaque hemorrhage, direct effect of circulating lipids, and iatrogenic causes such as balloon angioplasty. Following the initial endothelial disruption, the ensuing fibrin platelet–collagen interaction and adhesion of platelets to the connective tissue elements stimulates the platelet release reaction, liberating adenosine diphos-

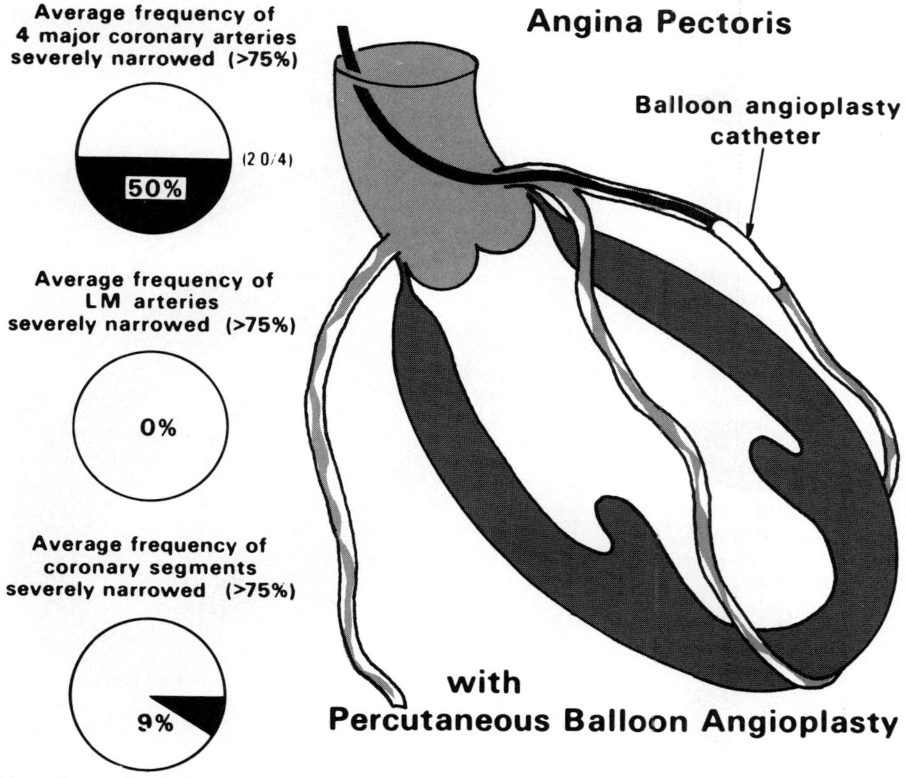

Figure 3–27. Extent and degree of coronary atherosclerosis at necropsy in patients with *angina pectoris who underwent percutaneous transluminal balloon angioplasty*. Pie diagrams as described in Figure 3–20.

phate (ADP), serotonin, and a variety of vasoactive agents.[108] ADP results in intense local aggregation of platelets with the development of microthrombi. Fibrin deposition, which enhances growth and stabilization of the platelet thrombus, is initiated via activation of intrinsic and extrinsic coagulation pathways. Thrombus formation is intensified by platelet-derived thromboxane A_2—an aggregating and vasoconstrictor agent. The thrombus is altered further by prostacyclin (an inhibitor of aggregation and a vasodilator) derived from endothelial or smooth muscle cells (PGI_2). Focal vasoconstriction is a feature of the hemostatic plug formation in response to injury and may promote arterial spasm with exacerbation of ischemia associated with the process of thrombosis even in the absence of complete occlusion. The thrombus resulting from the cascade of events involving platelet–collagen interactions, the platelet release reaction, and activation of the blood coagulation pathways results in a nonhomogenous mass, comprising a selective accumulation of platelets and leukocytes with variable numbers of erythrocytes in a stabilizing network of fibrin.[108] Its laminated structure reflects both its episodic growth and the influence of blood flow characteristics on thrombogenesis. Both the proteolytic enzymes secreted by the accumulating neutrophils and plasminogen activator derived from activated monocytes

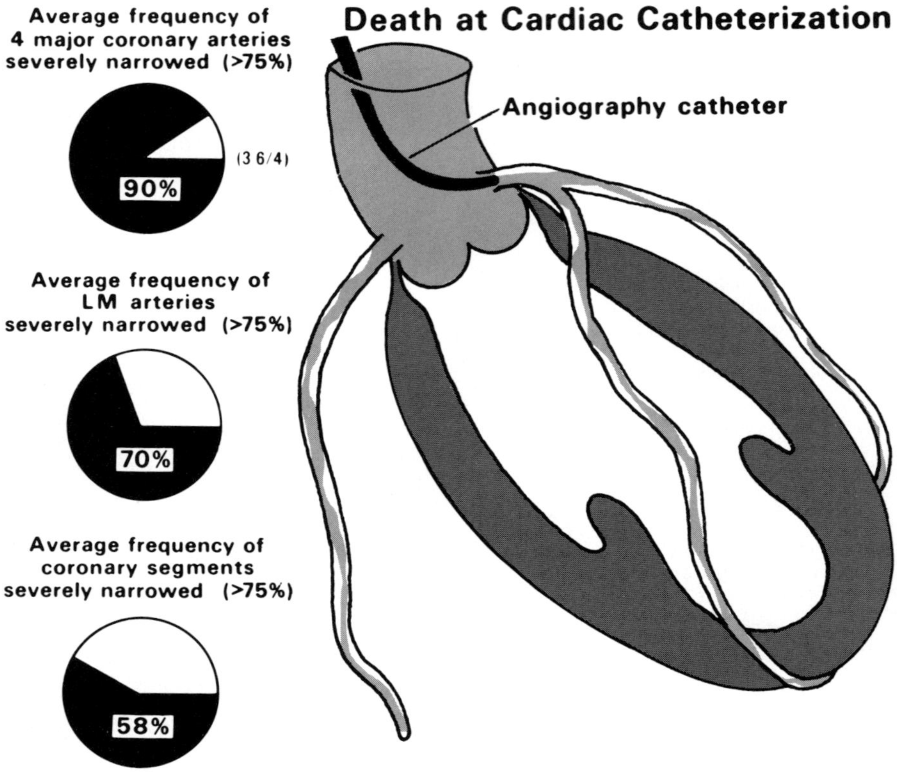

Figure 3–28. Extent and degree of coronary atherosclerosis at necropsy in patients with *death during cardiac catheterization.* Pie diagrams as described in Figure 3–20.

within the thrombus may influence the composition and extent of thrombi via fibrinolysis.[108]

Although the occurrence at necropsy of occlusive coronary artery thrombi in patients with fatal AMI has been long known (Table 3–3), the frequency of this finding has been quite variable.[113–137] Systemic analysis of the necropsy frequency of coronary artery thrombus started with the work of Friedberg and Horn in 1939.[113] Later, Blumgart and colleagues[138,139] established that thrombotic occlusion of a major coronary artery was not inevitably associated with myocardial infarction if the collateral circulation was extensive, but that when an infarct was present, it was usually associated with a thrombus occluding the epicardial artery supplying the zone of necrosis. From 1912 with Herrick's paper[110] to the late 1960s, coronary artery thrombosis was thought to *precipitate* AMI. The impression that coronary thrombus was the result of myocardial infarction rather than a precipitating event was probably first proposed by Branwood and Montgomery in 1956.[115] In the early 1970s a few prominent investigators[126,127] championed the view that *thrombosis was a secondary event* and often an epiphenomenon associated with infarction. This view "obviously precluded unabashed enthusiasm for attempts at coronary thrombolysis"[107] and actually set back the clinical use of thrombolytic therapy for evolving AMI by 10 years. In the late 1970s and early

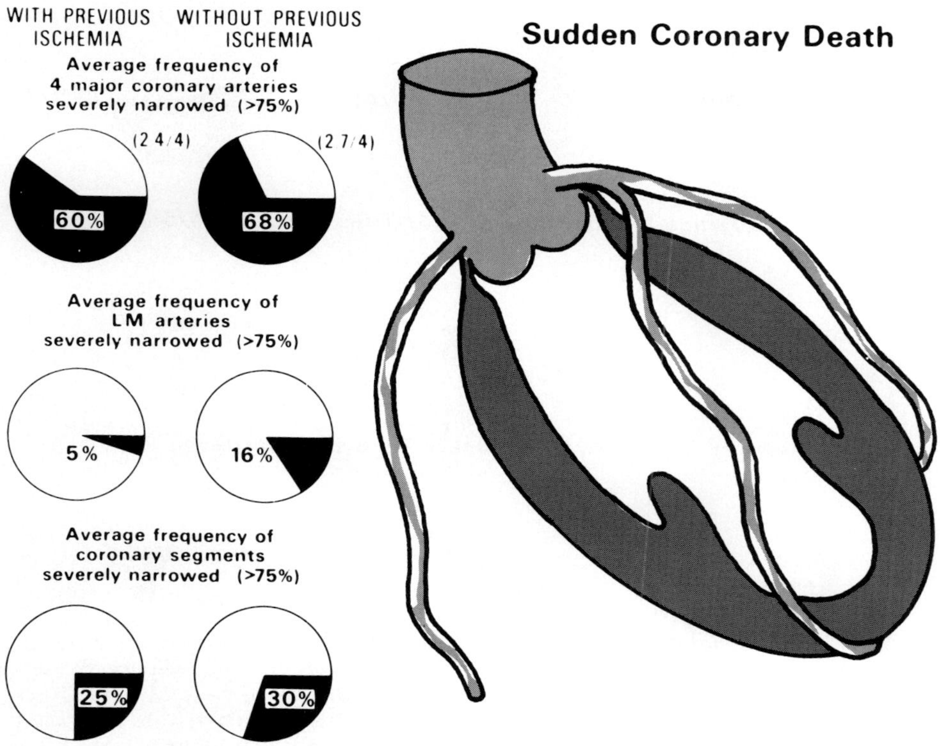

Figure 3–29. Extent and degree of coronary atherosclerosis at necropsy in patients with *sudden coronary death with or without previous clinical ischemia.* Pie diagrams as described in Figure 3–20.

1980s, reports of a high frequency of coronary thrombi observed in patients with evolving AMI[136] and angiographic demonstrations that coronary recanalization could be accomplished by thrombolytic agents[140,141] swung the pendulum toward aggressive intervention in patients with evolving AMI (Fig. 3–38).

Several factors may explain the differences in frequencies of occlusive coronary artery thrombus observed at necropsy over the last 60 years: *differences in patient populations* studied at necropsy, *definitions of transmural and nontransmural infarction, definitions of AMI and sudden death,* the *histologic recognition of early AMI,* and *laboratory techniques* in evaluation of the coronary arterial tree (cross-sectional analysis versus longitudinal coronary artery dissection).

Status of the Infarct-Artery Following Attempts at Mechanical, Pharmacologic, or Combined Forms of Reperfusion Therapy

Intense interest has focused on the status of the infarct artery following attempts at reperfusion for evolving AMI. Nonsurgical attempts to salvage jeopardized myocardium have employed methods of rapid restoration of coronary blood flow using *purely pharmacologic* (streptokinase, urokinase, tissue-plasminogen activator), *purely mechanical* (percutaneous transluminal balloon angioplasty, guide wire perforation) or *combined* types of reperfusion therapy. Waller

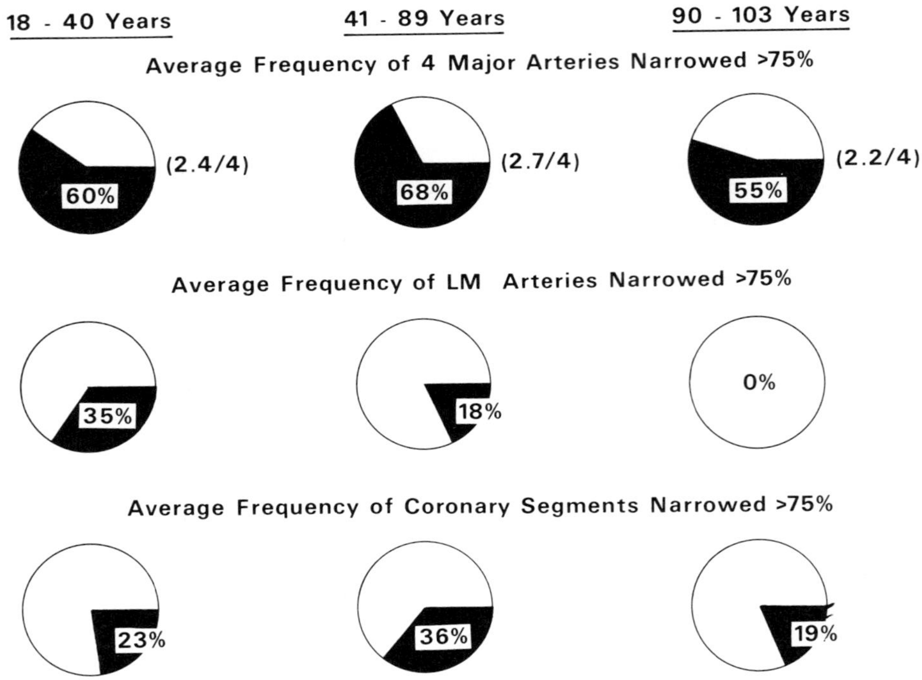

Figure 3–30. Diagram showing amounts of coronary atherosclerotic plaque in relation to age at necropsy in patients with fatal coronary events. The top set of pie diagrams indicates the average number (percent) of the four major coronary arteries severely narrowed by plaque. The middle set of pie diagrams indicates the average frequency of left main (LM) arteries severely diseased, and the lower set of pie diagrams indicates the average frequency of coronary segments (serially cut in 1 to 5 mm sections; see Table 3–2) severely narrowed by plaques.

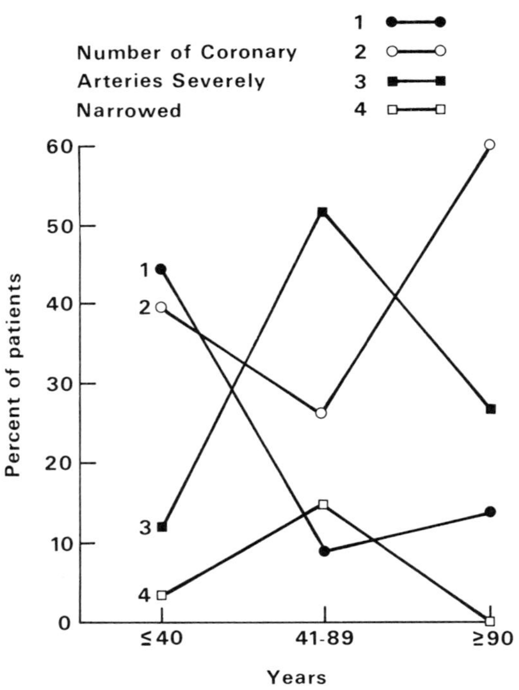

Figure 3–31. Comparison of age at death from coronary heart disease and the number of major epicardial coronary arteries severely narrowed by atherosclerotic plaques. "Single vessel" disease is most frequent in the young (≤40 years); "double vessel" disease is common in the elderly (≥90 years); and "triple vessel" disease is most common in the middle-aged group (41 to 89 years). Four-vessel disease (i.e., severe left main disease) is rarely seen in the very elderly patient.

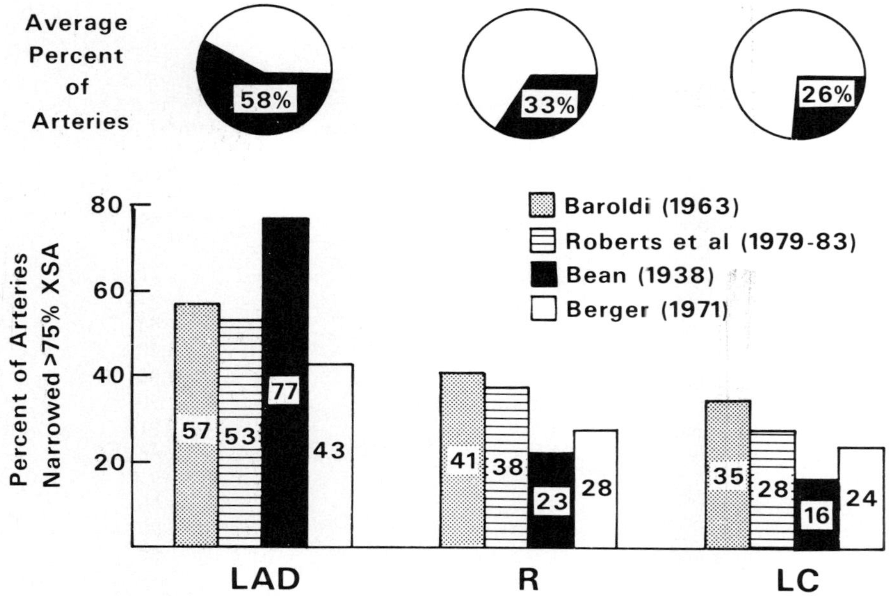

Figure 3–32. Diagram showing the frequency of severe coronary luminal narrowing of the left anterior descending (LAD), left circumflex (LC), and right (R) coronary arteries at necropsy in patients with fatal coronary heart disease. The pie diagrams indicate the average percent of the respective arteries severely narrowed.

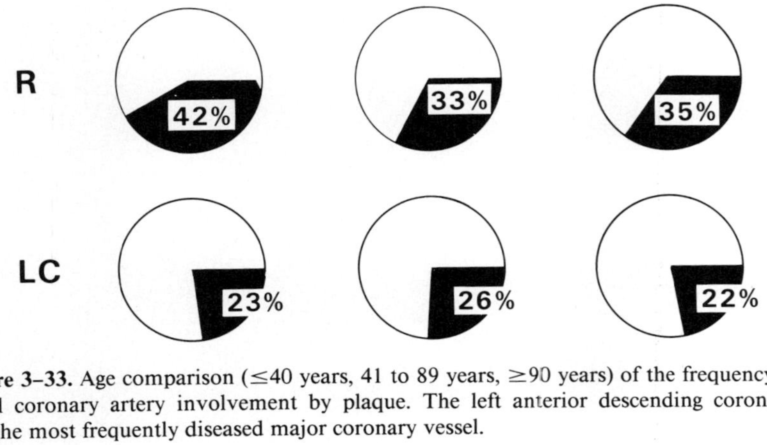

Figure 3–33. Age comparison (≤40 years, 41 to 89 years, ≥90 years) of the frequency of major epicardial coronary artery involvement by plaque. The left anterior descending coronary artery remains the most frequently diseased major coronary vessel.

Table 3–3. Frequency of Occlusive Coronary Artery Thrombi in Necropsy Patients with Fatal Transmural (T) or Nontransmural (NT) Acute Myocardial Infarction

		Frequency of Thrombus(%)		
First Author	Year Published	T	NT	Total
Friedberg[113]	1939	—	—	59
Miller[114]	1951	90	20	66
Branwood[115]	1956	—	—	21
Spiekerman[116]	1962	—	—	32
Mitchell[117]	1963	86	—	86
Ehrlich[118]	1964	—	10	50
Harland[119]	1966	86	71	90
Kagan[120]	1968	—	—	50
Chapman[121]	1968	—	—	91
Hackel[122]	1969	(General ward)		68
		(Coronary care unit)		94
Bouch[31]	1970	—	—	66
Spain[47]	1970	—	—	90
Sinapius[125]	1972	96	55	89
Roberts[126]	1972	54	0	39
Baroldi[127]	1974	38	0	38
Davies[128]	1976	92	13	95
Ridolfi[129]	1977	—	—	96
Bulkley[130]	1977	—	—	95
Horie[131]	1978	—	—	92
Branwood[132]	1978	82	20	36
Barrillon[133]	1979	—	—	90
Tanaka[134]	1979	—	27	69
Silver[135]	1980	55	—	45
DeWood[136]	1980	70	—	70
Lie[137]	1987	61	12	39
	TOTALS	74	28	70

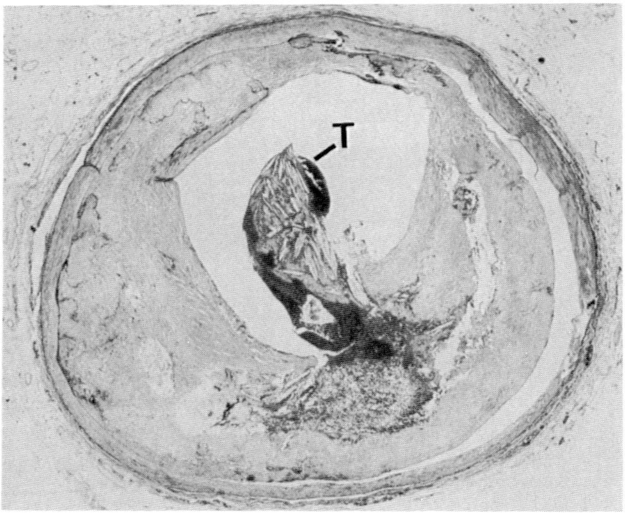

Figure 3–34. Early formation of coronary artery thrombus. Cross-section of epicardial coronary artery showing intimal fissure and formation of fibrin-platelet thrombus (T).

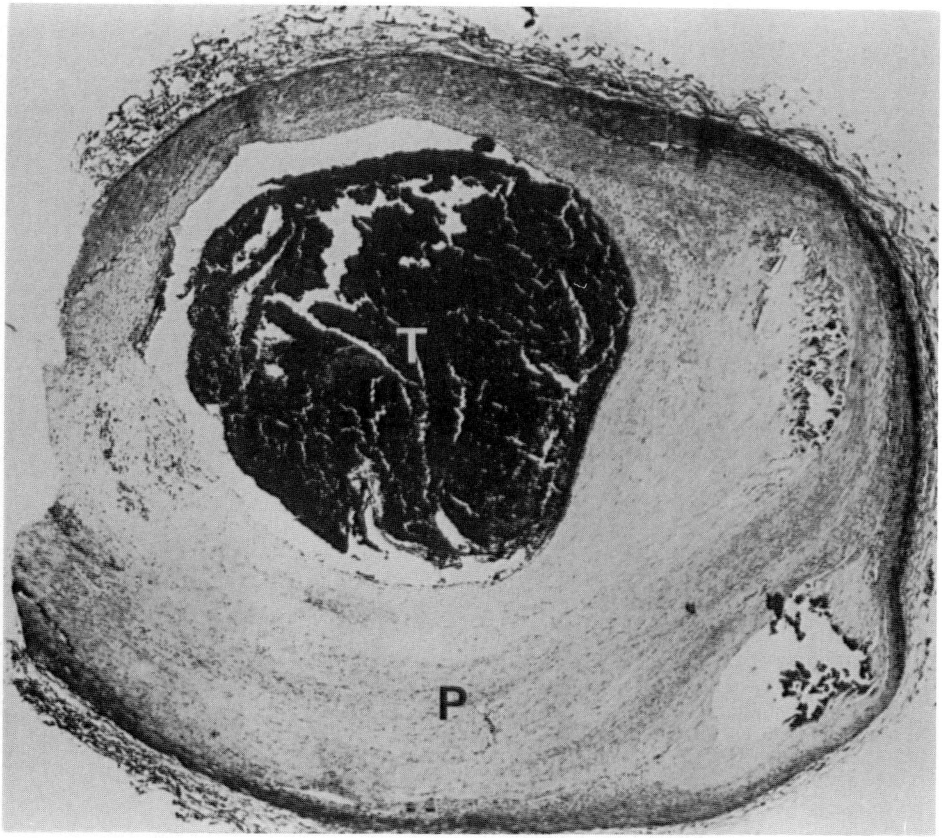

Figure 3–35. Occlusive coronary artery thrombus (T) in proximal left anterior descending coronary artery superimposed on severe atherosclerotic plaque (P).

and colleagues[142A] recently reported morphologic findings in the infarct-related coronary artery in 19 necropsy patients undergoing various forms of acute recanalization therapy (Table 3–4). Gross and histologic observations in the infarct-related reperfused coronary artery separated the 19 necropsy patients into two distinct groups: *those patients treated with and those without coronary angioplasty.*[142] Of the 19 necropsy patients, 9 (47 percent) underwent acute balloon angioplasty and had morphologic evidence of plaque "cracks," "fractures," and medial dissection that appeared to increase the coronary luminal cross-sectional area in eight of the nine arteries dilated. Of the nine dilation sites, eight had a reduction of 51 percent to 75 percent in luminal cross-sectional area and one had a 76 percent to 100 percent narrowing in cross-sectional area by atherosclerotic plaque. In contrast, 9 of the 10 remaining infarct coronary arteries from patients with thrombolytic therapy without balloon angioplasty had no morphologic evidence of plaque cracks or localized medial dissection, and the 9 sites of previous occlusion were narrowed 76 percent to 100 percent in cross-sectional area by atherosclerotic plaque. *Thus, in patients treated with acute angioplasty reperfusion therapy, the sites of previous total occlusion had less luminal cross-sectional area reduction by residual atherosclerotic plaque than did the sites of previous total occlusion in patients treated with thrombolytic agents.*

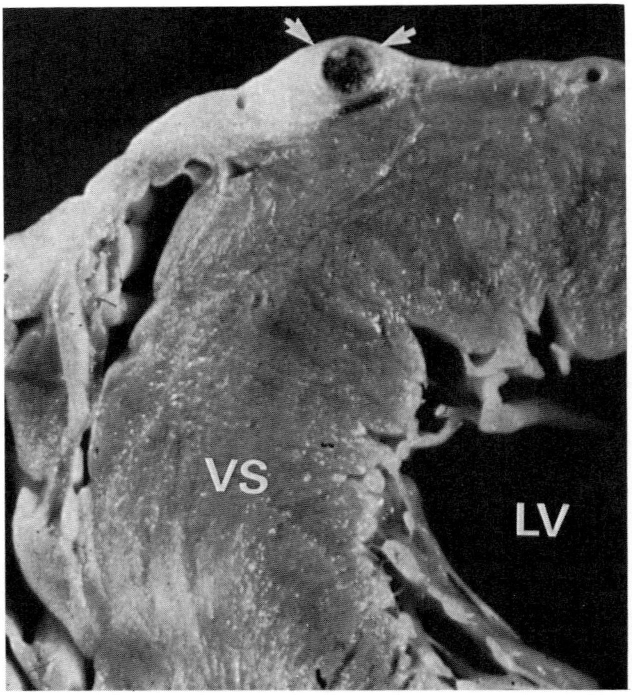

Figure 3–36. Acute coronary artery thrombosis. Photograph of occluded proximal left anterior descending coronary artery *(arrows)* by atherosclerotic plaque and thrombus. The patient had a fatal acute myocardial infarction. LV = left ventricle; VS = ventricular septum.

Table 3–4. Infarct Coronary Artery Observations in 19 Necropsy Patients with Acute Myocardial Infarction Undergoing Various Forms of Acute Reperfusion Therapy

Observation	S Only (N = 9)	PTCA Only (N = 5)	PTCA + S (N = 3)	S + Guidewire (N = 1)	r-Tissue-Plasminogen Activator + PTCA (N = 1)
Artery involved					
LAD	6	3	3	0	1
R	2	2	0	0	0
LC	1	0	0	0	0
LM	0	0	0	1	0
Residual thrombus	8	4	3	1	0
Occlusive	5	3	1	0	0
Degree of underlying atherosclerotic plaque: (% XSA)					
51–75%	1	5	2	0	1
>75%	8	0	1	1	0
Intraplaque Hemorrhage	0	0	3	0	1
"Crack"					
Occlusive	0	0	1	0	0
Intimal-medial tear	0	5	3	0	1*

*Coronary artery rupture with extension of medial "crack" to adventitia.

LAD = left anterior descending; LC = left circumflex; LM = left main; R = right; XSA = cross sectional area; S = streptokinase; PTCA = percutaneous transluminal coronary angioplasty.

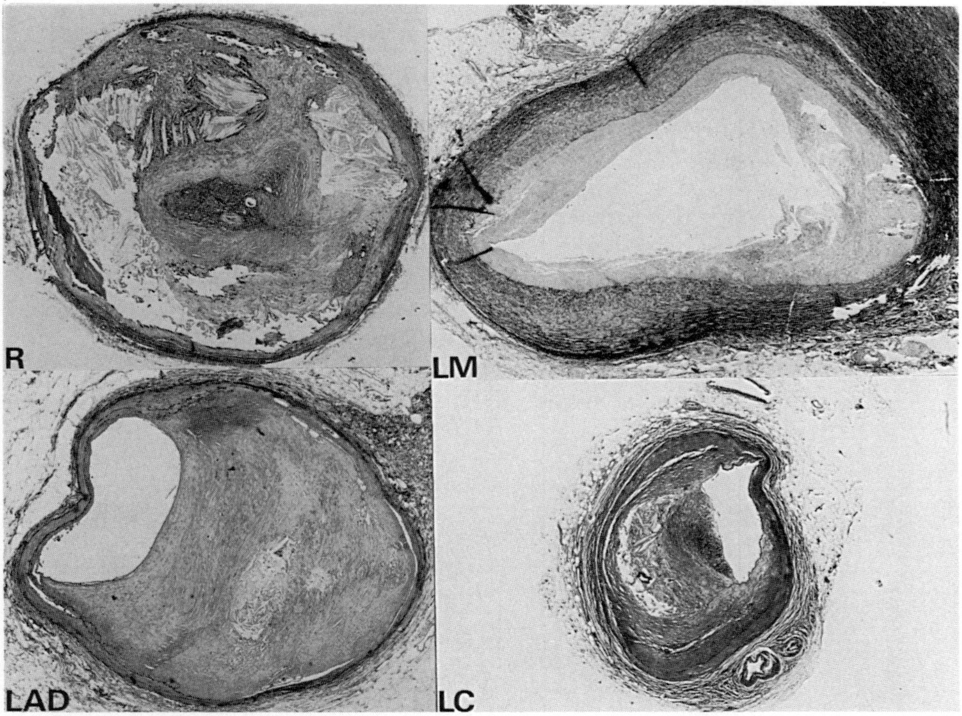

Figure 3–37. Composite of cross-sections of coronary arteries at sites of maximal luminal narrowing of the right (R), left main (LM), left anterior descending (LAD), and left circumflex (LC) coronary arteries. Recent thrombus occludes the severely narrowed R coronary artery.

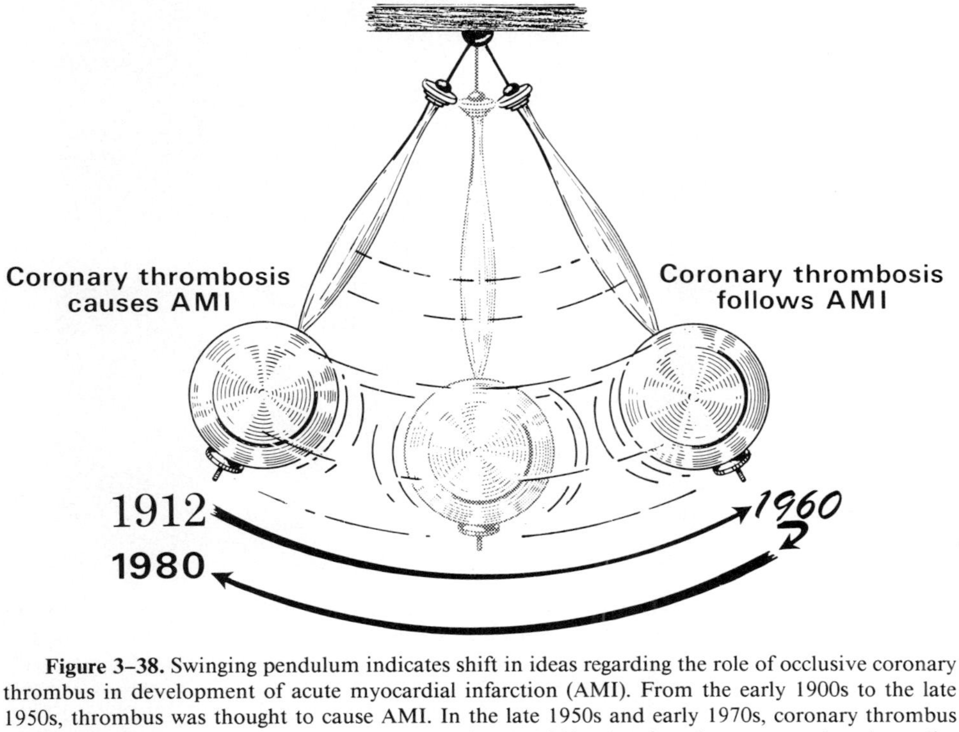

Figure 3–38. Swinging pendulum indicates shift in ideas regarding the role of occlusive coronary thrombus in development of acute myocardial infarction (AMI). From the early 1900s to the late 1950s, thrombus was thought to cause AMI. In the late 1950s and early 1970s, coronary thrombus was thought to follow AMI. In the late 1970s and early 1980s, the views have returned to the earlier beliefs.

Intraplaque Hemorrhage in the Infarct-Related Artery

The nine patients receiving acute angioplasty reperfusion therapy also can be separated into two distinct subgroups: those patients treated with angioplasty alone and those treated with angioplasty and thrombolytic agents (see Table 3–4).[142] In the five patients treated with angioplasty alone, the site of angioplasty had plaque "fractures" and "cracks" *without* intimal or medial hemorrhage. In contrast, in the four patients treated with angioplasty plus thrombolytic therapy, the site of angioplasty had plaque "fractures" and "cracks" with *hemorrhage* involving the intimal, medial, and adventitial layers of the coronary artery (Figs. 3–39 and 3–40). In one patient, the hemorrhage was so extensive that it narrowed the coronary lumen at the angioplasty site (see Figs. 3–39 and 3–40). In the 10

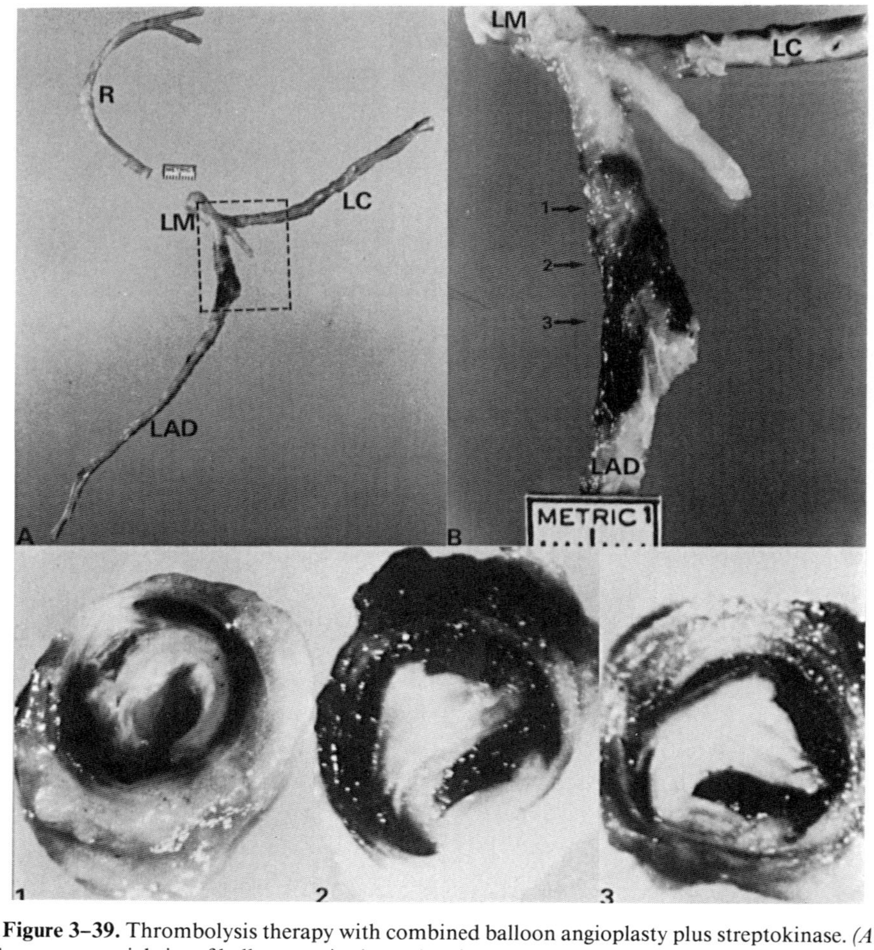

Figure 3–39. Thrombolysis therapy with combined balloon angioplasty plus streptokinase. *(A and B)* Coronary arterial site of balloon angioplasty showing marked adventitial hemorrhage. Numbers in *B* indicate sites of cross-sections (1 to 3) shown below. (*1*) Prominent atherosclerotic plaque "crack" with surrounding hemorrhage. *(2 and 3)* Marked bleeding into area of angioplasty severely narrows the coronary lumen. LAD = left anterior descending; LC = left circumflex; LM = left main; R = right. (From Waller,[142A] with permission.)

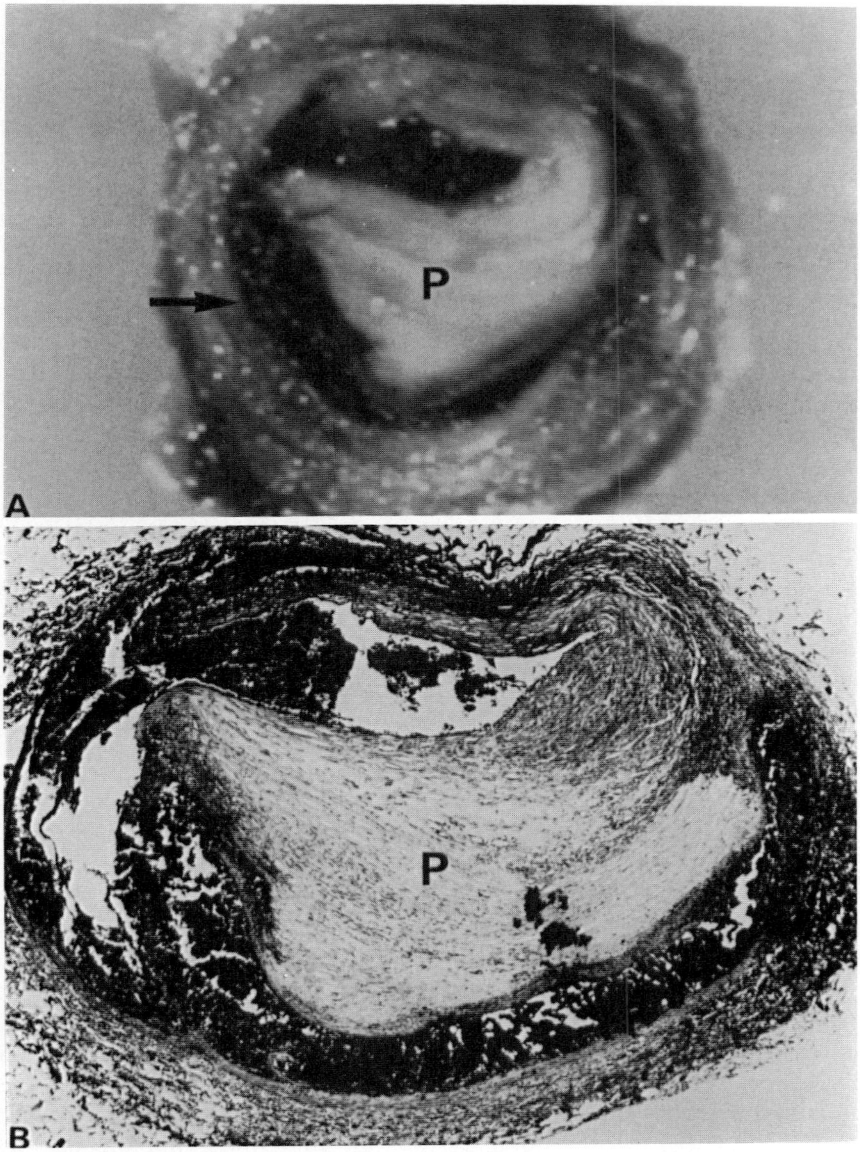

Figure 3–40. Close-up of angioplasty site shown in Figure 3–38. (*A*) Prominent plaque (P) "crack" with surrounding hemorrhage *(arrow)*. (*B*) Histologic section of segment shows medial dissection and extensive adventitial blood. (From Waller,[142A] with permission.)

patients receiving streptokinase therapy alone, intraplaque hemorrhage was absent. Thus, *the use of combined angioplasty and thrombolytic agents in acute reperfusion therapy may produce localized bleeding at the angioplasty site, and the bleeding may produce additional coronary luminal narrowing.*

NONATHEROSCLEROTIC CORONARY ARTERY DISEASE

Although atherosclerotic disease of the coronary arteries is the most common cause of coronary luminal narrowing and acute myocardial infarction, there are several nonatherosclerotic causes of severe luminal narrowing and subsequent clinical coronary event (angina pectoris, acute myocardial infarction, sudden death) (see Table 3–1). This portion of the chapter will briefly describe some of these conditions.

Congenital Coronary Artery Anomalies

Variation in the origin, course, or distribution of the epicardial coronary arteries are found in 1 percent to 2 percent of the population.[144] Certain types of these anomalies (ostial lesions, passage of a major artery between the walls of the pulmonary trunk and aorta, origin of a major artery from the pulmonary trunk, myocardial "bridges") may be more likely to produce ischemia with subsequent myocardial infarction.[145]

Origin of Both Right and Left Coronary Arteries from the Same Sinus of Valsalva. When either the right or left coronary artery arises from the left or right sinus of Valsalva, respectively, the anomalous vessel transverses the base of the heart in a course anterior to the pulmonary trunk, posterior to the aorta, or between the aorta and pulmonary trunk (Figs. 3–41 and 3–42). At least 43 necropsy patients have been reported with the origin of the left (left main) coronary artery from the right sinus and passage between the aorta and pulmonary trunk,[146] and, in 34 (79 percent), death was related to the anomaly (sudden death, AMI). At necropsy, 5 of 26 patients aged <20 years had myocardial infarcts.[146] Origin of the right coronary artery from the left sinus of Valsalva and passage between the aorta and pulmonary trunk also may be associated with symptoms of myocardial ischemia, infarction, or sudden death.[146] Of 12 necropsy patients with this anomaly reported by Roberts and associates,[147] 3 died suddenly and 2 had angina or syncope. At necropsy, transmural ventricular scars (healed infarction) were seen in 2.

The mechanism of ischemia, infarction, and/or sudden death in this coronary anomaly appears related to the shape of the coronary ostium of the anomalous vessel (Fig. 3–41 through 3–44). Normally, the coronary ostia are round to oval in shape, but, in this anomaly, the coronary artery has an acute takeoff angle that makes the ostium slit-like in shape. With increased cardiac output (e.g., exercise), the aorta dilates and upon aortic wall stretching, this slit-like ostium becomes severely narrowed (see Figs. 3–41 through 3–44). It is unlikely that "compression" of the anomalous coronary artery by the aorta and pulmonary trunk occurs, in view of the marked differences in diastolic pressures. At best, there would be an anterior shift of the anomalous vessel rather than a vice-like compression.

Single Coronary Artery. Origin of the entire coronary circulation from a single aortic ostium has been termed "single coronary artery." This anomaly is

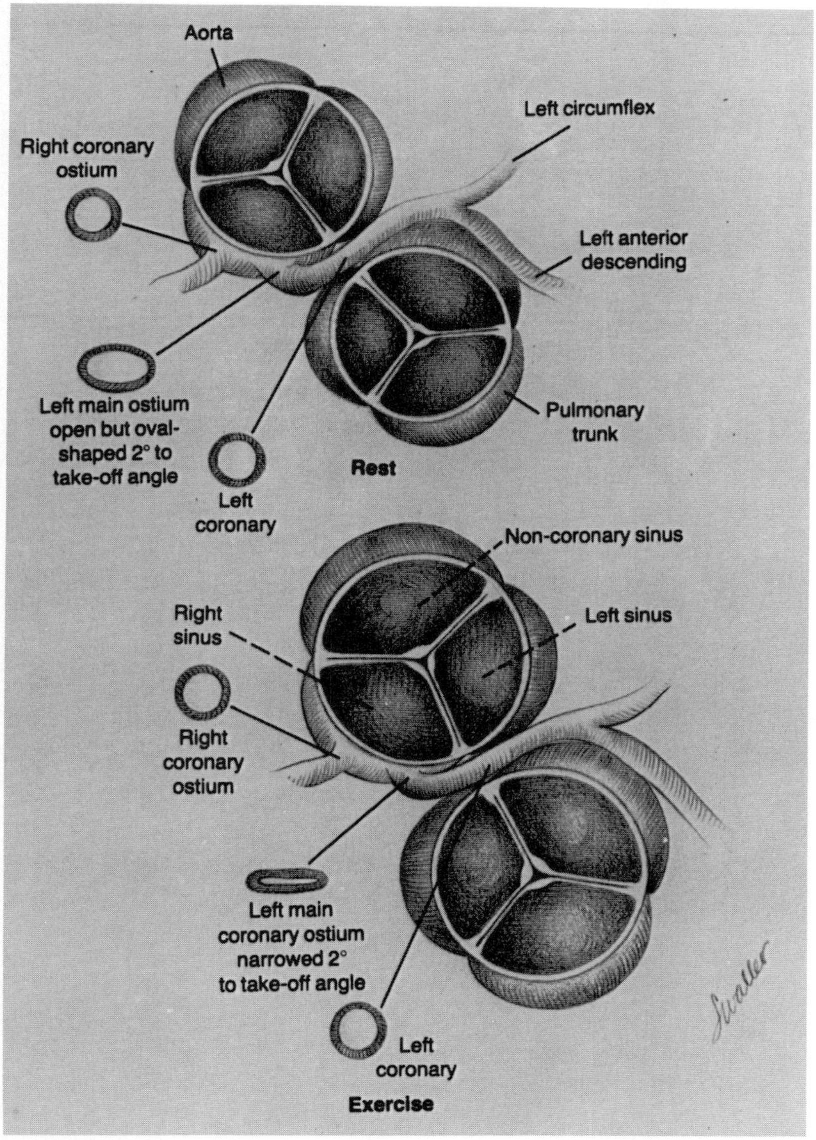

Figure 3–41. Diagram showing the proposed mechanism of myocardial ischemia produced by anomalous origin of the left coronary artery from the right sinus of Valsalva. With exercise, the aorta and pulmonary trunk dilate, thereby reducing the already narrowed coronary ostium of the anomalous left coronary. (From Waller,[233] with permission.)

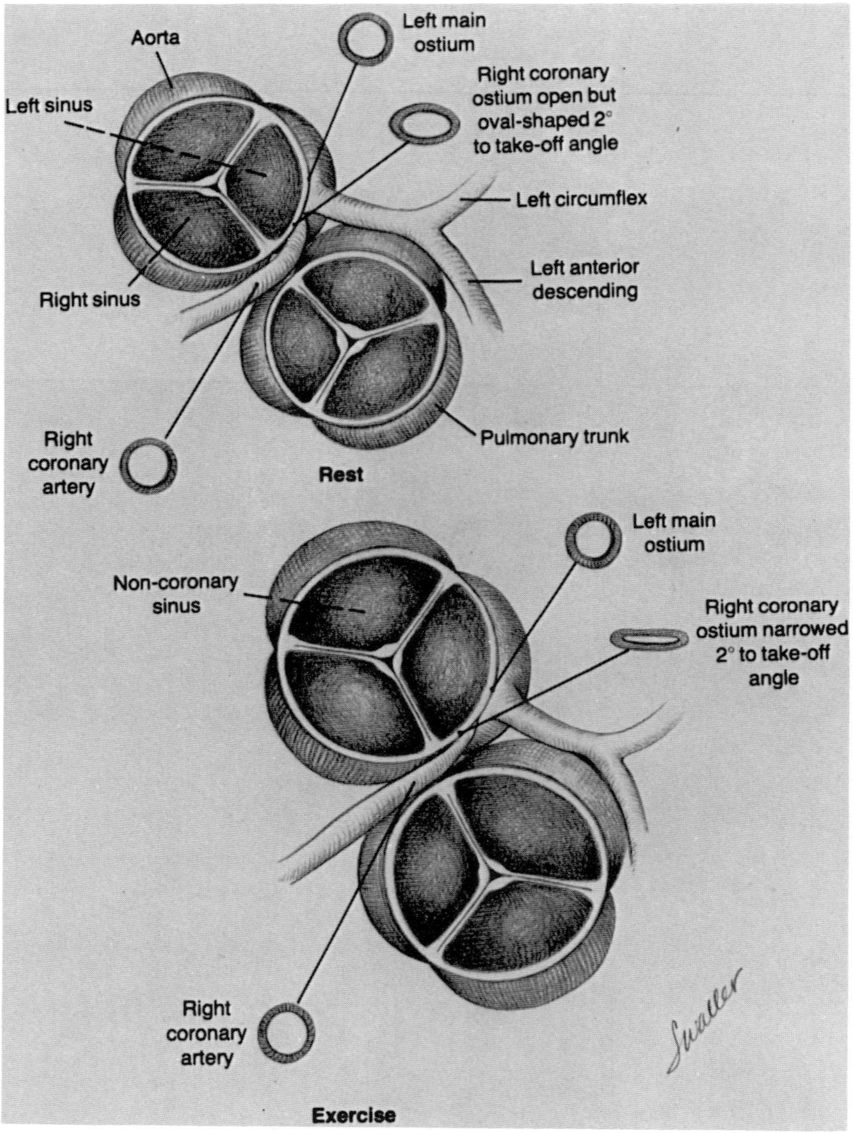

Figure 3–42. Diagram showing the proposed mechanism of myocardial ischemia produced by anomalous origin of the right coronary artery from the left sinus of Valsalva. With exercise, the aorta and pulmonary trunk dilate, thereby reducing the already narrowed coronary ostium of the anomalous right coronary. (From Waller,[233] with permission.)

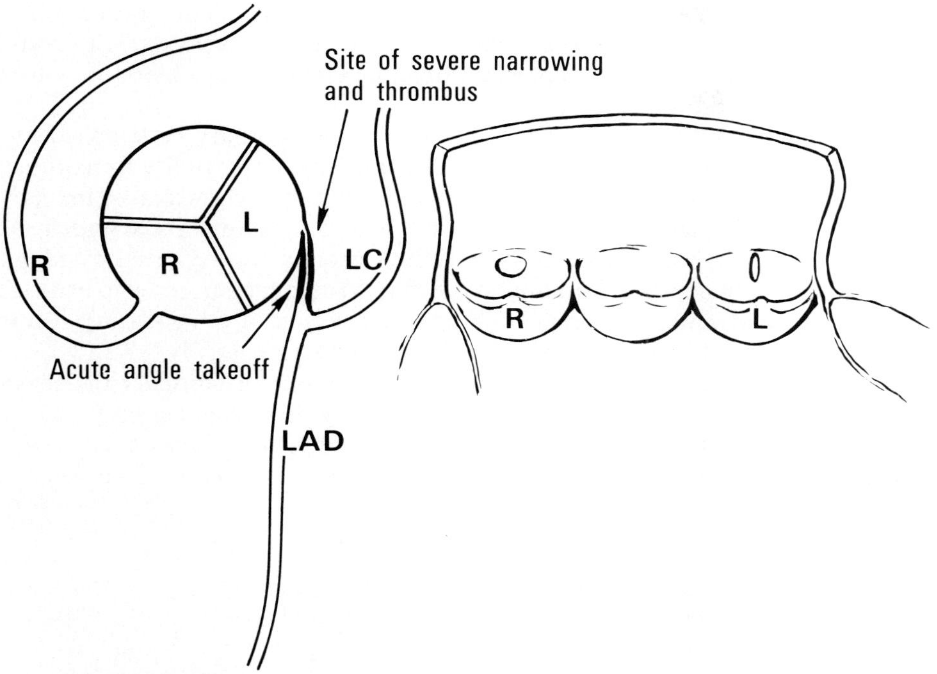

Figure 3–43. Diagram showing acute angle takeoff of the left main coronary artery with ostial ridge and slit-like orifice. The proximal left main is occluded by atherosclerotic plaque and thrombus, but the remaining vessels are normal. Accelerated coronary atherosclerosis may result from the acute angle takeoff malformation. Ao = aorta; L = left cusp; L = left main; LC = left circumflex; LAD = left anterior descending; R = right cusp; RC = right coronary. (From Menke, et al,[234] with permission.)

rare in the absence of other associated anomalies of the heart. One or more branches of the single artery may cross the base of the heart in a fashion described above and thus may be exposed to the risks of ischemia owing to acute angulation.[143] Angina pectoris and myocardial lactate production have been demonstrated in patients with single coronary arteries in whom coronary atherosclerosis or anomalous coronary artery passage were not present.[148]

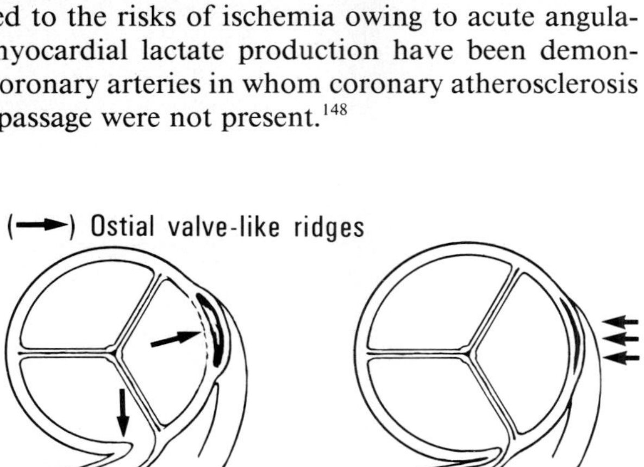

Figure 3–44. Diagram illustrating ostial valve-like ridges and the proposed mechanism of ostial compression with aortic root dilation. (From Virmani, et al,[152A] with permission.)

Coronary Artery Atresia. Atresia of one of the two main coronary ostia may be associated with myocardial ischemia/infarction in infancy or childhood.[143] The involved vessel becomes dependent on collateral coronary blood flow from the contralateral coronary artery.

High-Takeoff Coronary Ostia. Normally, the coronary ostia are located within the sinuses of Valsalva, which permits maximal opportunity for coronary artery diastolic filling. Location of the ostia in the tubular portion of the aorta (i.e., high-takeoff position) may be associated with decreased coronary perfusion (Fig. 3–45). Morphologic evidence of chronic ischemia was reported by Menke and associates[149] in a patient with high-takeoff right coronary artery who had right and left ventricular wall scarring. High-takeoff position of the coronary ostium also has been postulated as a cause of sudden coronary death.[150]

Ostial Fibrous Ridges. Nonatherosclerotic causes of coronary ostial narrowing include syphilis,[103] homozygous Type II hyperlipoproteinemia,[99] Takayasu's disease (pulseless disease),[151] fibromuscular hyperplasia associated with methysergide therapy,[152] aortic valve surgery with or without coronary artery can-

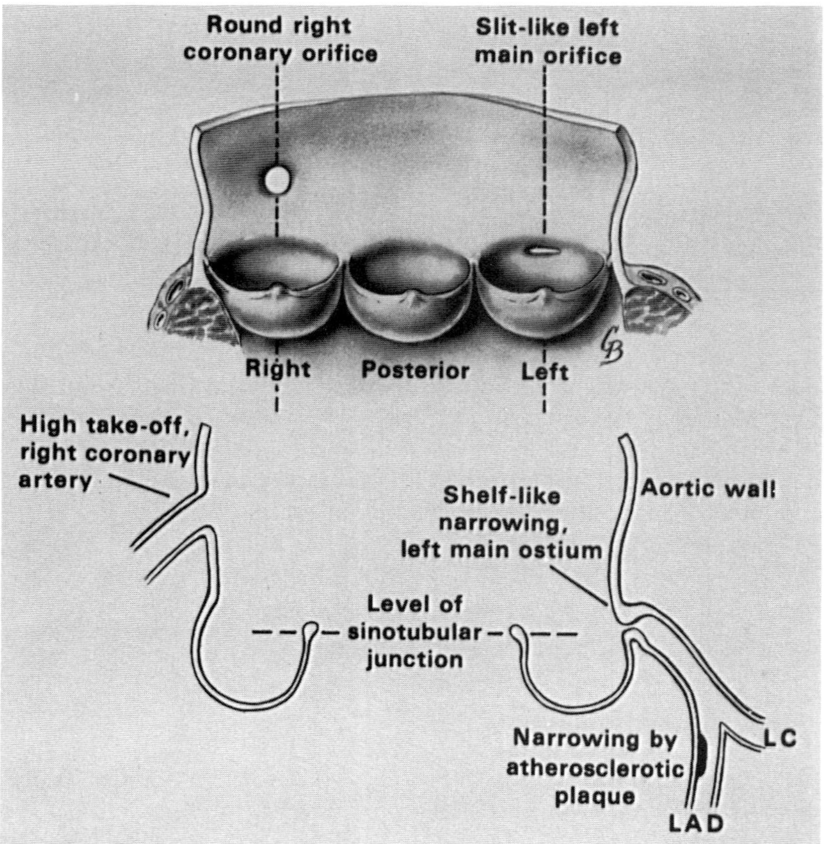

Figure 3–45. Diagram showing high takeoff position of the right coronary artery and the nonatherosclerotic fibrous ridge occluding the left main coronary ostium. LAD = left anterior descending; LC = left circumflex. (From Foster and Waller,[102] with permission.)

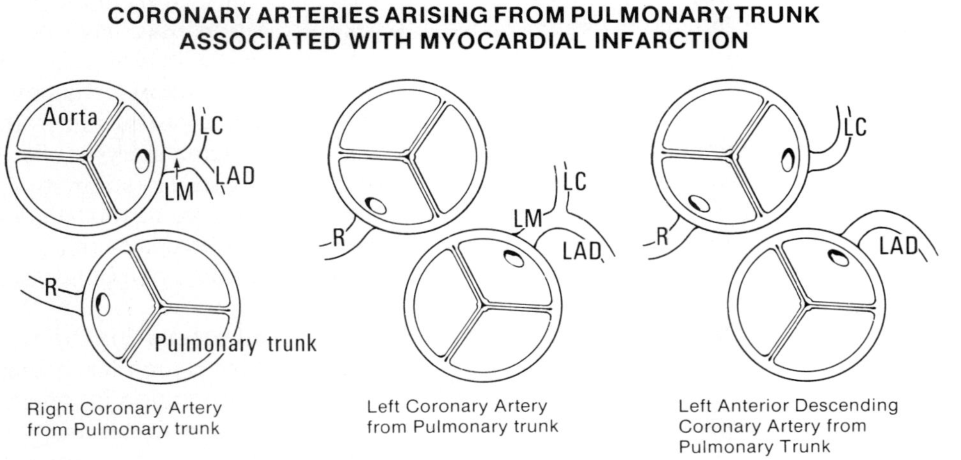

Figure 3–46. Anomalous origin of one or two major epicardial coronary arteries from the pulmonary trunk.

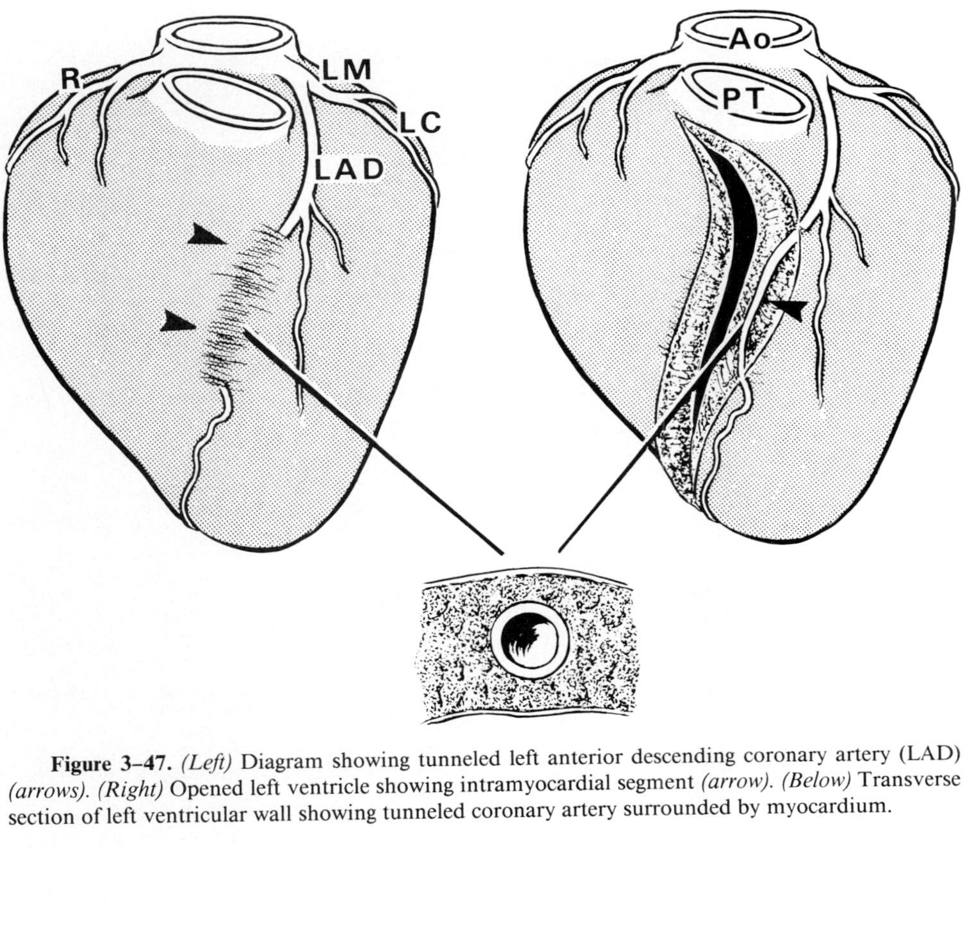

Figure 3–47. *(Left)* Diagram showing tunneled left anterior descending coronary artery (LAD) *(arrows)*. *(Right)* Opened left ventricle showing intramyocardial segment *(arrow)*. *(Below)* Transverse section of left ventricular wall showing tunneled coronary artery surrounded by myocardium.

nulation,[102] and ostial valve-like ridges (see Fig. 3–44). Foster and Waller[102] reported a nonatherosclerotic fibrous shelf-like ridge that projected from the wall of aorta into the left main ostium. This ridge-like projection may have been responsible for chronic ischemia and recent myocardial necrosis in a 56-year-old woman. Other rare diseases that may narrow or occlude the coronary ostia have been summarized by Baroldi[22]: (1) a nonatheromatous, calcific protrusion from the sinotubular junction into the right or left ostium; (2) saccular aneurysm of the aorta; (3) aortic dissection extending into the coronary ostium (right ostium more common than left); (4) supravalvular aortic stenosis with severe intimal thickening; (5) oblisteration of the ostium due to adhesion of the free edge of an aortic cusp to the aortic wall above the coronary ostium; (6) occlusion by embolus (see below); and (7) occlusive fibroelastosis.

Anomalous Origin of One or Two Coronary Arteries from the Pulmonary Trunk. Anomalous origin of a coronary artery from the pulmonary trunk (Fig. 3–46) may be responsible for myocardial ischemia and infarction in infants and chidren. In more than 90 percent of cases,[143,146] the left main is the anomalous artery, and thus the anteroseptal and anterolateral left ventricular myocardium may be at jeopardy for injury. Asymptomatic older patients with this coronary anomaly usually are discovered by having an abnormal electrocardiogram, by having a precordial murmur, or by the occurrence of sudden death.[146] The peri-

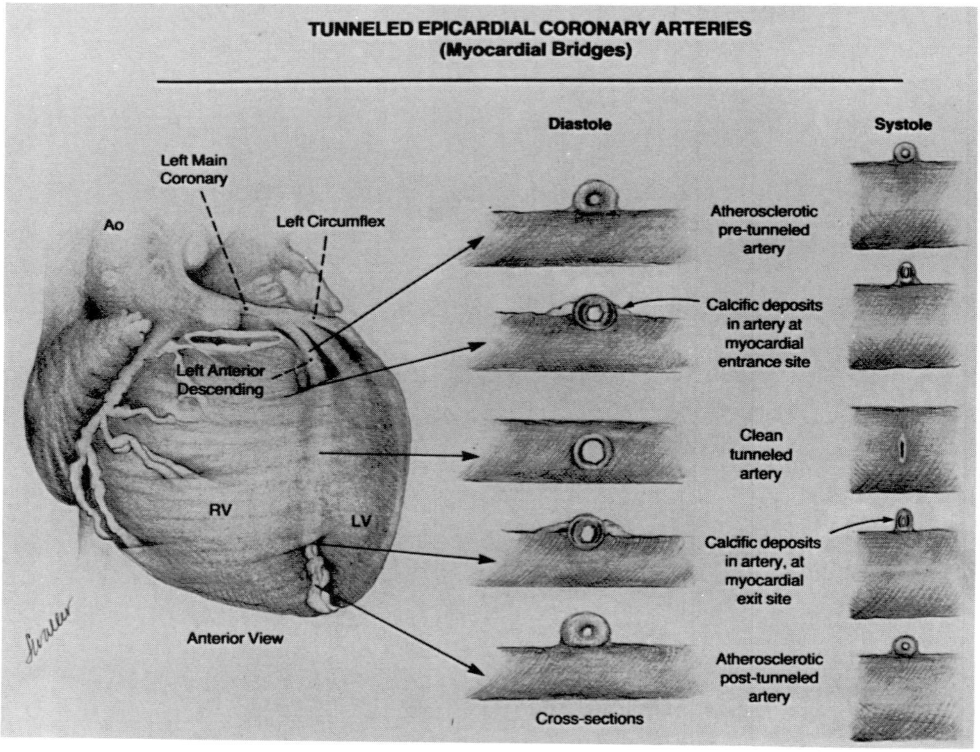

Figure 3–48. Diagram showing segments of tunneled and nontunneled epicardial coronary artery with changes during ventricular systole and diastole. Ao = aorta; LV = left ventricle; RV = right ventricle. (From Waller,[233] with permission.)

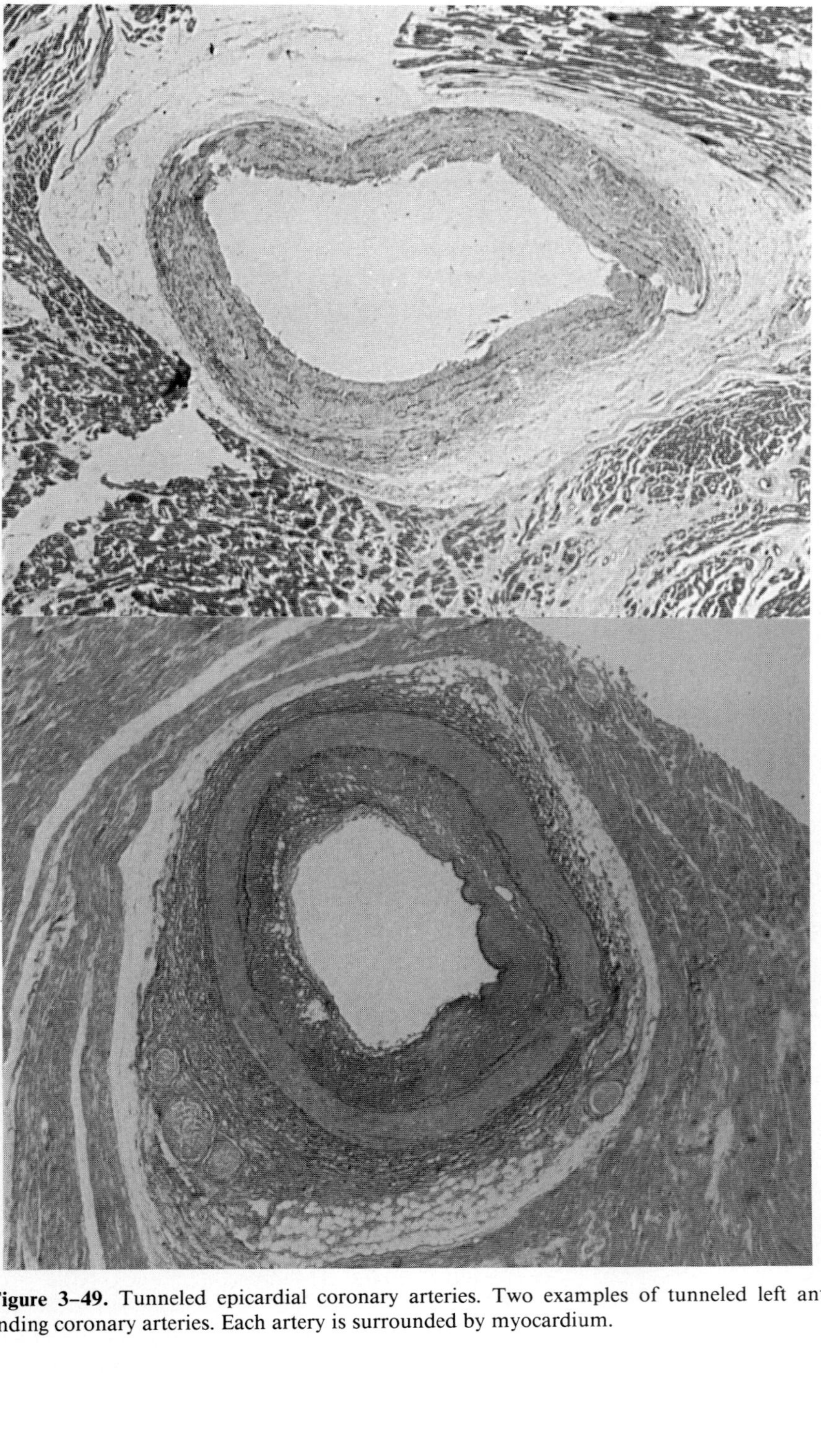

Figure 3–49. Tunneled epicardial coronary arteries. Two examples of tunneled left anterior descending coronary arteries. Each artery is surrounded by myocardium.

cardial murmur and abnormal electrocardiogram are the result of papillary muscle and/or anteroseptal myocardial wall damage.

Coronary Artery Fistula. Direct connection between a major epicardial coronary artery and a cardiac chamber or major vessel (vena cava, coronary sinus, pulmonary artery) is the most common hemodynamically significant coronary artery anomaly.[143] Fistulas from the right coronary artery are more common than from the left. Over 90 percent of the fistulas drain into the venous circulation.[143] Myocardial ischemia has been documented in some patients with coronary artery fistulas who have no evidence of coronary atherosclerosis.[143]

Myocardial Bridges ("Tunneled" Epicardial Coronary Artery). The coronary arteries, which normally course over the epicardial surface of the heart, may dip into the myocardium to travel for varying lengths and then reappear on the heart's surface (Figs. 3–47 through 3–55). The muscle overlying the intramyocardial segment of the epicardial coronary artery is termed a "myocardial bridge," and the artery coursing within the myocardium is called a "tunneled" artery (see Figs. 3–47 through 3–49). Tunneled coronary arteries have been recognized anatomically for more than two centuries,[153] but recent reports indicating an association with myocardial ischemia and myocardial bridges have heightened clinical relevance.[154,155] Tunneled coronary arteries have been presumed congenital in origin. Visscher and colleagues[156] reported a tunneled left anterior descending artery in a 42-day-old infant, supporting the presumption that myocardial bridging of coronary arteries existed since birth. At least three factors have been postulated to account for differences between the high frequency of tunneled major coronary arteries observed at necropsy (5 percent[157] to 86 percent[158]), and

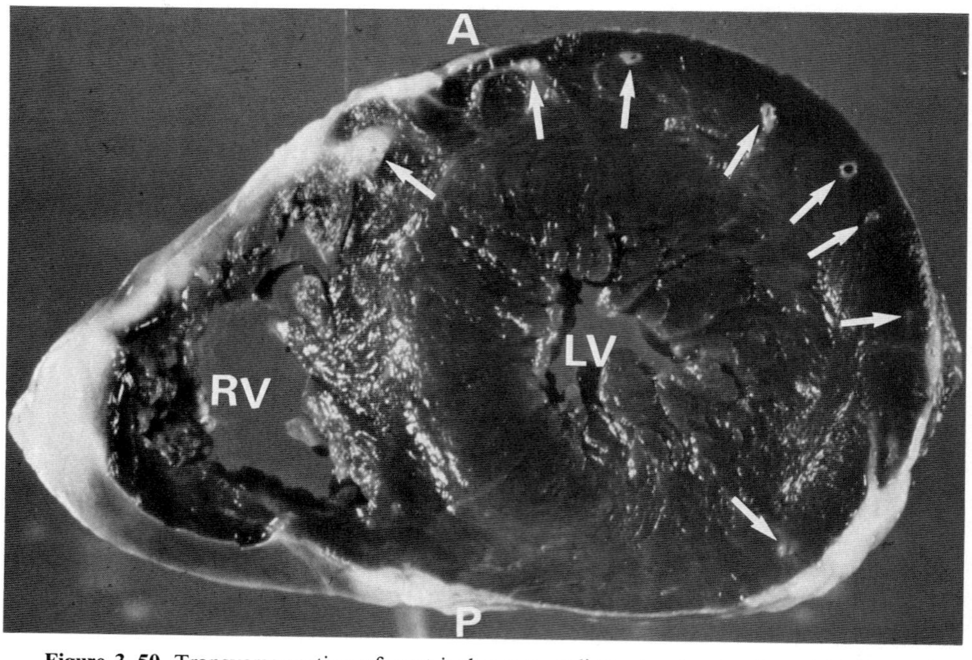

Figure 3–50. Transverse section of ventricular myocardium showing the "arcade" of tunneled epicardial coronary arteries *(arrows)*. A = anterior; LV = left ventricle; RV = right ventricle; P = posterior.

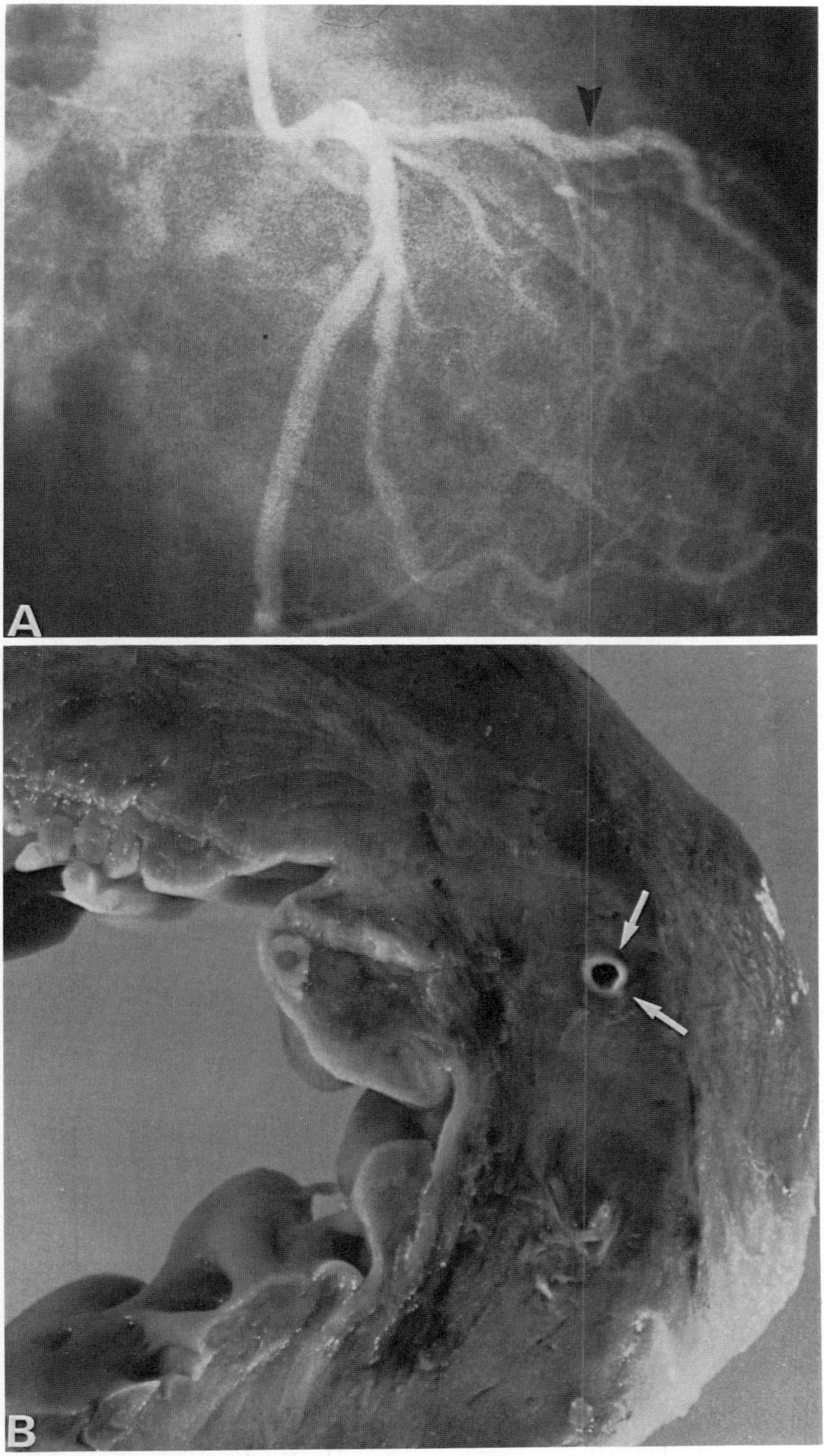

Figure 3–51. Tunneled epicardial coronary artery. (*A*) Coronary angiogram show tunneled segment of epicardial coronary artery. (*B*) Corresponding segment of tunneled left circumflex coronary artery *(arrow)*.

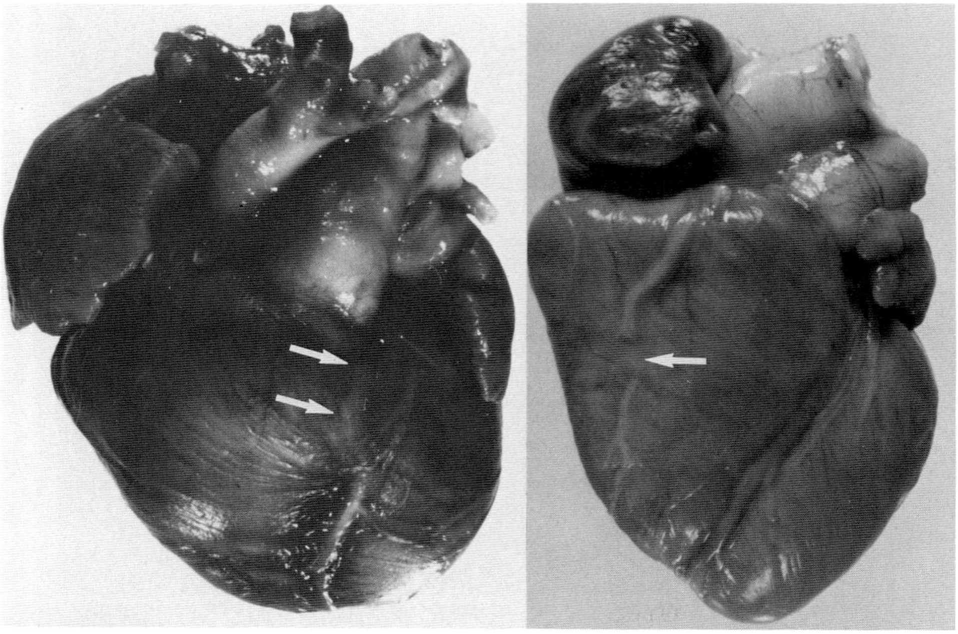

Figure 3–52. Tunneled left anterior epicardial coronary arteries from two newborn infants. *(Left)* Tunneled left anterior descending. *(Right)* Tunneled marginal branch of right coronary artery.

the lower frequency of tunneled coronary arteries observed angiographically (0.5 percent[154] to 12 percent[151]) or associated with symptoms of myocardial ischemia (18 percent[159]): (1) *length* of the tunneled coronary segment, (2) degree of *systolic compression,* and (3) *heart rate.* Isolated reports have suggested that *longer tunneled segments* of coronary arteries,[155] *more severe systolic diameter narrowing* of the tunneled segment,[155] and *tachycardia*[160] are contributing factors in the production of myocardial ischemia in association with myocardial bridging (see Figs. 3–53 and 3–54). The length of coronary tunneling may not be an important factor

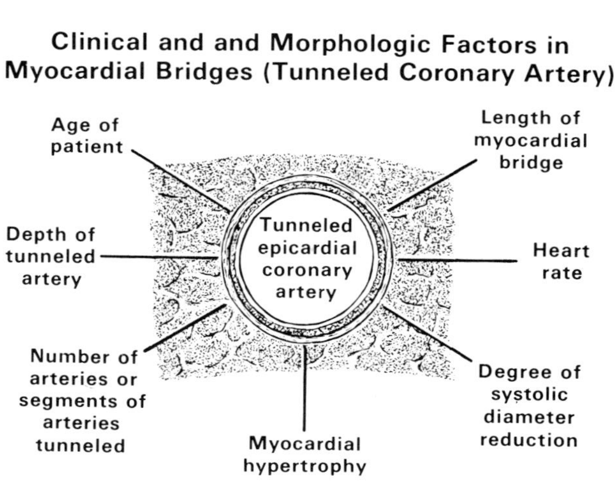

Figure 3–53. Diagram shows some of the clinical and anatomic factors in a tunneled epicardial coronary artery.

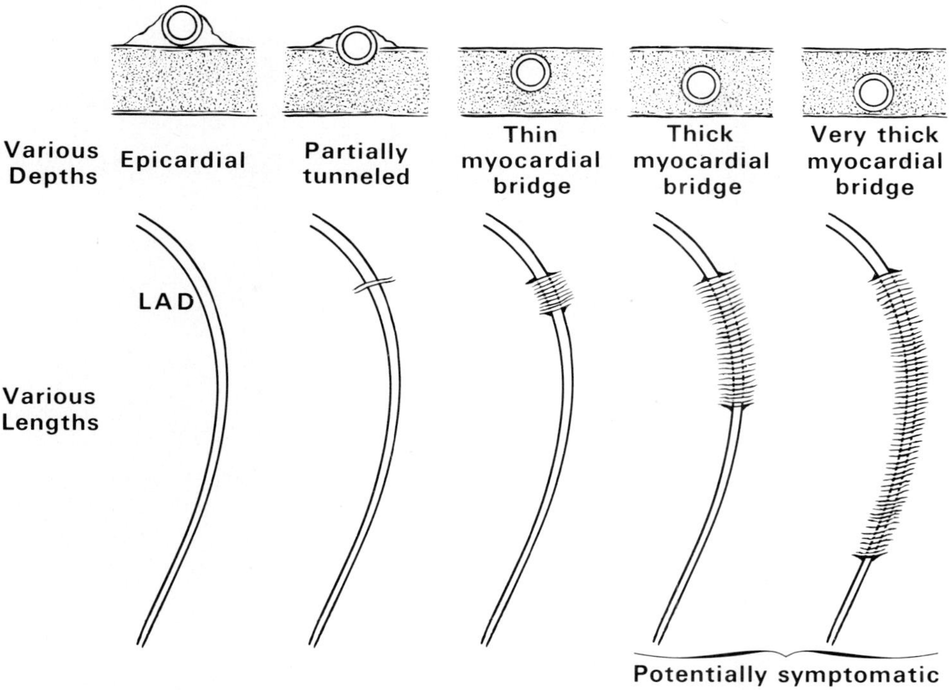

Figure 3–54. Diagram showing morphologic variations in tunneling (length of tunneled segment, depth of tunneled segment).

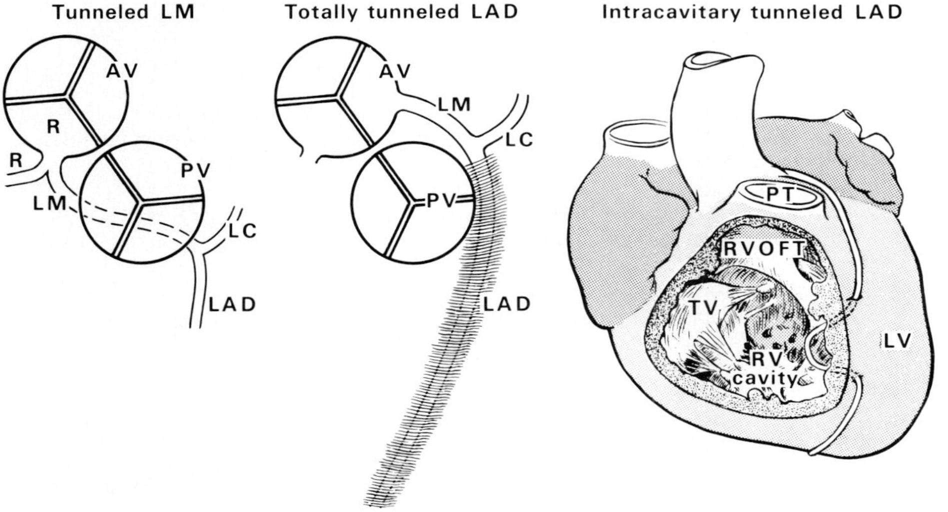

Figure 3–55. Diagram showing extremes of tunneled coronary arteries: left main (LM) tunneled through the ventricular septum, total length of the left anterior descending (LAD) located within the myocardium, tunneled segment of LAD becoming intracavitary. AV = aortic valve; LAD = left anterior descending; LC = left circumflex; LM = left main; LV = left ventricular; PT = pulmonary trunk; PV = pulmonary valve; RVOFT = right ventricular outflow tract; RV = right ventricle; TV = tricuspid valve.

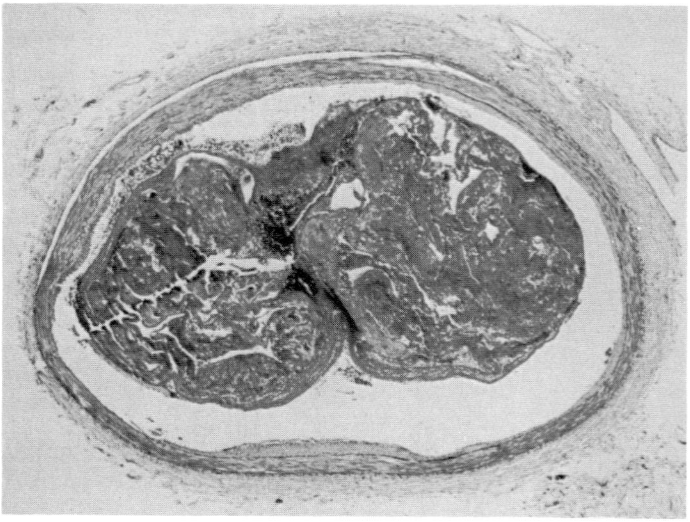

Figure 3–56. Coronary artery embolus. Fibrin-platelet thrombus occluding the left anterior descending coronary artery. The source of the embolus was not established, but the patient recently underwent cardiac surgery.

Table 3–5. Etiology of Coronary Artery Emboli

1. Natural
   - A. Vegetation
     1. Active infective endocarditis (native valve)
     2. Active infective endocarditis (prosthetic valve)
     3. Mural endocarditis
     4. Noninfective (marantic) endocarditis
   - B. Calcific deposit
     1. Aortic valve stenosis
     2. Mitral valve stenosis
   - C. Intracardiac thrombus
     1. Left ventricle (myocardial infarction, cardiomyopathy, fibroelastosis with mural thrombus, ventricular aneurysm)
     2. Left atrium—appendage (low cardiac output states)
     3. Left atrium—body (mitral stenosis, native or prosthetic)
     4. Pulmonary veins (mitral stenosis)
   - D. Intracardiac tumor
     1. Primary (myxoma)
     2. Secondary (extension from pulmonary veins, lymphatic extension, direct extension)
   - E. Coronary artery
     1. Plaque rupture
     2. Thrombus dislodgement
2. Iatrogenic
   - A. Cardiac surgery (ostial cannalization, prosthetic valve, patch repair)
   - B. Cardiac catheterization and angiography (catheter thrombus, catheter fragments)
   - C. Coronary angioplasty and thrombolysis
   - D. Prosthetic valves (thrombus, vegetation, occluders, leaflets, cloth covering, struts)
   - E. Cardioversion (left atrial thrombus, left ventricular thrombus)
   - F. Cardiac resuscitation (thrombus)
3. "Paradoxical"
   - A. Congenital heart disease (atrial septal defect, ventricular septal defect)
   - B. Probe patent foramen ovale defect (thrombophlebitis, right atrial catheters)
   - C. Pulmonary hypertension (acquired atrial septal defect)

in causing myocardial ischemia, as evidenced by two recent reports.[161,162] The authors of these reports describe three men with intramyocardial tunneling of greater than 40 mm of the left main coronary artery. Although the left main coronary artery was tunneled, none of the patients had clinical or morphologic evidence of myocardial ischemia (see Fig. 3–55).

Coronary Aneurysms. Congenital coronary artery aneurysms are found most commonly in the right coronary artery.[163] Abnormal flow patterns within the aneurysm may lead to thrombus formation with subsequent vessel occlusion, distal thromboembolization, and myocardial infarction.[164] In general, angina pectoris or acute myocardial infarction present in young patients (under 20 years of age) should prompt suspicion of a congenital coronary artery anomaly or a congenital coronary artery aneurysm.[163]

Coronary Artery Emboli

Coronary arterial emboli (Figs. 3–56 through 3–59) are clinically suspected in patients who develop severe chest pain (acute myocardial infarction) under the following circumstances: in the presence of a prosthetic left-sided valve, active infective endocarditis, native left-sided valve stenosis, atrial fibrillation, left ventricular aneurysm, dilated cardiomyopathy, known cardiac tumor, or during cardiac catheterization or cardiac surgery. The etiology of coronary emboli can be classified as *natural causes, iatrogenic causes,* and *"paradoxical" causes* (Table 3–

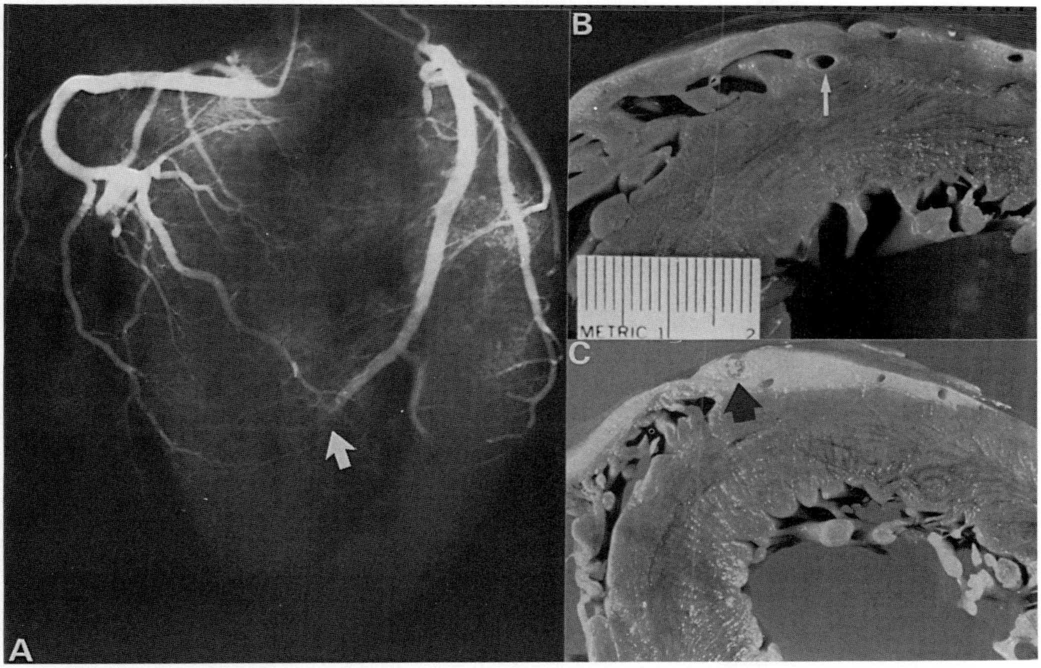

Figure 3–57. Coronary artery embolus. (*A*) Postmortem coronary angiogram showing normal epicardial coronary arteries except for sudden cutoff of the distal third of the left anterior coronary artery *(arrow)*. (*B*) Portion of anterior left ventricle and proximal left anterior descending coronary artery showing normal artery. (*C*) Site *(arrow)* of embolic occlusion of the left anterior descending coronary artery. The remaining distal left anterior descending, right, left circumflex, and left main coronary arteries were normal.

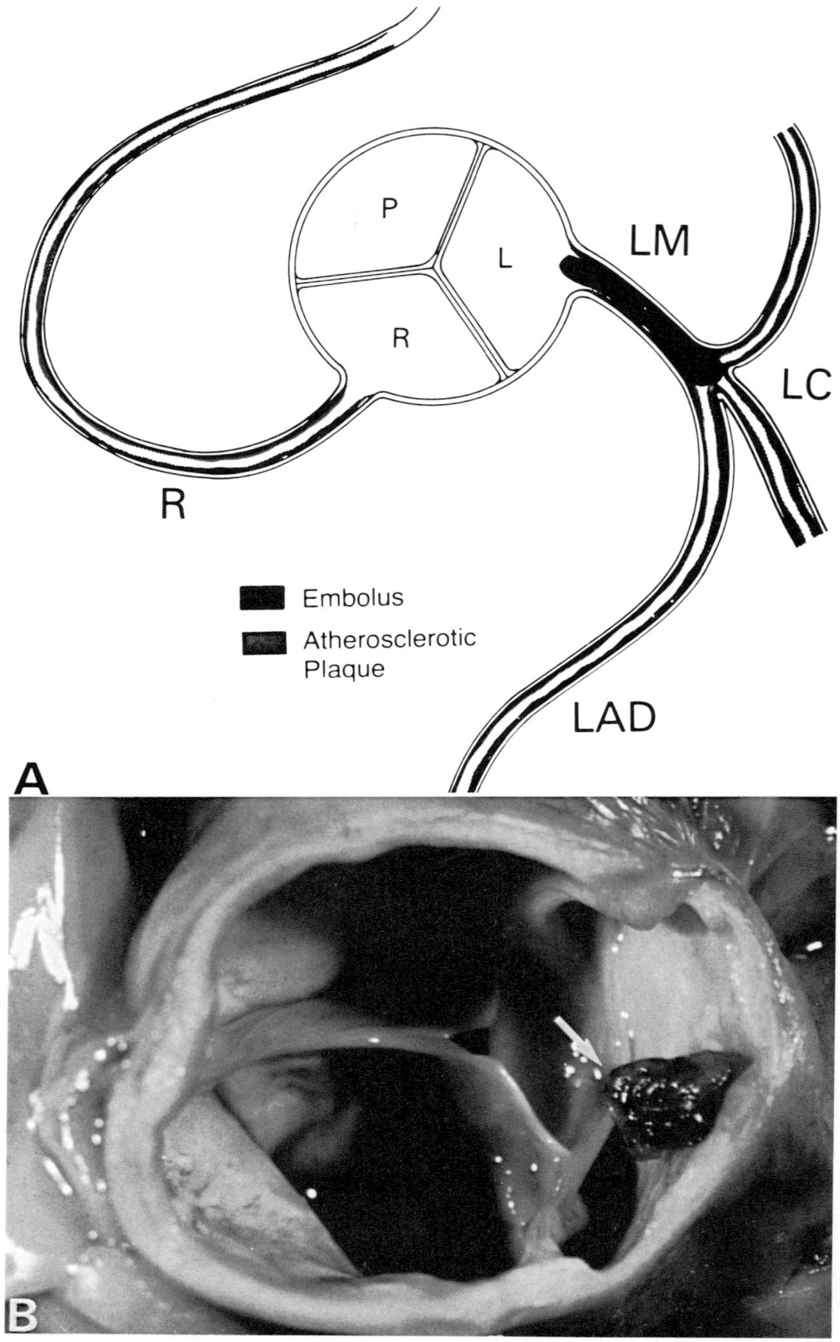

Figure 3–58. Coronary artery embolism. (*A*) Diagram showing location and extent of occlusion of the left main (LM) coronary artery by an embolus. (*B*) Photograph of aortic root showing embolus protruding from the LM coronary ostium *(arrows)*. LAD = left anterior descending; LC = left circumflex; R = right. (From Waller, et al,[166] with permission.)

5) (see Figs. 3–56 through 3–58). Coronary embolism most often involves the left anterior descending coronary artery.[163] Coronary embolism is suspected as the cause of acute myocardial infarction when at necropsy, the zone of necrosis is large but discrete (i.e., little time to develop effective collaterals). Embolic coronary artery lesions can resolve completely and spontaneously and are one of the explanations for angiographically normal coronary arteries several months following an acute myocardial infarction.[163]

The consequences of coronary embolism depend on two major factors (see Fig. 3–59): *size of the embolus* and the *size of the lumen of the artery in which it becomes impacted.*[165,166] The smaller the embolus, the greater the chance that it will travel distally to a small coronary arterial segment and the less the likelihood of myocardial infarction or fatal arrhythmia.[165,166] An embolus so small that it travels distally and impacts in a single intramural vessel is probably clinically silent and observed only at necropsy.[165,166] The status of the coronary lumen before the embolus also determines the subsequent myocardial consequences. An

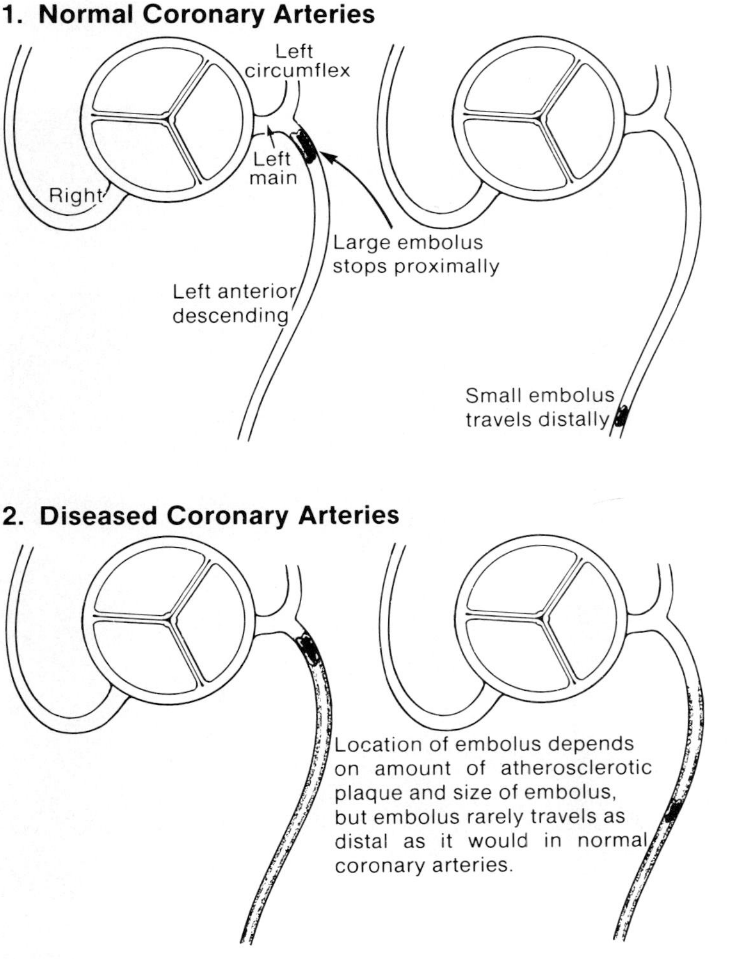

Figure 3–59. Coronary emboli in normal and diseased coronary arteries.

embolus to a previously normal coronary artery is likely to migrate distally and may result in localized myocardial infarction because of absence of collaterals. An embolus traveling to a previously diseased coronary artery is more likely to impact proximally. Emboli to the left main coronary arteries are rare but usually fatal (see Fig. 3–58).[166]

Coronary Artery Dissection

Separation of the media by hemorrhage with or without an associated intimal tear is termed coronary artery dissection. The medial separation forces the intimal-medial layer (wall of true channel) toward the true coronary lumen and produces distal myocardial ischemia/infarction (Figs. 3–60 through 3–62). Coronary artery dissections may be *primary* or *secondary*. Secondary coronary artery dissections are more frequent, especially those associated as an extension from aortic root dissection.[143] Primary coronary artery dissections may occur as a consequence of coronary angiography, cardiac surgery, chest trauma, or spontaneously. Most spontaneous coronary artery dissections occur in women (postpartum commonly) and may be associated with coronary arterial wall eosinophils.[167] The left anterior descending artery is the most frequently involved artery. Systemic hyper-

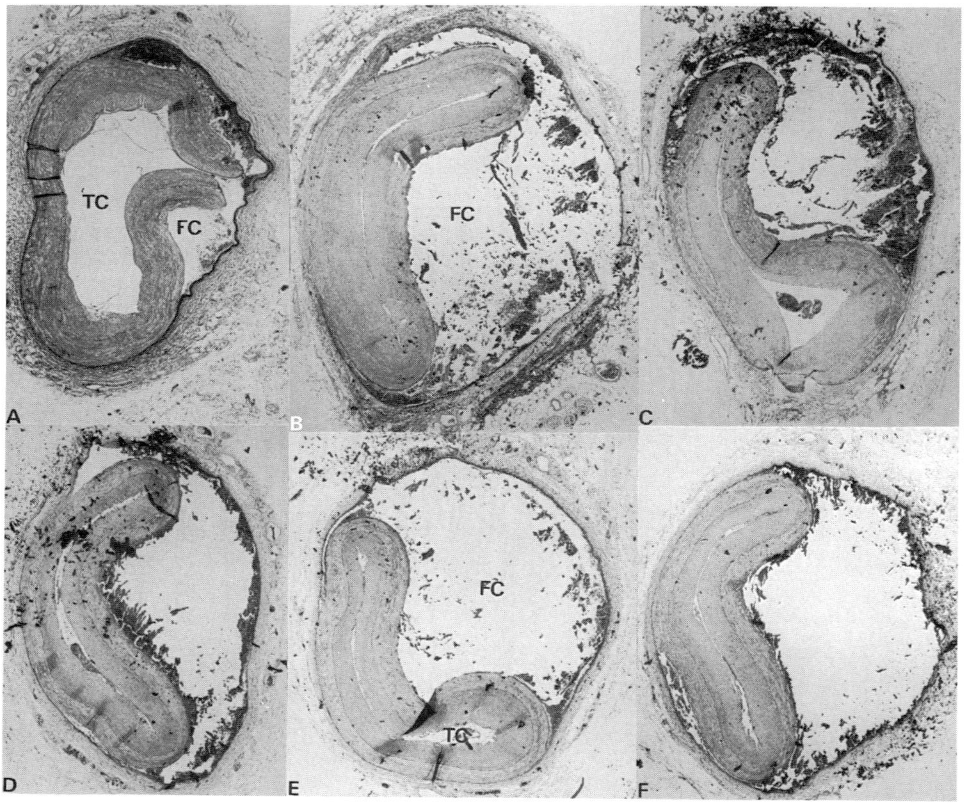

Figure 3–60. Coronary artery dissection. Serial cross-sections (*A–F*) showing dissection of the left anterior descending coronary artery. The true channel (TL) is severely compromised by external compression from the false channel (FC) ("dissection channel").

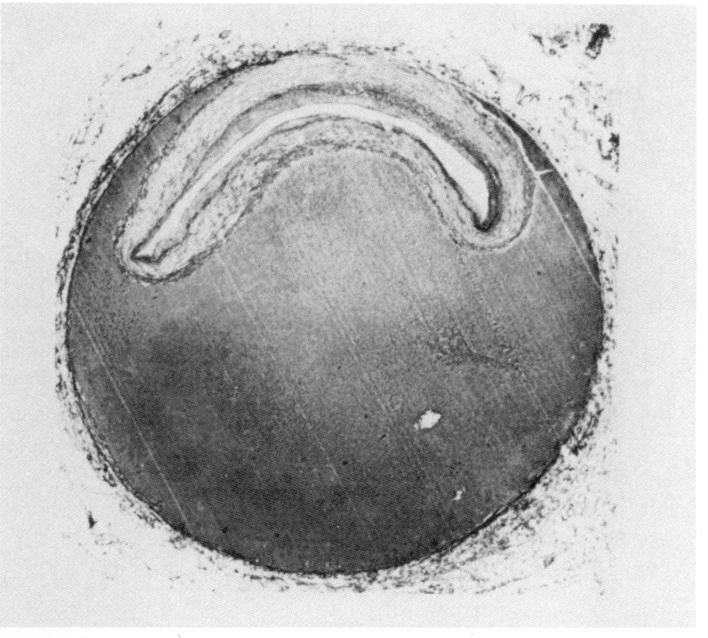

Figure 3–61. Coronary artery dissection of the left anterior descending coronary artery. The false channel is filled with blood and severely narrows the true channel. (From Roberts,[18] with permission.)

tension does not appear to be a significant risk factor.[163] Spontaneous coronary artery dissection may result in sudden death or acute myocardial infarction and subsequent death. Parenthetically, localized and limited coronary artery dissection (i.e., intimal-media tear) appears necessary for a clinically successful coronary artery balloon angioplasty procedure.[168]

Coronary Artery Spasm

Coronary artery luminal narrowing produced by spasm has been associated with angina pectoris, acute myocardial infarction, and sudden death. Despite the extensive clinical information about coronary artery spasm, relatively few necropsy data are available from these patients[169–180] (Table 3–6). Contraction of the smooth-muscle cells in the coronary artery wall may contract in response to various neurologic and pharmacologic stimuli and temporarily reduce the vessel lumen (see Figs. 3–16 and 3–17). Various postulates exist as to the exact mechanism of spasm, but the specific pathogenesis of this disorder is unknown.[180A] Enhanced alpha-adrenergic tone[181] and various vasoactive substances (histamine, catecholamines, prostaglandins, thromboxane A_2)[182,183] are presently thought to be relevant factors. Roberts and colleagues[179] and Isner[180] have reviewed the necropsy findings in 13 previously reported cases and in 3 new cases (see Table 3–6) (Figs. 3–63 and 3–64). Most of the 13 previous patients with clinical evidence of spasm had significant fixed coronary luminal narrowing due to atherosclerotic plaque, although coronary angiograms during life did not recognize these lesions which were later identified at necropsy.[180] In one of the original patients described by Prinzmetal and colleagues,[169] both major epicardial coronary arteries were

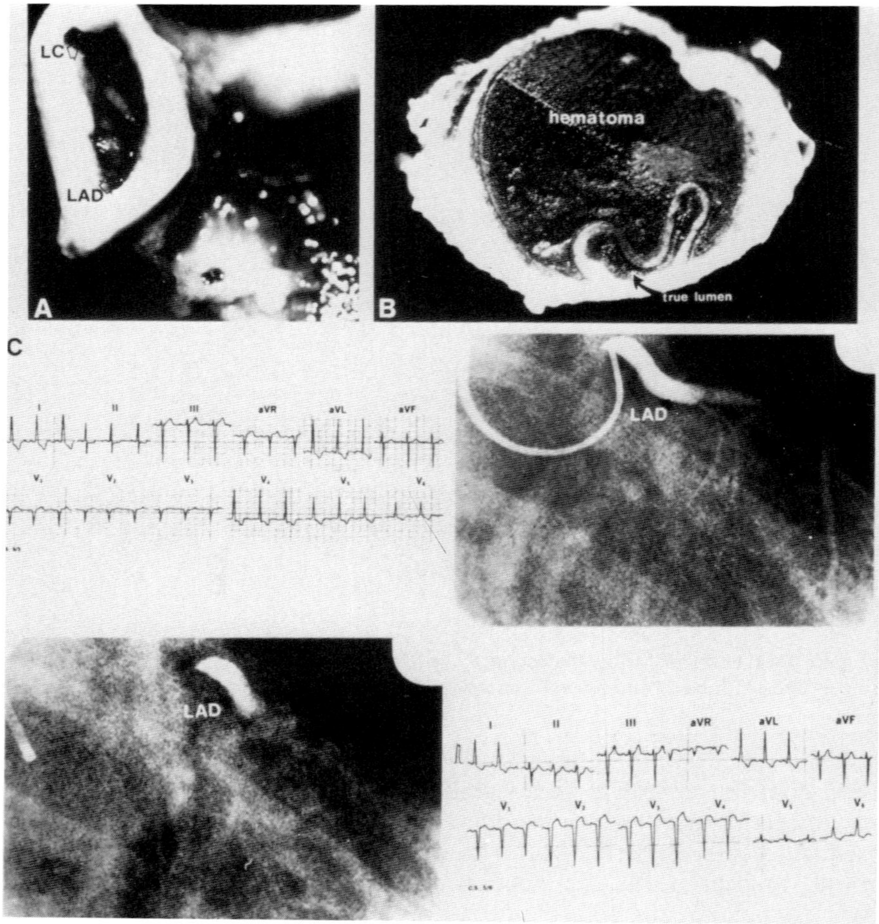

Figure 3–62. Coronary artery dissection. Occlusion of the left anterior descending (LAD) artery due to dissection. (*A*) The LAD and left circumflex (LC) are seen through the left main artery. (*B*) Cross-section shows hematoma in false channel severely narrows native (true channel) unobstructed lumen. (*C*) Sequential electrocardiograph and angiographic findings. (From Isner and Donaldson,[180] with permission.)

"markedly sclerotic," and the "posterior coronary artery" was 80 percent narrowed. Of the subsequent 12 necropsy patients, 10 had at least one major artery severely narrowed by atherosclerotic plaque at necropsy (see Table 3–6). In the three necropsy patients with clinical spasm described by Roberts and colleagues,[179,180] all three had severe luminal coronary narrowing by atherosclerotic plaque at necropsy in at least the artery in which spasm had been demonstrated during life (see Fig. 3–63). In two of these patients, the coronary arteries were devoid of calcific deposits. In the remaining patient, histologic sections of the left anterior descending artery at the site of spasm disclosed luminal *concentric* plaque that had a predominance of smooth muscle cells. These findings suggest that the plaque may have been responsive to pharmacologic and neurologic stimuli compared with "garden-variety" fibrotic and calcified atherosclerotic plaque

Table 3–6. Previous Necropsy Findings in Patients with Coronary Artery Spasm

	Clinical Findings				Necropsy Findings				
			Evidence of Spasm		Coronary Narrowing			Myocardial	
Author	*Sex*	*Age*	*ECG*	*Angio*	*R*	*LAD*	*LC*	*Necrosis*	*Fibrosis*
Prinzmetal[169]	M	58	I	—	80	—	—	0	0
Peretz[170]	M	50	AS	—	0			?VS	0
Gianelly[171]	F	49	I	0		←mild→		0	VS
Silverman[172]	M	40	A	—	0	100	0	VS	
Dhurandhar[173]	M	52	IL	R	75	0	0	0	0
Cosby[174]	F	46	I	0	67	0	0	—	—
Cheng[175]	M	60	A	0	0	0	0	0	0
Donsky[176]	F	44	I	0		←severe→		0	0
Wiener[177]	F	67	I	R	R	0	0	PW	PW
	M	48	A	LAD	0	0	0	AW	0
Bharati[178]	F	33	I	0	R	0	0	0	0
Maseri[178A]	M	52	A	LC	0	100	90	0	PW
	M	52	A	0	50	80	40	0	APW
Roberts[179]	F	32	+	LAD	>75	>75	<50	0	0
	M	57	+	LAD	<75	>75	<25	0	0
	M	61	+	R	>75	>75	<75	0	0

A = anterior; Angio = angiography; AS = anteroseptal; AW = anterior free wall; ECG = electrocardiography; F = female; I = inferior; IL = inferolateral; LAD = left anterior descending; LC = left circumflex; M = male; PW = posterior wall; R = right; VS = ventricular septum; 0 = none.

(From Isner,[180] with permission.)

(see Fig. 3–64). El-Maraghi and Sealey[184] reported a patient with normal angiograms and documented myocardial infarction who had "intimal ridges" observed on postmortem angiography. These authors interpreted these ridges as "necropsy evidence of spasm." Isner[185] has observed similar ridges at necropsy in a patient with coronary artery spasm. Histologic examination of the ridges disclosed that they were typical atherosclerotic plaque.[185] These clinical pathologic findings suggest that varying degrees of dynamic muscular contraction may be superimposed upon fixed atherosclerotic lesions. The ability and extent of "dynamic augmentation" of the coronary wall to contract is presumably related to the amount of smooth muscle present.[180] The demonstration by Isner and colleagues[186] that coronary artery smooth muscle depletion ("medial attenuation") accompanies advanced degrees of luminal narrowing by atherosclerotic plaque suggests that the potential for augmentation of coronary wall tone at the sites of severe luminal narrowing is diminished (see Figs. 3–16 and 3–17). Factor and colleagues[187] have recently suggested that medial "contraction" bands may represent a morphologic–histologic marker for arteries that have spasm during life.

As previously described, eccentric atherosclerotic plaques have a segment of disease-free wall that has preserved media and presumably has the potential for spasm. This form of stenosis has recently been evaluated by Hangartner and colleagues[188] in relation to patients with clinical coronary spasm, unstable and stable angina pectoris, and episodes of silent myocardial ischemia. Of 448 segments nar-

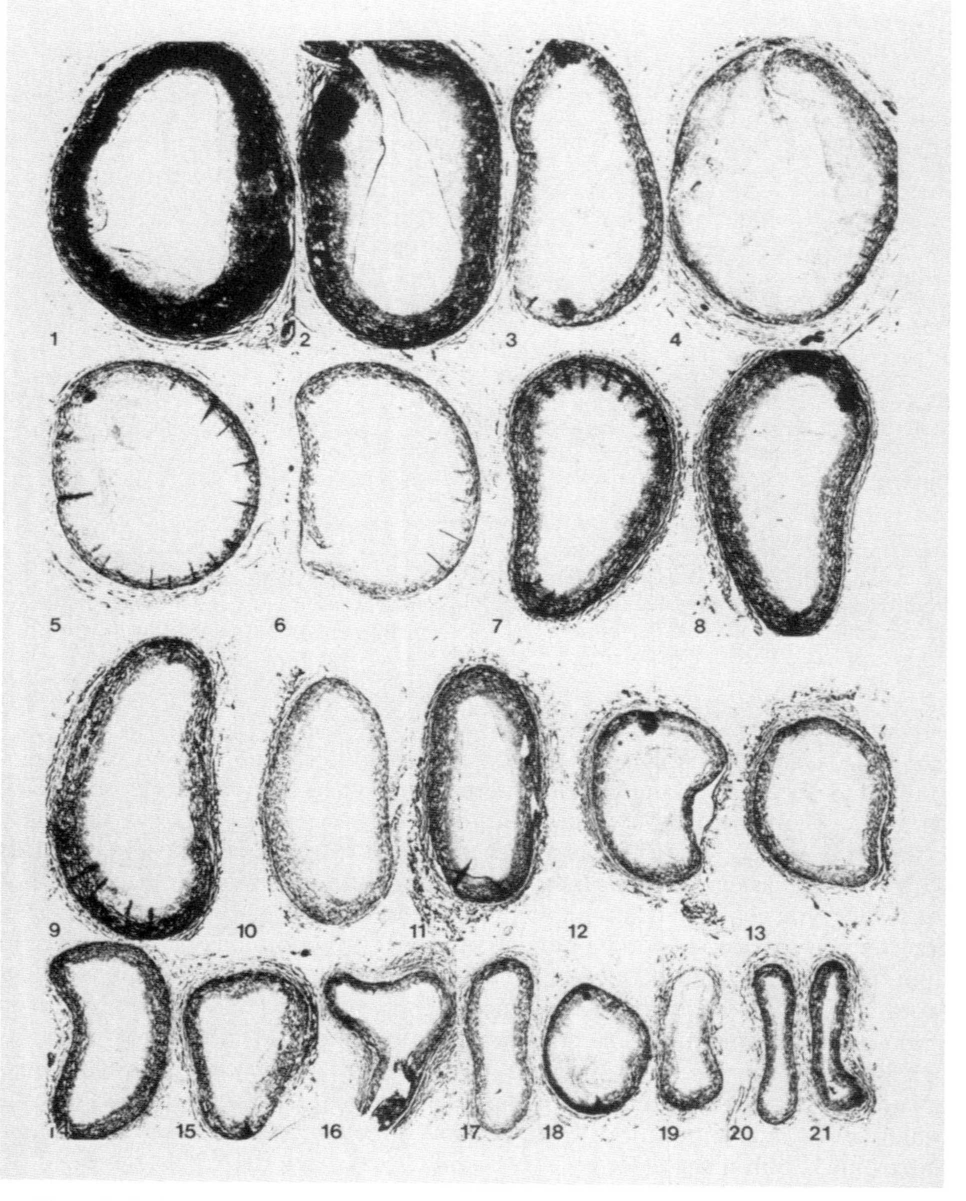

Figure 3–63. Coronary artery spasm. Composite of coronary artery cross-sections of a patient with coronary spasm during life. Clinical spasm involved segments 3–7. Severe atherosclerotic plaque is seen in 8 of the 21 segments. (From Roberts, et al,[179] with permission.)

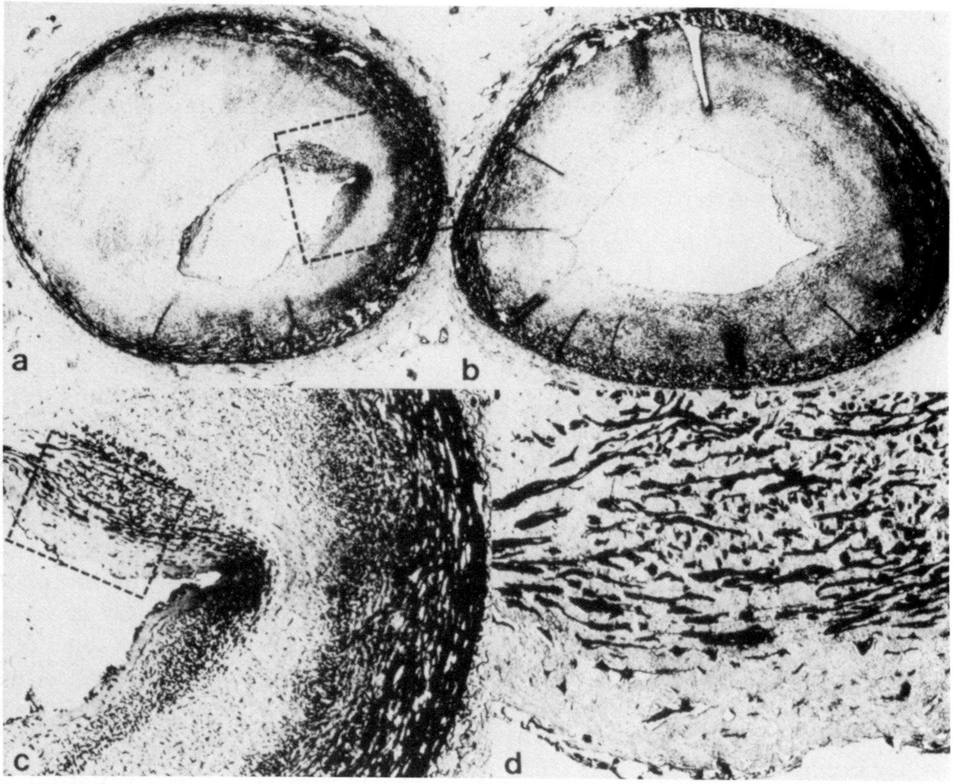

Figure 3–64. Coronary artery spasm. (*a* and *b*) Histology sections of the left anterior descending coronary artery at the approximate site of spasm showing severe luminal narrowing. (*c* and *d*) Higher magnifications of the internal plaque showing the predominance of smooth muscle cells. (From Roberts, et al,[179] with permission.)

rowed >75 percent in cross-sectional area by plaques, 15 percent had a variable arc of disease-free wall (normal media) (≥16 percent of the perimeter of the residual lumen). This is similar to figures reported by Quyyumi and colleagues[189] (15 percent) and Hort and associates[190] (20 percent) but contrasts to studies by Freudenberg[190A] and Saner[24] in which an arc of disease-free wall was found in 70 percent of cases. This disease-free coronary segment represents a site of "vasospastic potential" and could convert a hemodynamically insignificant (<50 percent cross-sectional area) lesion or borderline significant (70% cross-sectional area) lesion to a hemodynamically significant (>75 percent) lesion (see Figs. 3–16 and 3–17).

Coronary Artery Trauma

Coronary artery trauma may produce myocardial ischemia and/or acute myocardial infarction. Traumatic injury may result from nonpenetrating blunt chest wall injury (e.g., steering wheel injury), penetrating trauma (e.g., laceration from stab wound or bullet), or during cardiac surgery (e.g., inadvertent ligation, laceration, intimal dissection) or during coronary angiography (e.g., laceration, dissection, embolus). Nonpenetrating trauma may produce coronary injury and subsequent myocardial infarction as a result of coronary dissection, contusion and thrombosis, fistula formation and/or coronary artery aneurysm formation.[143] Extensive coronary artery dissections appear more likely to occur as the result of catheter or cannula injury in normal or nearly normal arteries as opposed to coronary arteries with severe atherosclerotic plaque.

Coronary Artery Arteritis (Vasculitis)

Epicardial coronary arteries (vasculitis) is a rare event that has been reported in several conditions (Table 3–7) (Fig. 3–65). The resulting coronary injury may directly lead to myocardial ischemia/infarction with or without associated coronary artery thrombosis. Baroldi[22] provides a useful classification of the arteritis conditions based upon type of coronary artery route of entry. Coronary arteritis may result from *direct extension* from adjacent organ or tissue infections (e.g., epicardial or myocardial abscess from aortic valve endocarditis, pericardial tuberculosis) (see Fig. 3–65). In this situation, the coronary artery adventitial layer is initially involved. Coronary arteritis may result from a *hematogenous spread* through the coronary lumen or through vasa vasorum. In this situation, the intimal layer is initially involved. In other vasculitides, the exact mechanism of vascular origin is not understood. Baroldi[22] also considers the following morphologic–histologic findings as "signs" of coronary arteritis: (1) focal artery necrosis with or without calcification; (2) acute coronary artery thrombosis or recanalized thrombus *unassociated* with underlying atherosclerotic plaque; (3) rupture of the vessel wall unassociated with trauma or an interventional procedure; (4) coronary artery wall thickening with secondary luminal narrowing; and (5) wall thinning with aneurysm formation.[191] Specific coronary lesions also may be seen in specific systemic diseases (e.g., polyarteritis nodosa).

TUBERCULOSIS. Tuberculosis arteritis is seen chiefly in patients with pericardial or myocardial lesions. Specific coronary artery granuloma may involve the adventitia, the intima, or the entire wall.[22,192]

Table 3–7. Some Conditions Associated with Coronary Artery Arteritis (Vasculitis)

Tuberculosis[22,142,192]
Polyarteritis nodosa[22,92,142,143,193,194]
Giant cell[22,92,195,196]
Rheumatic fever[22,197,200]
Systemic lupus erythematosus[22,142,143,163,198,199,201,202,202A]
Burger's disease (thrombo-angiitis obliterans)[22,203,204]
Wegener's granulomatosis[143,198,205]
Salmonella[142,208]
Leprosy[142]
Mucocutaneous lymph node syndrome[212–214]
Takayasu's disease[142,200,215,216]
Typhus[209]
Infective endocarditis[207]
Rheumatoid arthritis[163,216,217]
Amylosing spondylitis[218]
Syphilis[143,163,206]

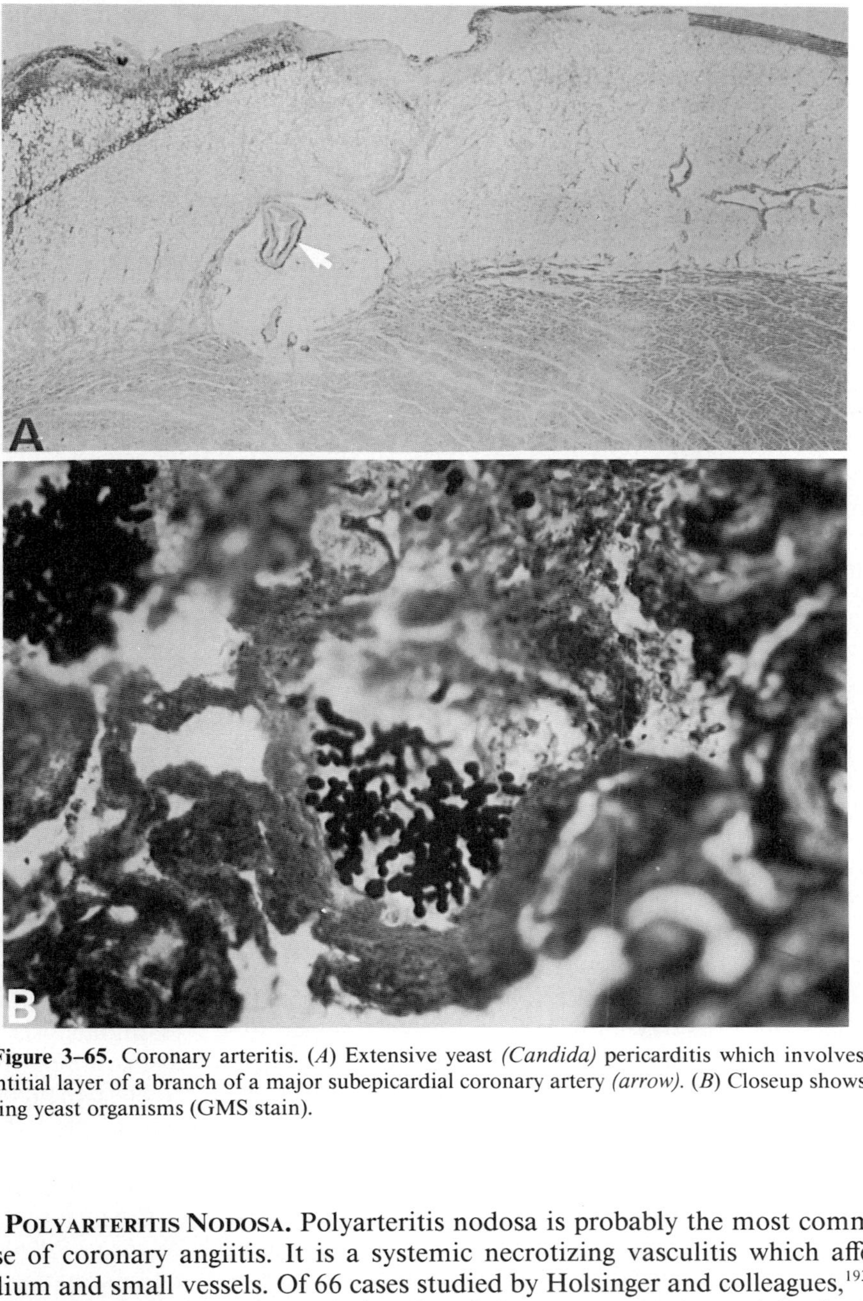

Figure 3–65. Coronary arteritis. (*A*) Extensive yeast *(Candida)* pericarditis which involves the adventitial layer of a branch of a major subepicardial coronary artery *(arrow)*. (*B*) Closeup shows the budding yeast organisms (GMS stain).

Polyarteritis Nodosa. Polyarteritis nodosa is probably the most common cause of coronary angiitis. It is a systemic necrotizing vasculitis which affects medium and small vessels. Of 66 cases studied by Holsinger and colleagues,[193] 41 (62 percent) had involvement of the epicardial coronary arteries and 41 also had myocardial infarcts of varying size. The coronary lesions resemble the necrotizing vascular lesions elsewhere with an acute cellular phase with destruction of the media and internal elastic membrane and subsequent intimal proliferation and scar in the healed phase. The coronary artery may dilate to form small berry-like aneurysms, become occluded by thrombus, or rupture (producing fatal pericardial tamponade).[194]

Giant Cell Arteritis. Giant cell arteritis affects chiefly the temporal and other cranial arteries, but coronary artery involvement and myocardial infarction have been reported by Ainsworth and associates.[92,195] The arterial wall lesion is a granulomatous inflammation with giant cells found along a degenerated internal elastic membrane.[92] The intima becomes greatly thickened, and ultimately the vessel is converted into a fibrous cord. Luminal thrombus may also be present. Of 16 cases of temporal arteritis reported by Harrison,[196] only 1 case involved the epicardial coronary arteries.

Systemic Lupus Erythematosus. Pericardial and myocardial involvement are common complications in systemic lupus erythematosus. Several young patients with lupus and absent coronary atherosclerosis have suffered acute myocardial infarction.[198,199,201,202] Necropsy examination of the coronary arteries in these patients showed intimal fibrous proliferation, which may represent healed arteritis. In a 16-year-old girl with lupus studied by Bonfiglio and colleagues,[201] acute myocardial infarction was associated with recent thrombotic occlusion of all three major arteries. Tsakraklides and colleagues[202A] studied a 29-year-old woman with lupus and fatal acute myocardial infarcation who had severe coronary atherosclerosis. This case suggested that lupus and other conditions causing arteritis may predispose to premature coronary atherosclerosis. Smaller intramyocardial coronary arteries are involved frequently in the diffuse vasculitis with fibrinoid necrosis and fibrosis.[163]

Burger's Disease (Thromboangiitis Obliterans). In a few patients with Burger's disease, the epicardial coronary arteries have shown focal polymorphonuclear infiltrates, histiocytes, and giant cells with or without coronary artery thrombosis[203] or with only coronary thrombosis.[204] In 30 cases studied by Saphir,[203] only 1 patient had coronary involvement, whereas in 19 cases studied by Averbuck and Silbert,[204] 6 patients had coronary thrombosis.

Wegener's Granulomatosis. Wegener's granulomatosis is a necrotizing vasculitis commonly affecting renal and pulmonary systems. Fibrinoid necrosis of the small and medium-sized coronary arteries has been reported by Parrillo and Fauci.[198] Larger epicardial coronary artery occlusion and myocardial infarction was reported by Gatenby and colleagues.[205]

Infectious Diseases. Various infectious diseases have been associated with coronary arteritis: syphilis,[163,206] infective endocarditis,[207] salmonellosis,[142,208] typhus,[209] and leprosy.[142] Syphilis is stated to be one of the most common infectious diseases affecting the coronary arteries.[143] Up to one quarter of patients with tertiary syphilis may have ostial stenosis.[206] The first 3 to 4 mm of the left and right coronary arteries may be involved with an obliterative arteritis.[163] Rarely does a coronary artery contain a gumma.[163] Angina and acute myocardial infarction may result from syphilic coronary disease.[206] Malarial parasites and parasitized red blood cells also may plug larger coronary arteries.[210] *Schistosoma hematobium* has been found in a major epicardial coronary artery unassociated with myocardial infarction.[211]

Mucocutaneous Lymph Node Syndrome (Kawasaki's Disease). This acute febrile illness affects infants and young children. In about 20 percent of patients, a vasculitis of the coronary vasa vasorum leads to coronary arterial aneurysm formation, thrombosis, and myocardial infarction. Death may result from myocardial infarction or ventricular arrhythmia in 1 percent to 2 percent. Late presentation with myocardial infarction secondary to dislodged aneurysmal thrombus may also occur.[212,213] Occasional death may result from coronary artery aneurysm rupture.

TAKAYASU'S DISEASE (PULSELESS DISEASE). This disease results in granulomatous panarteritis and fibrosis of the aorta and its large branches, which in turn leads to luminal narrowing.[143] Involvement of the coronary artery ostia and proximal main coronary artery segments has been described in several patients.[200,215,216] Angina pectoris and acute myocardial infarction may result from these coronary lesions.

RHEUMATOID DISEASES. Rarely, arteritis and intimal thickening associated with rheumatoid disease severely narrow major epicardial coronary arteries. More commonly, diffuse arteritis involves smaller coronary arteries (including conduction system vessels) in 10 percent to 20 percent of necropsy patients with rheumatoid arthritis.[216,217] Small myocardial vessels may also be narrowed severely in patients with ankylosing spondylitis. Grismer and colleagues have described a patient with ankylosing spondylitis who had occlusion of the left main ostium.[218]

Metabolic Disorders Narrowing Coronary Arteries

Specific metabolic substances may accumulate in the walls of large and small coronary arteries as a result of inborn errors of metabolism. The deposition of this material may severely narrow the coronary artery lumen and produce acute myocardial infarction.[143] Inherited inborn errors of metabolism that are known to affect *major epicardial coronary* arteries include Hunter's and Hurler's diseases (mocopolysaccharidoses).[219–221] The involvement of the coronary arteries in these disorders may be so severe as to occlude totally the vessel and to produce myocardial ischemia/infarction. Other disorders of metabolism such as primary oxalosis,[222] Fabry's disease,[163] Sandhoff's disease (gangliosidoses),[223] and homocystinuria may affect smaller coronary vessels by severe intimal proliferation.

Intimal Proliferation

Fibrous hyperplasia of the coronary arteries may severely narrow the lumen and produce myocardial ischemia/infarction. The process may be associated with mediastinal irradiation,[225] fibromuscular hyperplasia of the renal arteries,[143] the use of methysergide,[226] ostial cannulation during cardiac surgery, or following aortic valve replacement.[227,228] Up to 50 percent of patients undergoing cardiac transplantation develop significant epicardial coronary artery luminal narrowing or total occlusion by intimal fibrous proliferation within 3 to 5 years after transplantation.[229] Myocardial infarction and sudden death may result from this "chronic rejection" process. Fibrosis of the intramural vessels may also occur. Intimal damage from immunologic rejection is believed to be the basis for the accelerated intimal fibrous hyperplasia involving the coronary arteries.

A similar histologic picture of intimal fibrous proliferation is seen in epicardial coronary arteries late after undergoing percutaneous balloon angioplasty (Fig. 3–66).[168] Waller and colleagues[230] recently reported intimal fibrous proliferation of the left main coronary artery occurring late after balloon angioplasty of a lesion in the proximal left anterior descending coronary artery. They postulated that the left main intimal reaction (identical to that seen at the left anterior descending coronary artery angioplasty site) resulted from balloon rubbing of the intimal surface and/or extension of the fibrous process from the angioplasty dilation site.

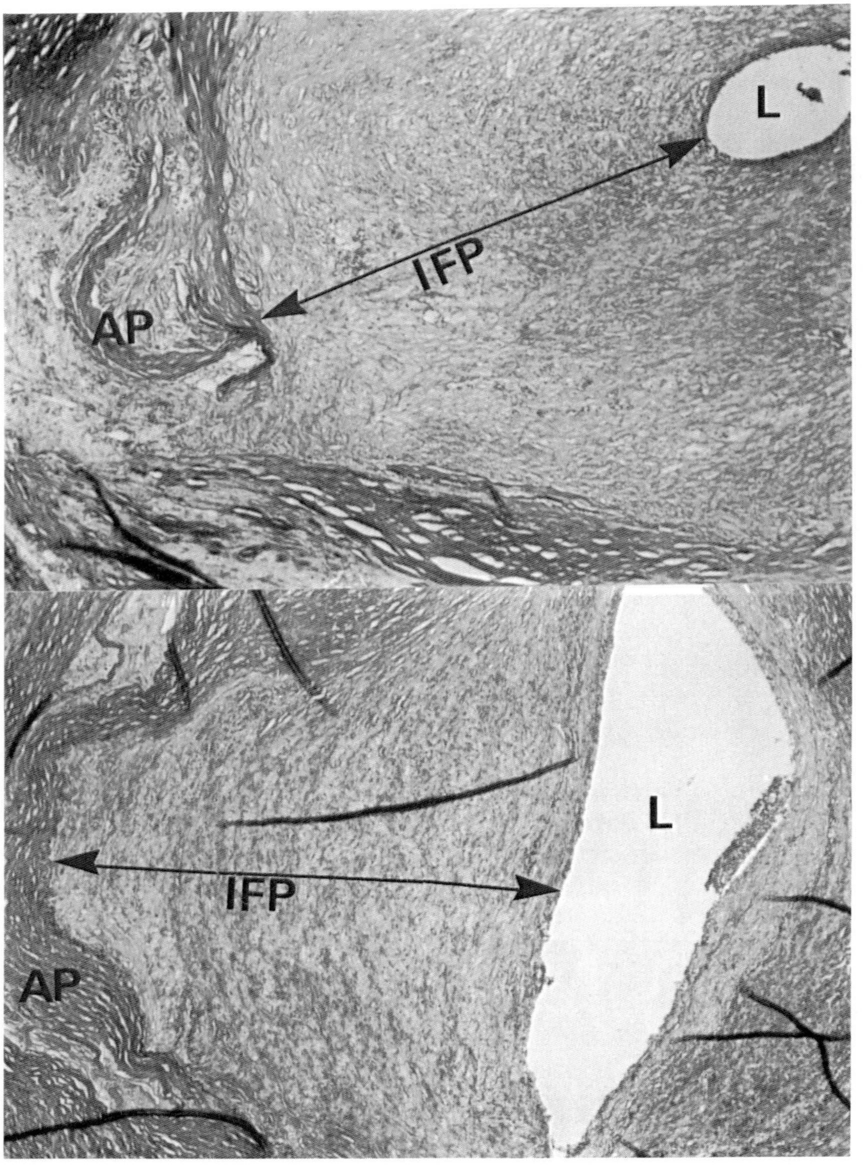

Figure 3–66. Intimal fibrous proliferation. Severe luminal narrowing of the left anterior descending coronary artery by intimal fibrous proliferation (IFP) several months after percutaneous balloon angioplasty. The IFP superimposes underlying atherosclerotic plaque (AP). L = lumen.

External Compression

External compression of the epicardial coronary arteries may result in severe luminal narrowing and progressive myocardial ischemia. External compression of a major epicardial coronary artery has been reported in patients with sinus of Valsalva aneurysms and epicardial tumor metastases.[231,232] Myocardial bridging (external muscle compression during ventricular systole) has been reviewed earlier.

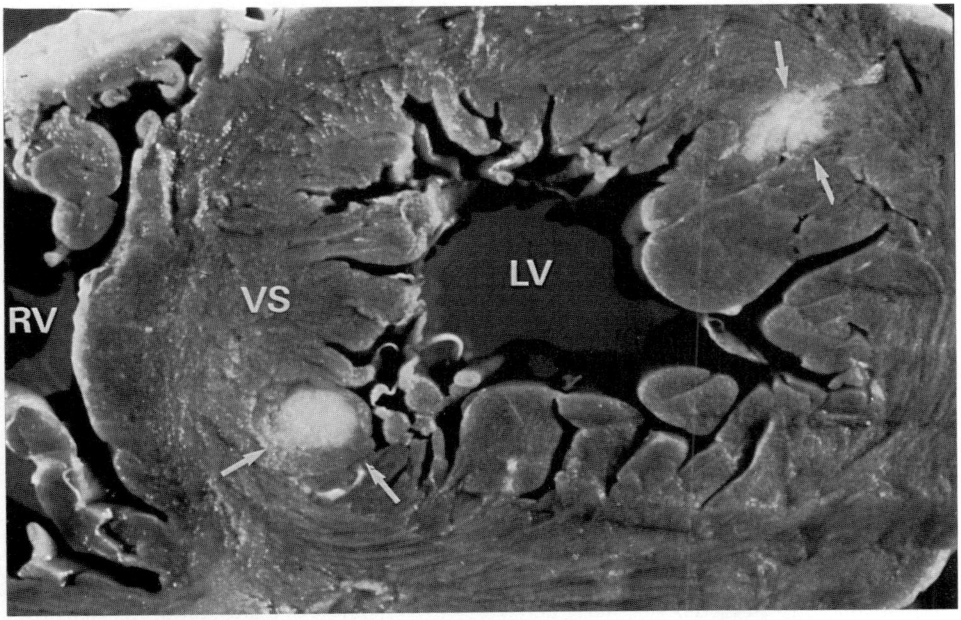

Figure 3–67. Metastatic deposits mimicking myocardial infarction. Transverse section of cardiac ventricle showing two discrete myocardial metastatic deposits of lymphoma. These whitish deposits may be mistakenly interpreted as healed myocardial infarctions in a patient with clean epicardial coronary arteries. LV = left ventricle; RV = right ventricle; VS = ventricular septum.

Metastatic Implants

Myocardial metastatic lesions from various tumurs (carcinomas, sarcomas, lymphomas) may mimic a healed myocardial infarct at necropsy (Fig. 3–67). The discrete location or locations of these metastatic deposits generally are unrelated to specific coronary arterial supply zones, and the lesions are usually surrounded by normal myocardium. These two gross observations suggest the lesions are metastatic tumor implants rather than healed myocardial infarcts.

Coronary Artery Thrombosis Without Underlying Atherosclerotic Plaque (Thrombosis In-Situ)

Thrombotic occlusion of the coronary system unassociated with underlying atherosclerotic plaque may be seen with several hematologic diseases: thrombocytopenia purpura,[163] leukemia,[235] polycythemia vera,[236] sickle cell anemia,[163] and primary thrombocytosis.[237] Occasionally, acute myocardial infarction may be the initial manifestation of these hematologic disorders. A main factor responsible for the myocardial ischemia in these conditions is blockage of small intramural coronary vessels by platelet aggregates.[238] These platelet aggregates initially may form in the major coronary arteries and then embolize distally.

Myocardial Oxygen Demand–Supply Disproportion[142]

In this category are disease states in which there is *failure to deliver adequate oxygen* to the myocardium over a prolonged period or *increased myocardial wall tension requiring increased oxygen supply.* The classic example of the first situation is carbon monoxide poisoning,[142] which has been associated with extensive nontransmural infarction in the presence of normal epicardial coronary arteries. Prolonged shock (from any cause) can also result in extensive nontransmural necrosis and frequently is associated with transmural necrosis of the papillary muscles. The classic example of the situation in which there is increased myocardial wall tension requiring increased coronary oxygen supply is aortic valve stenosis.[142] In the face of increased oxygen demand (increased muscle mass), coronary blood supply is limited by poor perfusion resulting from the lower coronary arterial pressure. In addition, poor perfusion results from the high coronary resistance caused by increased wall pressure on the intramural coronary arteries and the high left ventricular end-diastolic pressure from a stiff ventricle.[142] Excessive myocardial oxygen demand exceeding supply (resulting in myocardial ischemia/infarction) may also be seen in thyrotoxicosis.[239]

Intramural Coronary Artery Disease (Small Vessel Disease)

Acute myocardial infarction may result from abnormally thickened or totally occluded intramural coronary arteries in the presence of normal extramural (epicardial) coronary arteries. A few of the conditions in this category include: (1) hypertrophic cardiomyopathy, (2) diabetes mellitus, (3) amyloid heart disease, (4) neuromuscular disorders (Friedreich's ataxia; progressive muscular dystrophy), (5) cardiac transplantation, (6) rheumatoid arthritis, (7) collagen-vascular disorders (scleroderma; systemic lupus erythematosus), (8) metabolism abnormalities (mucopolysaccharidoses; gangliosidoses), and (9) polyarteritis nodosa.

Normal Epicardial Coronary Arteries

Relatively few necropsy reports have evaluated patients with acute myocardial infarction who had angiographic normal coronary arteries and normal coronary arteries at necropsy.[3,90,240,241] Of 100 consecutive necropsy cases of AMI studied by Baroldi and colleagues,[2] 7 percent had infarcts without evidence of coronary luminal narrowing. Eliot and colleagues[3] studied 10 necropsy patients who died with a typical picture of AMI within 25 days of onset of symptoms. The coronary arterial systems showed minimal or no luminal narrowing by atherosclerosis. No thrombotic material was observed in the coronary arteries despite the fact that the AMI was 2 days old in five patients and 3 to 4 days old in three other patients. Numerous theories have been proposed to explain the occurrence of AMI in these patients: coronary artery spasm; coronary artery disease in vessels too small to be visualized angiographically (i.e., small vessel disease); coronary artery thrombosis or embolus with subsequent clot lysis, retraction or recanalization; congenital coronary anomalies; and myocardial oxygen supply–demand disproportion.

ACKNOWLEDGMENT

I wish to thank George Buckley for his many diagrams and figures.

REFERENCES

1. Alpert, JS and Braunwald, E: Acute myocardial infarction: Pathological, pathophysiological and clinical manifestations. In Braunwald, E (ed): Heart Disease. A Textbook of Cardiovascular Medicine, Vol 2. WB Saunders, Philadelphia, 1984, p 1262.

2. Baroldi, G, Radice, F, Schmid, G, and Leone, A: Morphology of acute myocardial infarction in relation to coronary thrombosis. Am Heart J 87:65, 1974.
3. Eliot, RS, Baroldi, G, and Leone, A: Necropsy studies in myocardial infarction with minimal or no coronary luminal reduction due to atherosclerosis. Circulation 49:1127, 1974.
4. Waller, BF: Unpublished data, 1986.
5. Fuster, V and Kottke, BA: Atherosclerosis. Pathogenesis, pathology and presentation of atherosclerosis. In Brandenburg, RO, Fuster, V, Guiliani, ER, et al (eds): Cardiology. Fundamentals and Practice. Year Book, Chicago, 1987, p 951.
6. von Rokitansky, C: A Manual of Pathological Anatomy, Vol 4. (Translated by GE Day.) Sydenham Society, London, 1852, p 261.
7. Virchow, R: Cellular Pathology: As Based upon Physiological and Pathological Histology. (Translated from the second German edition by F Chance.) Dover Publications, New York, 1971.
7A. Bean, WB: Infarction of the heart. III. Clinical course and morphological findings. Ann Intern Med 12:71, 1938.
7B. Blumgart, HL, Schlesinger, M, and Davis, D: A study of marked coronary arteriosclerosis in patients with and without angina pectoris and related conditions. Am Heart J 18:600, 1939.
7C. Crawford, T: The pathogenesis of myocardial infarction. In Trounce, JR (ed): Second Symposium on Advanced Medicine. Pitman, London, 1966.
8. Davies, MJ and Thomas, T: The pathological basis and microanatomy of occlusive thrombus formation in human coronary arteries. Philos Trans R Soc Lond (Biol) 294:225, 1981.
9. Falk, E: Plaque rupture with severe pre-existing stenosis precipitating coronary thrombosis: Characteristics of coronary atherosclerotic plaques underlying fatal occlusive thrombi. Br Heart J 50:127–134, 1983.
10. Davies, MJ, Fulton, WFM, and Robertson, WB: The relation of coronary thrombosis to ischemic myocardial necrosis. J Pathol 127:99–110, 1979.
10A. Davies, MJ and Thomas, T: Plaque fissuring—the cause of acute myocardial infarction, sudden ischemic death and crescendo angina. Br Heart J 53:363, 1985.
11. Davies, MJ and Thomas, AC: Thrombosis and acute coronary artery lesions in sudden cardiac ischemic death. N Engl J Med 310:1137–1140, 1984.
12. Willerson, JT, Campbell, WB, Winniford, MD, et al: Conversion from chronic to acute coronary artery disease: Speculation regarding mechanisms. Am J Cardiol 54:1349, 1984.
13. Ambrose, JA, Winters, SL, Arora, RR, et al: Angiographic evolution of coronary artery morphology in unstable angina. J Am Coll Cardiol 7:472, 1986.
14. Ambrose, JA, Winters, SL, Stern, A, et al: Angiographic morphology and the pathogenesis of unstable angina pectoris. J Am Coll Cardiol 5:609, 1985.
15. Ambrose, JA, Winters, SL, Arora, RR, et al: Coronary angiographic morphology in myocardial infarction: A link between the pathogenesis of unstable angina and myocardial infarction. J Am Coll Cardiol 6:1233, 1985.
16. Levin, DC and Fallon, JT: Significance of the angiographic morphology of localized coronary stenosis: Histopathologic correlations. Circulation 66:316, 1982.
17. Vetrovec, GW, Cowley, MJ, Overton, H, and Richardson, DW: Intracoronary thrombus in syndromes of unstable myocardial ischemia. Am Heart J 102:1202, 1981.
18. Roberts, WC: The status of the coronary arteries in fatal ischemic heart disease. In Brest, A, Wenger, N, Chung, E, and Kasparian, H (eds): Innovations in the Diagnosis and Management of Acute Myocardial Infarction. FA Davis, Philadelphia, 1975, p 1.
19. Vlodaver, Z, Amplatz, K, Burchell, HB, and Edwards, JE: Coronary Heart Disease: Clinical, Angiographic and Pathologic Profiles. Springer-Verlag, New York, 1976.
19A. Isner, MJ and Donaldson, RF: Coronary angiographic–morphologic correlation. In Waller, BF (ed): Cardiac Morphology. WB Saunders, Philadelphia, 1984, p 571.
20. Waller, BF: Coronary luminal shape and the arc of disease free wall: Morphologic observations and clinical relevance. J Am Coll Cardiol 6:1100, 1985.
21. Vlodaver, Z and Edwards, JE: Pathology of coronary atherosclerosis. Prog Cardiovasc Dis 14:256, 1971.
22. Baroldi, G: Diseases of the coronary arteries. In Silver, MD (ed): Cardiovascular Pathology. Churchill Livingstone, New York, 1983, p 341.
23. Waller, BF: Unpublished data, 1987.
24. Saner, HE, Gobel, FL, Salomonowitz, E, et al: The disease-free wall in coronary atherosclerosis: Its relation to degree of obstruction. J Am Coll Cardiol 6:1096, 1985.

25. Spears, JR, Sandor, T, Baim, DS, and Paulin, S: The minimum error in estimating coronary luminal cross-sectional area from cineangiographic diameter measurements. Cathet Cardiovasc Diagn 9:119, 1983.
26. Isner, JM, Fortin, AH, and Fortin, RV: Repletion of smooth muscle from the media of atherosclerotic coronary arteries: A potential factor in the pathogenesis of myocardial ischemia and the variable response to antianginal therapy (abstr). Clin Res 31:193A, 1983.
26A. Waller, BF: Pathology of new interventions used in the treatment of coronary heart disease. Curr Probl Cardiol 11(12):1, 1986.
27. Gregg, DE: Coronary Circulation in Health and Disease. Lea & Febiger, Philadelphia, 1950.
28. Olson, EGJ: Ischemic diseases of the myocardium and its complications. In Silver, MD (ed): Cardiovascular Pathology, Vol 1. Churchill Livingstone, New York, 1983, p 393.
29. Baroldi, G: Myocardial infarct and sudden coronary death in relation to coronary occlusion and collateral circulation. Am Heart J 71:826, 1966.
30. Blumgart, HL and Zoll, PM: Pathologic physiology of angina pectoris and acute myocardial infarction. Circulation 22:301, 1960.
31. Bouch, DC and Montgomery, GL: Cardiac lesions in fatal cases of recent myocardial ischemia from a coronary care unit. Br Heart J 32:795, 1970.
32. Branwood, AW and Montgomery, GL: Observation on the morbid anatomy of coronary artery disease. Scottish Med J 1:367, 1956.
33. Crawford, T, Dexter, D, and Teare, RD: Coronary-artery pathology in sudden death from myocardial ischemia. A comparison by age-groups. Lancet 1:181, 1961.
34. Chapman, I: Morphogenesis of occluding coronary artery thrombosis. Arch Pathol 80:256, 1965.
35. Croce, L, Noseda, V, Bertelli, A, et al: Sudden and unexpected death from heart disease. Epidemiologic, anatomo- and physiopathologic aspects. A study of 1047 cases. Cardiologia 37:331, 1960.
36. DeCoursey, E: Coronary occlusion and sudden death. A study based upon a review of 345 necropsies performed at the board of health laboratory, Ancon, Canal Zone, between April 15, 1932 and April 15, 1933. J Lab Clin Med 19:1272, 1934.
37. Duff, GL and McMillan, GC: Pathology of atherosclerosis. Am J Med 11:92, 195.
38. Ehrlich, JC and Shinohara, Y: Low incidence of coronary thrombosis in myocardial infarction. A restudy by serial block technique. Arch Pathol 78:432, 1964.
39. Foord, AG: Embolism and thrombosis in coronary heart disease. JAMA 168:1009, 1948.
40. Friedman, M and Van den Bovenkamp, GJ: The pathogenesis of a coronary thrombus. Am J Pathol 48:19, 1966.
41. Guthrie, RB, Vlodaver, Z, Nicoloff, DM, and Edwards, JE: Pathology of stable and unstable angina pectoris. Circulation 51:1059, 1975.
42. Hackel, DB, Estes, H, Walston, A, et al: Some problems concerning coronary artery occlusion and acute myocardial infarction. Circulation 39, 40 (Suppl. IV):31, 1969.
43. Halpert, B, Erickson, EE, and Gyorkey, F: Occlusion of a coronary artery. A study of one hundred ninety-five cases. Arch Pathol 62:391, 1956.
44. Harland, WA and Holburn, AM: Coronary thrombosis and myocardial infarction. Lancet 2:1158, 1966.
45. Holyoke, JB: Coronary arteriosclerosis and myocardial infarction as studied by an injection technic. Arch Pathol 39:268, 1945.
46. Horn, H and Finkelstein, LE: Arteriosclerosis of the coronary arteries and the mechanism of their occlusion. Am Heart J 19:655, 1940.
46A. Roberts, WC and Buja, LM: The frequency and significance of coronary artery thrombi and other observations in fatal acute myocardial infarction. A study of 107 necropsy patients. Am J Med 52:425, 1972.
47. Spain, DM and Bradess, VA: Sudden death from coronary heart disease. Survival time, frequency of thrombi and cigarette smoking. Chest 58:107, 1970.
48. Walston, A, Hackel, DB, and Estes, EH: Acute coronary occlusion and the "power failure" syndrome. Am Heart J 79:613, 1970.
49. Wartman, WB and Hellerstein, HK: The incidence of heart disease in 2000 consecutive autopsies. Ann Intern Med 28:41, 1948.
50. Yater, WM, Traum, AH, Brown, WG, et al: Coronary artery disease in men eighteen to thirty nine years of age. Report of eight hundred sixty-six cases, four hundred fifty with necropsy examination. Am Heart J 36:481, 1948.

51. Baroldi, G: Acute coronary occlusion as a cause of myocardial infarct and sudden coronary heart death. Am J Cardiol 16:859, 1965.
52. Baroldi, G and Mariani, F: Sudden coronary death. A postmorten study in 208 selected cases compared to 97 "control" subjects. Am Heart J 98:20, 1979.
53. Leary, T: Pathology of coronary sclerosis. Am Heart J 10:328, 1935.
54. Friedman, M: The coronary thrombus: Its origin and fate. Human Pathol 2:81, 1971.
55. Benson, RL: The present status of coronary arterial disease. Arch Pathol 2:876, 1926.
56. Leary, T: Coronary spasm as a possible factor in producing sudden death. Am Heart J 10:338, 1934.
57. Zak, FG and Elias, K: Embolization with material from atheromata. Am J Med Sci 218:510, 1949.
58. Roberts, WC: Coronary arteries in fatal acute myocardial infarction. Circulation 45:215, 1972.
59. Tjotta, E: The distribution of atheromatosis in the coronary arteries. J Atheroscler Res 3:253, 1963.
60. Rodriguez, FL, Robbins, SL, and Banasiewicz, M: Postmortem angiographic studies on the coronary arterial circulation. Incidence and topography of occlusive coronary lesions: Relation to anatomic pattern of large coronary arteries. Am Heart J 68:490, 1964.
61. Schlesinger, MJ and Zoll, PM: Incidence and localization of coronary occlusions. Arch Pathol 32:178, 1941.
62. Berger, RL and Stary, HC: Anatomic assessment of operability by the saphenous-vein bypass operation in coronary-artery disease. N Engl J Med 285:248, 1971.
63. Schlesinger, MJ: Relation of anatomic pattern to pathologic conditions of the coronary arteries. Arch Pathol 30:403, 1941.
64. Pitt, B, Zoll, PM, Blumgart, HL, and Freiman, DG: Location of coronary arterial occlusions and their relation to the arterial pattern. Circulation 28:35, 1963.
65. Ravin, A and Geever, EF: Coronary arteriosclerosis, coronary anastomoses and myocardial infarction. A clinicopathologic study based on an injection method. Arch Intern Med 78:125, 1946.
66. Wearn, JT: Thrombosis of the coronary arteries, with infarction of the heart. Am J Med Sci 165:250, 1923.
67. Crawford, T: Some aspects of the pathology of atherosclerosis. Proc Roy Soc Med 59:9, 1960.
68. White, NK, Edwards, JE, and Dry, TJ: The relationship of the degree of coronary atherosclerosis with age, in men. Circulation 1:645, 1950.
69. Schwartz, CJ and Mitchell, JRA: The relation between myocardial lesions and coronary artery disease. An unselected necropsy study. Br Heart J 24:761, 1962.
70. Clawson, BJ: Coronary sclerosis. An analysis of nine hundred and twenty-eight cases. Am Heart J 17:387, 1939.
71. Bean, WB: Infarction of the heart. II. Clinical course and morphological findings. Ann Intern Med 12:71, 1938.
72. Appelbaum, E and Nicholson, GHB: Occlusive disease of the coronary arteries. An analysis of the pathological anatomy in one hundred sixty eight cases, with electrocardiogram correlations in thirty-six of these. Am Heart J 10:662, 1935.
73. Ackerman, RF, Dry, TJ, and Edwards, JE: Relationship of various factors to the degree of coronary atherosclerosis in women. Circulation 1:1345, 1950.
74. Lenegre, J and Himbert, J: Critical study of the relationship between angina pectoris and coronary atherosclerosis. Am Heart J 58:539, 1976.
75. Roberts, WC: The coronary arteries and left ventricle in clinically isolated angina pectoris. A necropsy analysis. Circulation 54:338, 1976.
76. Blumgart, JJ, Schlesinger, MJ, and Zoll, PM: Angina pectoris, coronary failure and acute myocardial infarction. The role of coronary occlusions and collateral circulation. JAMA 116:91, 1941.
77. Bulkley, BH and Roberts, WC: Atherosclerotic narrowing of the left main coronary artery. A necropsy analysis of 152 patients with fatal coronary heart disease and varying degrees of left main narrowing. Circulation 53:832, 1976.
78. Cabin, HS and Roberts, WC: True left ventricular aneurysm and healed myocardial infarction. Clinical and necropsy observations including quantification of degrees of coronary narrowing. Am J Cardiol 46:754, 1980.
79. Cabin, HS and Roberts, WC: Fatal cardiac arrest during cardiac catherterization for angina pectoris: Analysis of 10 necropsy patients. Am J Cardiol 48:1, 1981.

80. Roberts, WC and Jones, AA: Quantitation of coronary arterial narrowing at necropsy in sudden coronary death: Analysis of 31 patients and comparison with 25 control subjects. Am J Cardiol 44:39, 1979.
81. Roberts, WC and Jones, AA: Quantification of coronary arterial narrowing at necropsy in acute transmural myocardial infarction: Analysis and comparison of findings in 27 patients and 22 controls. Circulation 61:786, 1980.
82. Virmani, R and Roberts, WC: Quantification of coronary arterial narrowing and of left ventricular myocardial scarring in healed myocardial infarction with chronic, eventually fatal, congestive cardiac failure. Am J Med 68:831, 1980.
83. Virmani, R and Roberts, WC: Non-fatal healed transmural myocardial infarction and fatal non-cardiac disease. Qualification and quantification of coronary arterial narrowing and of left ventricular scarring in 18 necropsy patients. Br Heart J 45:434, 1981.
84. Waller, BF, McManus, BM, Gorfinkel, HJ, et al: Status of the major epicardial coronary arteries 80 to 150 days after percutaneous transluminal coronary angioplasty. Analysis of 3 necropsy patients. Am J Cardiol 51:81, 1983.
85. Fulton, WFW: The Coronary Arteries. Microanatomy and Pathogenesis of Obliterative Coronary Artery Disease. Charles C Thomas, Springfield, Illinois, 1965.
86. Osborn, GR: The Incubation Period of Coronary Thrombosis. Buttersworth, London, 1963.
87. Vlodaver, Z and Edwards, JE: Pathology of coronary atherosclerosis. Prog Cardiovasc Dis 14:256, 1971.
88. Liberthson, RR, Nagel, EL, Hirschman, JC, et al: Pathophysiologic observations in prehospital ventricular fibrillation and sudden cardiac death. Circulation 49:790, 1974.
89. Friedman, M, Manwaring, JH, Rosenman, RH, et al: Instantaneous and sudden death. Clinical and pathological differentiation in coronary artery disease. JAMA 225:1319, 1973.
90. Baroldi, G, Scomazzoni: Coronary Circulation in the Normal and Pathologic Heart. US Government Printing Office, American Registry of Pathology, Armed Forces Institute of Washington, DC, 1967.
91. Baroldi, G, Falzi, G, and Mariani, F: Sudden coronary death. A post-mortem study in 208 selected cases to 97 "control" subjects. Am Heart J 98:20, 1979.
92. Crawford, T: Pathology of Ischemic Heart Disease. Buttersworth, London, 1977.
93. Berger, RL and Story, HC: Anatomic assessment of operability by the coronary artery disease. N Engl J Med 285:248, 1971.
94. Bean, WB: Infarction of the heart. II. Clinical course and morphologic findings. Ann Intern Med 12:71, 1938.
95. Perper, JA, Kuller, LH, and Cooper, M: Arteriosclerosis of coronary arteries in sudden, unexpected deaths. Circulation 52 (Suppl 3):27, 1975.
96. Vlodaver, Z and Edwards, JE: The pathologist approachs clinical coronary disease. Hum Pathol 3:3, 1972.
97. Roberts, WC: Examining the pericardium and heart. Chest 57:567, 1970.
98. Pomerance, A and Davies, MJ: The Pathology of the Heart. Blackwell, Oxford, 1975.
99. Roberts, WC: Cardiovascular pathology in hyperlipoproteinemia: Anatomic observations in 42 necropsy patients with normal or abnormal serum lipoprotein patterns. Am J Cardiol 31:557, 1973.
100. Waller, BF, Palumbo, PJ, Lie, JT, and Roberts, WC: Status of the coronary arteries at necropsy in diabetes mellitus with onset after age 30 years. Analysis of 229 diabetic patients with and without clinical evidence of coronary heart disease. Am J Med 69:498, 1980.
101. Waller, BF and Roberts, WC: Diabetes mellitus—a frequent finding in necropsy patients with severe (>75%) narrowing of the left main coronary artery: Comparison of 275 diabetic to 229 nondiabetic patients. Circulation 66 (Suppl 4):II-283, 1982.
102. Foster, L and Waller, BF: Nonatherosclerotic fibrous ridges: A previously unrecognized cause of ostial left main stenosis. J Indiana Med Assoc 76:682, 1983.
103. Holt, S: Syphilitic ostial occlusion. Br Heart J 39:469, 1977.
104. Heggtveit, HA: The role of coronary ostial stenosis in the etiology of myocardial infarction. Pathol Microbiol 30:716, 1967.
105. Crawford, T: The pathogenesis of myocardial infarction. In Trounce, JR (ed): Second Symposium on Advanced Medicine. Pitman, London, 1966.
106. Ford, S and Silver, MD: Thrombosis and the coronary arteries. In Kalsner, S (ed): The Coronary Artery. Oxford University Press, New York, 1982, pp 596–618.

107. Tiefenbrunn, AJ and Sobel, BE: Factors contributing to the emergence of coronary thrombolysis. In Sobel, BE (ed): Thrombolysis and the Heart, Cardiology Clinics, #5(1). WB Saunders, Philadelphia, 1987, pp 49–53.
108. Staffitz, JE and Schwartz, CJ: Coronary atherosclerosis and thrombolysis underlying acute myocardial infarction. In Sobel, BE (ed): Thrombolysis and the Heart, Cardiology Clinics, # 5(1). WB Saunders, Philadelphia, 1987, pp 21–30.
109. Lie, JT: Coronary thrombosis and acute myocardial infarction. In Waller, BF (ed): Contemporary Issues in Cardiovascular Pathology. FA Davis, Philadelphia, 1987, pp 23–40.
110. Herrick, JB: Clinical features of sudden obstruction of the coronary arteries. JAMA 59:2015, 1912.
111. Blumgart, HL, Schlesinger, MJ, and Davis, D: Studies on the relation of the clinical manifestations of angina pectoris, coronary thrombosis, and myocardial infarction to the pathologic findings with particular reference to significance of collateral circulation. Am Heart J 19:1, 1941.
112. Blumgart, HL, Schlesinger, JM, and Zoll, PM: Angina pectoris, coronary failure and acute myocardial infarction: Role of coronary occlusion and collateral circulation. JAMA 16:91, 1941.
113. Friedberg, CK and Horn, H: Acute myocardial infarction not due to coronary artery occlusion. JAMA 112:1675, 1939.
114. Miller, RP, Burchell, HB, and Edwards, JE: Myocardial infarction with and without acute coronary artery occlusion: A pathologic study. Arch Intern Med 88:597, 1951.
115. Branwood, AW and Montgomery, GL: Observations on the morbid anatomy of coronary artery disease. Scot Med J 1:367, 1956.
116. Spiekerman, RE, Brandenburg, JT, Achor, RWB, et al: Spectrum of coronary heart disease in a community of 30,000: A clinicopathologic study. Circulation 25:57, 1962.
117. Mitchell, JRA and Schwartz, CJ: The relation between myocardial lesions and coronary artery disease. II. A selected group of patients with massive cardiac necrosis or scarring. Br Heart J 25:1, 1963.
118. Ehrlich, JC and Shinohara, Y: Low incidence of coronary thrombus in myocardial infarction. A restudy by sterial block technique. Arch Pathol 78:432–435, 1964.
119. Harland, WA and Holburn, AM: Coronary thrombosis and myocardial infarction. Lancet 2:1158–1159, 1966.
120. Kagan, A, Livsic, AM, Sternby, N, et al: Coronary artery thrombosis and the acute attack of coronary heart disease. Lancet 2:1199, 1968.
121. Chapman, I: Relationships of recent coronary artery occlusion and acute myocardial infarction. J Mt Sinai Hosp 35:149, 1968.
122. Hackel, DB, Estes, EH, Walston, A, et al: Some problems concerning coronary artery occlusion and acute myocardial infarction. Circulation 39–40 (Suppl IV):317, 1969.
123. Hackel, DB and Montgomery, GL: Cardiac lesions in fatal cases of recent myocardial ischemia from a coronary care unit. Br Heart J 32:795, 1970.
124. Spain, DM and Bradess, VA: Relationships of coronary thrombosis to coronary atherosclerosis and ischemic heart disease (a necropsy study covering 25 years). Am J Med Sci 241:701, 1960.
125. Sinapius, D: Beziehungen Zwishchen Koronarthrombosen und Myockardinfarction. Deut Med Wochenschr 97:443, 1972.
126. Roberts, WC and Buja, LM: The frequency and significance of coronary arterial thrombi and other observations in fatal acute myocardial infarction. Am J Med 52:425, 1972.
127. Baroldi, G, Radice, F, Schmid, F, and Leone, A: Morphology of acute myocardial infarction in relation to coronary thrombosis. Am Heart J 87:65, 1974.
128. Davies, MJ, Woolf, N, and Robertson, WB: Pathology of acute myocardial infarction with special reference to occlusive coronary thrombi. Br Heart J 38:659, 1976.
129. Ridolfi, RL and Hutchins, GM: The relationship between coronary artery lesions and myocardial infarcts: Ulceration of atherosclerotic plaques precipitating coronary thrombosis. Am Heart J 93:468, 1977.
130. Bulkley, BH and Hutchins, GM: Coronary thrombosis: The major cause of acute myocardial infarction in atherosclerotic coronary artery disease. Circulation 55–56 (Suppl 3):64, 1977.
131. Horie, T, Sekiguchi, M, and Hirosawa, K: Coronary thrombosis in pathogenesis of acute myocardial infarction. Histopathologic study of coronary arteries in 108 necropsied cases using serial section. Br Heart J 40:153–161, 1978.

132. Branwood, AW: The development of coronary thrombosis following myocardial infarction. Lipids 13:378, 1978.
133. Barrillon, A, Kusmierek, J, and Gerbaux, A: Occlusive coronary thrombosis and oral anticoagulants. Thromb Hemostas 41:255, 1979.
134. Tanaka, K, Nakagahi, K, and Ishii, Y: Coronary thrombosis and its role in the development of myocardial infarction. In Proceedings of Florence International Meeting on Myocardial Infarction, Vol 2. Excerpta Medica, Amsterdam, 1979, p 735.
135. Silver, MD, Baroldi, G, and Mariano, F: The relationship between acute occlusive coronary thrombi and myocardial infarction studied in 100 consecutive patients. Circulation 61:219–227, 1980.
136. DeWood, MA, Sportes, J, Notske, R, et al: Prevalence of total coronary occlusion during the early hours of transmural myocardial infarction. N Engl J Med 303:897, 1980.
137. Lie, JT: Coronary thrombosis and acute myocardial infarction. In Contemporary Issues. In Waller, BF (ed): Cardiovascular Pathology. FA Davis, Philadelphia, 1987, p 23.
138. Blumgart, HL, Schlesinger, MJ, and Davis, D: Studies on the relation of the clinical manifestation of angina pectoris, coronary thrombosis, and myocardial infarction to the pathologic findings. Am Heart J 19:1940.
139. Blumgart, HL, Zoll, PM, and Wessler, S: Angina pectoris. Clinical pathologic study of 177 cases. Trans Assoc Am Physicians 63:262, 1950.
140. Ganz, W, Buchbinder, N, and Marcus, H: Intracoronary thrombolysis in evolving myocardial infarction. Am Heart J 101:4, 1981.
141. Rentrop, P, Blanke, H, and Karsch, KR: Acute myocardial infarction, intracoronary application of nitroglycerin and streptokinase. Clin Cardiol 2:354, 1979.
142. Davies, MJ and Thomas, T: The pathological basis and microanatomy of occlusive thrombus formation in human coronary arteries. Philos Trans R Soc Lond (Biol) 294:225, 1981.
142A. Waller, BF, Rothbaum, DA, Pinkerton, CA, et al: Status of the myocardium and infarct-related coronary artery in 19 necropsy patients with acute recanalization using pharmacologic (streptokinase, r-tissue plasminogen activator), mechanical (percutaneous transluminal coronary angioplasty) or combined types of reperfusion therapy. J Am Coll Cardiol 9:785, 1987.
142B. Cheitlin, MD, McAllister, HA, and de Castro, CM: Myocardial infarction without atherosclerosis. JAMA 231:951, 1975.
143. Baim, DS and Harrison, DC: Nonatherosclerotic coronary heart disease (including coronary artery spasm). In Hurst JW (ed): The Heart, 5th ed. McGraw-Hill, New York, 1982, p 1158.
144. Engel, HJ, Torres, C, and Page, HL Jr: Major variations in anatomical origin of the coronary arteries: Angiographic observations in 4,250 patients without associated congenital heart disease. Cathet Cardiovasc Diag 1:157, 1975.
145. Levin, DC, Fellows, KE, and Abrams, HL: Hemodynamically significant primary anomalies of the coronary arteries. Angiographic aspects. Circulation 58:25, 1978.
146. Roberts, WC: Major anomalies of coronary arterial origin seen in adulthood. Am Heart J 111:941, 1986.
147. Roberts, WC, Siegel, RJ, and Zipes, DP: Origin of the right coronary artery from the left sinus of Valsalva and its functional consequences: Analysis of 10 necropsy patients. Am J Cardiol 49:863, 1982.
148. Joswig, BF, Warren, SE, Vieweg, WV, et al: Transmural myocardial infarction in the absence of coronary arterial luminal narrowing in a young man with single coronary arterial anomaly. Cathet Cardiovasc Diag 4:297, 1978.
149. Menke, DM, Waller, BF, and Pless, JE: Hypoplastic coronary arteries and high takeoff position of the right coronary artery. Chest 88:299, 1985.
150. Vlodaver, Z, Amplatz, K, Burchell, HB, et al: Coronary Heart Disease. Clinical, Angiographic, and Pathologic Profiles. Springer-Verlag, New York, 1976, p 131.
151. Young, JA, Sengupta, A, and Khaja, FU: Coronary arterial stenosis, angina pectoris, and atypical coarctation of the aorta due to nonspecific arteritis: Treatment with aortocoronary bypass graft. Am J Cardiol 32:356–361, 1973.
152. Levin, DC, Fellows, KE, and Abrams, HL: Hemodynamically significant primary anomalies of the coronary arteries. Angiographic aspects. Circulation 58:25, 1978.
152A. Virmani, R, Chun, PKC, Goldstein, RE, et al: Acute takeoffs of the coronary arteries along the aortic wall and congenital coronary ostial valve-like ridges. Association with sudden death. J Am Coll Cardiol 3:766, 1984.

153. Reyman, HC: Disertatis de vasis cordis propiis. Bibl Anat 2:366, 1737.
154. Noble, J, Bourassa, MG, Petitclerc, R, et al: Myocardial bridging and milking effect of the left anterior descending coronary artery: Normal variant or obstruction? Am J Cardiol 37:933, 1976.
155. Farugui, AMA, Maloy, WC, Felner, JM, et al: Symptomatic myocardial bridging of the coronary artery. Am J Cardiol 41:1305, 1978.
156. Visscher, DW, Mildes, BM, and Waller, BF: Tunneled ("bridged") left anterior descending coronary artery in a newborn without clinical or morphological evidence of myocardial ischemia. Cath Cardiovasc Diag 9:493, 1983.
157. Edwards, JC, Burnsides, C, Swarm, RL, and Lansing, AI: Arteriosclerosis in the intramural and extramural portions of coronary arteries in the human heart. Circulation 13:235–241, 1956.
158. Polacek, P: Relation of myocardial bridges and loops on the coronary arteries to coronary occlusions. Am Heart J 61:44–52, 1961.
159. Kramer, JR, Kitazume, H, Proudfit, WL, and Sones, FM: Clinical significance of isolated coronary bridges: Benign and frequent condition involving the left anterior descending artery. Am Heart J 103:283–288, 1982.
160. Ishimori, T, Raizner, AE, Chahine, RA, et al: Myocardial bridges in man: Clinical correlations and angiographic accentuation with nitroglycerin. Cathet Cardiovas Diag 3:59–65, 1977.
161. Roberts, WC, Dicicco, BS, Waller, BF, et al: Origin of the left main from the right coronary artery or from the right aortic sinus with intramyocardial tunneling to the left side of the heart via the ventricular septum: The case against clinical significance of myocardial bridge or coronary tunnel. Am Heart J 104:303–305, 1982.
162. Schulte, MA, Waller, BF, Hull, MT, and Pless, JE: Origin of the left anterior descending artery from the right aortic sinus with intramyocardial tunneling to the left side of the heart via the ventricular septum: A case against clinical and morphologic significance of myocardial bridging. Am Heart J 110:499, 1985.
163. Wenger, NK: Nonatherosclerotic causes of myocardial ischemia and necrosis. In Hurst, JW (ed): The Heart, 4th ed. McGraw-Hill, New York, 1978, p 1345.
164. Glickel, SZ, Maggs, PR, and Ellis, FH Jr: Coronary artery aneurysm. Ann Thorac Surg 25:372, 1978.
165. Roberts, WC: Coronary embolism: A review of causes, consequences and diagnostic considerations. Cardiovasc Med 3:699, 1978.
166. Waller, BF, Dixon, DS, Kem, RW, et al: Embolus to the left main coronary artery. Am J Cardiol 50:658, 1982.
167. Robinowitz, M, Virmani, R, and McAllister, HA: Spontaneous coronary artery dissection and eosinophilic infiltration: A cause and effect relationship? Am J Med 72:923, 1982.
168. Waller, BF: Pathology of transluminal balloon angioplasty used in the treatment of coronary heart disease. Hum Pathol 18:476, 1987.
169. Prinzmetal, M, Kennamer, R, Merliss, R, et al: Angina pectoris. I. A variant form of angina pectoris. Preliminary report. Am J Med 27:375–388, 1959.
170. Peretz, DI: Variant angina pectoris of Prinzmetal. Can Med Assoc J 85:1101–1102, 1961.
171. Gianelly, R, Mugler, F, and Harrison, DC: Prinzmetal's variant of angina pectoris with only slight coronary atherosclerosis. California Med 108:129–132, 1968.
172. Silverman, ME and Flamm, MD Jr: Variant angina pectoris. Anatomic findings and prognostic implications. Ann Intern Med 75:339–343, 1971.
173. Dhurandhar, RW, Watt, DL, Silver, MD, et al: Prinzmetal's variant form of angina with arteriographic evidence of coronary arterial spasm. Am J Cardiol 30:902, 1972.
174. Cosby, RS, Giddings, JA, See, JR, et al: Variant angina. Case reports and critique. Am J Med 53:739, 1972.
175. Cheng, TO, Bashour, T, Kelser, GA Jr, et al: Variant angina of Prinzmetal with normal coronary arteriograms. A variant of the variant. Circulation 47:476, 1973.
176. Donsky, MS, Harris, MD, Curry, GC, et al: Variant angina pectoris: A clinical and coronary arteriographic spectrum. Am Heart J 89:571, 1975.
177. Wiener, L, Kasparian, H, Duca, PR, et al: Spectrum of coronary arterial spasm. Clinical, angiographic and myocardial metabolic experience in 29 cases. Am J Cardiol 38:945, 1976.
178. Bharati, S, Dhingra, RC, Lev, M, et al: Conduction system in a patient with Prinzmetal's angina and transient atrioventricular block. Am J Cardiol 39:120, 1977.

178A. Maseri, A, L'Abbate, A, Baroldi, G, et al: Coronary vasospasm as a possible cause of myocardial infarction. A conclusion derived from the study of "preinfarction" angina. N Engl J Med 299:1271, 1978.
179. Roberts, WC, Curry, RC Jr, Isner, JM, et al: Sudden death in Prinzmetal's angina with coronary spasm documented by angiography. Analysis of 3 necropsy patients. Am J Cardiol 50:203, 1982.
180. Isner, JM and Donaldson, RF: Coronary angiographic and morphologic correlation. In Waller, BF (ed): Cardiac Morphology, Cardiology Clinics. WB Saunders, Philadelphia, 1984, p 571.
180A. Brown, BG: Coronary vasospasm. Observations linking the clinical spectrum of ischemic heart disease to the dynamic pathology of coronary atherosclerosis. Arch Intern Med 141:716, 1981.
181. Hillis, LD and Braunwald, E: Coronary artery spasm. N Engl J Med 299:695, 1978.
182. Ginsburg, R, Birstow, MR, Harrison, DC, and Stinson, EB: Studies with isolated human coronary arteries: Some general observations, potential mediators of spasm, role of calcium antagonists. Chest 78:180, 1980.
183. Maseri, A, Severi, S, De Nes, M, et al: "Variant" angina. One aspect of a continous spectrum of vasospastic myocardial ischemia. Am J Cardiol 42:1019, 1978.
184. El-Maraghi, NRH and Sealey, BJ: Recurrent myocardial infarction in a young man with coronary arterial spasm demonstrated at autopsy. Circulation 61:199, 1980.
185. Isner, JM, Donaldson, RF, and Katsas, GG: Spasm at autopsy: A prospective study. Circulation 68:III-237, 1983.
186. Isner, JM, Fortin, AH, and Fortin, RV: Depletion of smooth muscle from the media of atherosclerotic coronary arteries: A potential factor in the pathogenesis of myocardial ischemia and the variable response to anti-anginal therapy. Clin Res 31:193A, 1983.
187. Factor, SM and Cho, S: Smooth muscle contraction bands in the media of coronary arteries: A postmorten marker of antemortem coronary spasm? J Am Coll Cardiol 6:1329, 1985.
188. Hangartner, JRW, Charleston, AJ, Davies, MJ, and Thomas, AC: Morphologic characteristics of clinically significant coronary artery stenosis in stable angina. Br Heart J 56:501, 1986.
189. Quyyumi, AA, Al-Rufaii, HK, Olsen, EGJ, et al: Coronary anatomy in patients with various manifestations of three vessel coronary artery disease. Br Heart J 54:362, 1985.
190. Hort, W, Moosdorf, R, Kalbfleisch, H, et al: Postmortale Untersuchungen uber Lokalisation und Form der starksten stenosen inden Koronararterien und ihre Beziehung Zu den Risikofaktoren. Z Kardiol 66:333, 1977.
190A. Freudenberg, H and Lichtlen, PR: Das Normale Wandsegment bei Koronarstenosen—ein postmortale Studie. Z Kardiol 70:863, 1981.
191. Manion, WC: Infectious angiitis. In Orbison, JL and Smith, DE (eds): The peripheral blood vessels. Williams & Wilkins, Baltimore, 1963, p 221.
192. Gouley, BA, Bellet, S, and McMillan, TM: Tuberculosis of the myocardium: Report of six cases, with observations on involvement of coronary arteries. Arch Intern Med 51:244, 1933.
193. Holsinger, DR, Osmundson, PJ, and Edwards, JE: The heart in periarteritis nodosa. Circulation 25:610, 1962.
194. Sinclair, W Jr and Nitsch, E: Polyarteritis nodosa of the coronary arteries. Report of a case with rupture of an aneurysm and intrapericardial hemorrhage. Am Heart J 38:898, 1949.
195. Ainsworth, RW, Gresham, GA, and Balmforth, GV: Pathologic changes in temporal arteries removed from unselected cadavers. J Clin Pathol 14:115, 1961.
196. Harrison, CV: Giant-cell or temporal arteritis: A review. Am J Clin Pathol 1:197, 1948.
197. Karsner, HT and Bayless, F: Coronary arteries in rheumatic fever. Am Heart J 9:557, 1934.
198. Parrillo, JE, and Fauci, AS: Necrotizing vasculitis, coronary angiitis and the cardiologist. Am Heart J 99:547, 1980.
199. Meller, J, Conde, CA, Deppisch, LM, et al: Myocardial infarction due to coronary atherosclerosis in three young adults with systemic lupus erythematosus. Am J Cardiol 35:309, 1975.
200. Heibel, RH, O'Toole, JD, Curtiss, EI, et al: Coronary arteritis in systemic lupus erythematosus. Chest 69:700, 1976.
201. Bonfiglio, TA, Botti, RE, and Hagstrom, JWC: Coronary arteritis, occlusion and myocardial infarction due to lupus erythematosus. Am Heart J 83:153, 1972.
202. Benisch, BM, and Pervez, N: Coronary artery vasculitis and myocardial infarction with systemic lupus erythematosus. NY State J Med 74:873, 1974.
202A. Tsakraklides, VG, Blieden, LC, and Edwards, JE: Coronary atherosclerosis and myocardial infarcation assiciated with lupus erythematosus. Am Heart J 87:637, 1974.

203. Saphir, O: Thromboangiitis obliterans of the coronary arteries and its relation to atherosclerosis. Am Heart J 25:521, 1936.
204. Averbuck, SH and Silbert, S: Thromboangiitis obliterans: Cause of death. Arch Intern Med 54:436, 1934.
205. Gatenby, PA, Lytton, DG, Bulteau, VG, et al: Myocardial infarction in Wegener's granulomatosis. Aust NZ J Med 6:336, 1976.
206. Holt, S: Syphilitic ostial occlusion. Br Heart J 39:469, 1977.
207. Saphir, O, Katz, LN, and Gore, I: The myocardium in subacute bacterial endocarditis. Circulation 1:1155, 1950.
208. Hennigar, GR, Thabet, R, Bundy, WE, and Sutton, LE Jr: Salmonellosis complicated by pancarditis. Report of a case with autopsy findings. J Pediatr 43:524, 1953.
209. Allen, AC and Spitz, S: A comparative study of the pathology of scrub typhus (Tsutsugamushi disease) and other rickettsial diseases. Am J Pathol 21:603, 1945.
210. Merkel, WC: *Plasmodium falciparum* malaria: The coronary and myocardial lesions observed in autopsy in two cases of acute fulminating *P. falciparum* infection. Arch Pathol 41:290, 1946.
211. Gazayerli, M: Unusual site of a schistosome worm in the circumflex branch of the left coronary artery. J Egypt Med Assoc 22:34, 1939.
212. Fukushige, J, Nihill, MR, and McNamara, DG: Spectrum of cardiovascular lesions in mucocutaneous lymph node syndrome. Am J Cardiol 45:98, 1980.
213. Kitamura, S, Kawashima, Y, Fujita, T, et al: Aorto-coronary bypass grafting in a child with coronary artery obstruction due to mucocutaneous lymph node syndrome. Report of a case. Circulation 53:1035, 1976.
214. Kato, H, Koike, S, Yamamoto, M, et al: Coronary aneurysms in infants and young children with acute febrile mucocutaneous lymph node syndrome. J Pediatr 86:892, 1975.
215. Cipriano, PR, Silverman, JF, Perlroth, MG, et al: Coronary arterial narrowing in Takayasu's aortitis. Am J Cardiol 39:744, 1977.
216. Young, JA, Sengupta, A, and Khaja, FU: Coronary arterial stenosis, angina pectoris, and atypical coarctation of the aorta due to nonspecific arteritis. Treatment with aortocoronary bypass graft. Am J Cardiol 32:356, 1973.
216A. James, TN: De Subitaneis Mortibus. XXIII Rheumatoid arthritis and ankylosing spondylitis. Circulation 55:669, 1977.
217. Hoffman, FG and Leight, L: Complete atrioventricular block associated with rheumatoid disease. Am J Cardiol 16:585, 1965.
218. Grismer, JT, Anderson, WR, and Weiss, L: Chronic occlusive rheumatic coronary vasculitis and myocardial dysfunction. Am J Cardiol 20:739, 1976.
219. Brosius, FC, and Roberts, WC: Coronary artery disease in the Hurler syndrome. Am J Cardiol 47:649, 1981.
220. Renteria, VG, Ferrans, VJ, and Roberts, WC: The heart in the Hurler syndrome. Gross histologic and ultrastructural observations in five necropsy cases. Am J Cardiol 38:487, 1976.
221. Lindsay, S: The cardiovascular system in gargoylism. Br Heart J 12:17, 1950.
222. Stauffer, M: Oxalosis. Report of a case with a review of the literature and discussion on pathogenesis. N Engl J Med 263:386, 1960.
223. Blieden, LC, Desnick, RJ, Carter, JB, et al: Cardiac involvement in Sandhoff's disease. An inborn error of glycosphingolipid metabolism. Am J Cardiol 34:83, 1974.
224. Blieden, LC, and Moller, JH: Cardiac involvement in inherited disorders of metabolism. Prog Cardiovasc Dis 16:615, 1974.
225. Brosius, FC III, Waller, BF, and Roberts, WC: Radiation heart disease. Analysis of 16 young (aged 15 to 33 years) necropsy patients who received over 3500 rads to the heart. Am J Med 70:519, 1981.
226. Brill, IC, Brodeur, MTH, and Oyama, AA: Myocardial infarction in two sisters less than 20 years old. JAMA 217:1345, 1971.
227. Yates, JD, Kirsh, MM, Sodeman, TM, et al: Coronary ostial stenosis: A complication of aortic valve replacement. Circulation 49:530, 1974.
228. Trimble, AS, Bigelow, WG, and Wigle, ED: Coronary ostial stenosis: A late complication of coronary perfusion in open-heart surgery. J Thorac Cardiovasc Surg 57:792, 1969.
229. Billingham, M: Personal communication, 1988.
230. Waller, BF, Pinkerton, CA, and Foster, LN: Morphologic evidence of accelerated left main coronary artery stenosis: A late complication of percutaneous transluminal angioplasty of the proximal left anterior descending coronary artery. J Am Coll Cardiol 9:1019, 1987.

231. Garcia-Rinaldi, R, Von Koch, L, and Howell, JF: Aneurysm of the sinus of Valsalva producing obstruction of the left main coronary artery. J Thorac Cardiovasc Surg 72:123, 1976.
232. Kopelson, G, and Herwig, KJ: The etiologies of coronary artery disease in cancer patients. Int J Radiat Oncol Biol Phys 4:895, 1978.
233. Waller, BF: Exercise-related sudden death in young (age $\leq$ 30 years) and old (age $>$ 30 years) conditioned athletes. In Wenger, NK (ed): Exercise and the Heart (ed 2), Cardiovascular Clinics. FA Davis, Philadelphia, 1985, p 9.
234. Menke, DM, Jordan, MD, Aust, CH, et al: Isolated and severe left main coronary atherosclerosis and thrombosis: A complication of acute angle takeoff of the left main coronary artery. Am Heart J 112:1319, 1986.
235. Fomina, LG: A case of myocardial infarct in acute leukemia. Sov Med 24:141, 1960.
236. Wirth, L: Mycardial infarction as the initial manifestation of polycythemia vera. Milit Med 125:544, 1960.
237. Spach, MS, Howell, DA, and Harris, JS: Myocardial infarction and multiple thrombosis in a child with primary thrombocytosis. Pediatrics 31:268, 1963.
238. James, TN: Pathology of the small coronary arteries. Am J Cardiol 20:679, 1963.
239. Kotter, MN, Michaélides, KM, and Bouchard, RJ: Myocardial infarction associated with thyrotoxicosis. Arch Intern Med 132:723, 1973.
240. Gross, H and Stenberg, WH: Myocardial infarction without significant lesions of coronary arteries. Arch Intern Med 64:249, 1939.
241. Friedberg, CK and Horn, H: Acute mycocardial infarction not due to coronary artery occlusion. JAMA 112:1675, 1939.

CHAPTER 4

Thrombosis/Platelets and Other Blood Factors in Acute Coronary Syndromes

Bernardo Stein, M.D.
Lina Badimon, Ph.D.
Douglas H. Israel, M.D.
Juan Jose Badimon, Ph.D.
Valentin Fuster, M.D., Ph.D.

Thrombus formation commonly occurs as a result of plaque fissure or rupture in an atherosclerotic coronary artery and plays a central role in the development of unstable angina, myocardial infarction, and ischemic sudden death. In the first part of this chapter we will analyze some of the basic concepts of thrombosis, including vessel wall injury, platelet and clotting activation, and natural inhibitors of thrombus formation. In the second part, we will discuss the pathogenetic mechanisms involved in the development of the acute coronary syndromes.

BASIC CONCEPTS OF THROMBOSIS

The arterial wall is composed of three layers: intima, media, and adventitia. The intima in the entire cardiovascular system is lined with endothelial cells joined by specialized junctional sites, which constitute a selectively permeable barrier. The endothelium lies on the basement membrane, which overlies connective tissue and smooth muscle cells. The internal elastic lamina separates the intima from the media, which is composed of smooth muscle cells, collagen, elastin, and mucopolysaccharides. The external elastic lamina separates the media from the adventitia, which is formed by fibroblasts, smooth muscle cells, loose collagen fibrils, and mucopolysaccharides. The normal vascular endothelium is thromboresistant.[1] Although the reasons for this thromboresistance are not entirely clear, there is increasing evidence that suggests that normal endothelium actively inhibits thrombosis.

Endothelial cells synthesize prostacyclin (PGI_2), which is a potent vasodilator and platelet inhibitor.[2,3] Experimental data suggest that PGI_2 is an important mediator of endothelial thromboresistance, particularly in situations in which its production is increased (i.e., during vessel wall damage).[4]

Additionally, the resistance to thrombus formation by intact endothelium can be mediated by the action of the endothelial cofactors thrombomodulin, heparan sulfate, and dermatan sulfate.[5,6] After binding thrombomodulin, the procoagulant and platelet-aggregating activity of thrombin is lost, but the complexed thrombin can still activate protein C, which is both an anticoagulant and a stimulus for the release of tissue plasminogen activator.[7,8] Therefore, the binding of thrombin to thrombomodulin results in both a reduction in thrombin's procoagulant effect and an increase in its antithrombotic activity via activated protein C. Thrombin also binds to other endothelial receptors, namely heparan sulfate and dermatan sulfate, which results in the activation of antithrombin III and heparin cofactor II, and subsequent inactivation of thrombin.[9] Furthermore, the endothelial production of a chemorepellent lipooxygenase metabolite coded LOX[10] or the mutual repulsion between endothelium and platelets by virtue of their negative electrical charges [11] may also, in part, explain the relative indifference of platelets to intact endothelium.

Injury to the vessel wall, in addition to hampering the thromboresistant activity of the endothelium, results in the exposure of the subendothelium and other components of the vessel wall to the circulating blood, which further promotes the formation of thrombus.

Vessel Wall Injury (Figs. 4–1 and 4–2)

Superficial Wall Injury (Fig. 4–1)

Once the endothelial lining of a vessel has been removed by a superficial injury, platelets immediately adhere to the subendothelium in a single or double layer. Adhesion of platelets to the subendothelium is dependent on three factors: exposure of subendothelial activating sites, the function of platelet membrane receptors, and the presence of adhesive glycoproteins.[12] After adhering to the subendothelium, platelets spread over its surface.

Two important factors that influence the arrival of platelets to the injured site are: the wall shear rate (the rate at which platelets are supplied to the affected area) and the platelet diffusivity (the ability of platelets to move across flow lines and reach their target).[13] We studied the rate of platelet deposition on deendothelialized aorta (which mimicks mild vessel injury), using a perfusion chamber in which different susbstrates were exposed to circulating blood at various shear rates.[14] At low shear rates of 106 to 424 sec^{-1} (typical of large arteries), platelet deposition increased in the first 5 to 10 minutes and reached a plateau. At higher shear rates of 1690 sec^{-1} (typical of arterioles and possibly of coronary stenoses), the rate of platelet deposition was significantly higher than at low shear rates, but also reached a plateau after 5 to 10 minutes. With continuous perfusion, platelet deposition decreased to values similar to those at lower shear rates, probably due to distal embolization of platelet aggregates from the exposed surface caused by flowing blood (see Fig. 4–1). Therefore, in cases of mild endothelial injury, platelet deposition occurs but is only transient and labile.

The observed transient thrombotic events in these experiments, which mimic mild vessel wall injury in an area of luminal stenosis, are clinically rele-

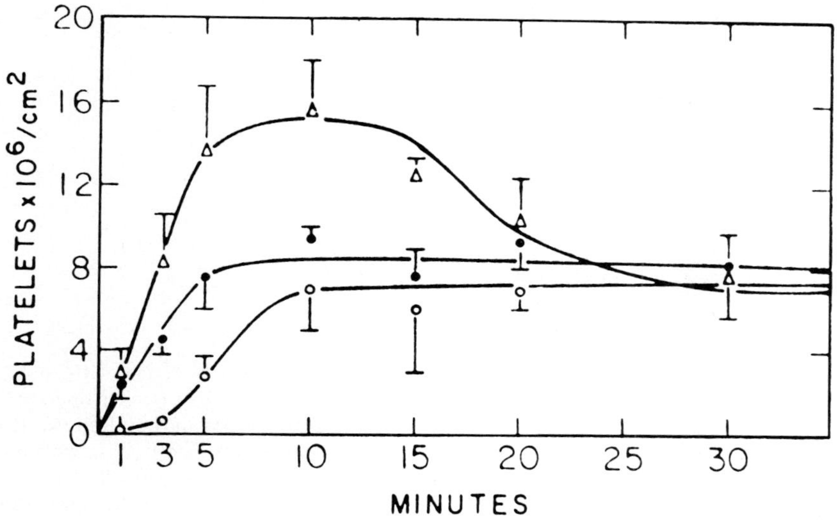

Figure 4–1. Platelet deposition on deendothelialized vessel wall (which mimics mild vessel injury) versus exposure time at different wall shear rates (sec^{-1}): △ = 1690; ● = 212; ○ = 106. Note that platelet deposition is highest at shear rates of 1690 sec^{-1} (typical of arterioles and possibly of coronary stenoses), but is transient and labile probably due to distal embolization of platelet aggregates. (From Badimon, et al,[14] with permission.)

vant with regards to the occurrence of episodic resting chest pain in patients with unstable angina, as will be discussed subsequently.

Deep Wall Injury (Fig. 4–2)

With deep vessel wall injury, such as during atherosclerotic plaque rupture or in some cases of angioplasty, fibrillar collagen (particularly type I) is exposed to the circulating blood. Exposed collagen is a powerful stimulus for platelet aggregation and thrombus formation.

In contrast to experiments using subendothelium as a substrate, when type I collagen from pig tendon (resembling collagen exposed during deep vessel wall injury) was used in the perfusion chamber,[14] we observed a substantial increase in platelet deposition both at low and at high shear rates. Platelet deposition increased with time even at high shear rates, which suggests that the platelet thrombus became fixed to the substrate and was not removed by high blood flow (see Fig. 4–2). These "ex vivo" studies support the concept that platelet deposition and thrombus formation not only occur more readily on exposed collagen than on subendothelium, but the thrombus remains fixed to the exposed surface. When an atherosclerotic plaque ruptures, collagen fibrils are exposed to circulating blood at high shear rates as a consequence of a reduction in the vessel lumen. Because shear stress is inversely proportional to the third power of the internal diameter of the vessel,[15] even small reductions in lumen produce large increases in shear. Thus both high shear rate at the area of plaque rupture and exposed collagen promote the rapid growth of platelet thrombi.

Furthermore, flowing blood is not only suddenly accelerated at the stenotic site, which enhances platelet deposition, but it immediately decelerates in the

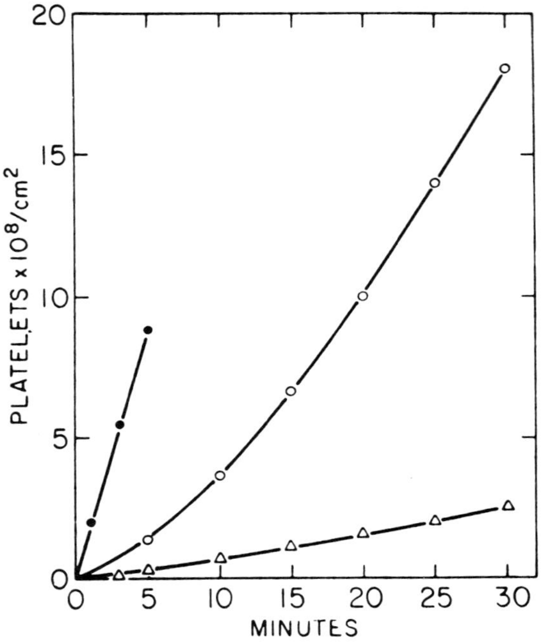

Figure 4–2. Platelet deposition on type I collagen (which resembles collagen exposed during deep vessel injury) versus exposure time at different shear rates (sec^{-1}): ● = 3380; ○ = 1690; △ = 212. Note that platelet deposition progressively increases with time; there is no loss of platelets even at high shear rates, which suggests that the thrombus is fixed and persistent. (From Badimon, et al,[14] with permission.)

poststenotic area. This deceleration produces flow separation and recirculation zones (vortices), which result in the deposition of fibrin. Thus, a fixed "head" of the thrombus formed mainly by platelets is seen in the area of stenosis and a "tail" formed by a large meshwork of fibrin and trapped erythrocytes is located in the poststenotic area.[16]

These findings are clinically important in the context of the pathogenesis of Q-wave myocardial infarction. In these patients, deep rupture of an atherosclerotic plaque, which is associated with increased shear rate, favors the formation of a permanent or fixed thrombotic vessel occlusion.[17] These concepts will be discussed later in more detail.

Platelets (Figs. 4–3 through 4–5)

Platelets are fragments of membrane-enclosed megakariocytic cytoplasm that travel as single elements in the bloodstream. Within the circulation, erythrocytes occupy a central position and platelets are forced to travel in the periphery, close to the endothelium.[13] As mentioned previously, platelets do not adhere to intact endothelium. Even after removal of the endothelium, platelets are minimally reactive to the exposed basement membrane. When deeper vessel wall injury occurs, platelets rapidly interact with exposed collagen, elastin, and microfibrils, but these structures soon become nonreactive to further platelet deposition. The neointima that is formed after deendothelialization remains thromboresistant.[7] If the neointima is damaged, significant platelet activation and aggregation occur, particularly when injured smooth muscle cells are exposed.[18,19]

Following endothelial or intimal vascular injury, several reactions may take place: platelet adhesion and spreading, secretion of granule contents and platelet

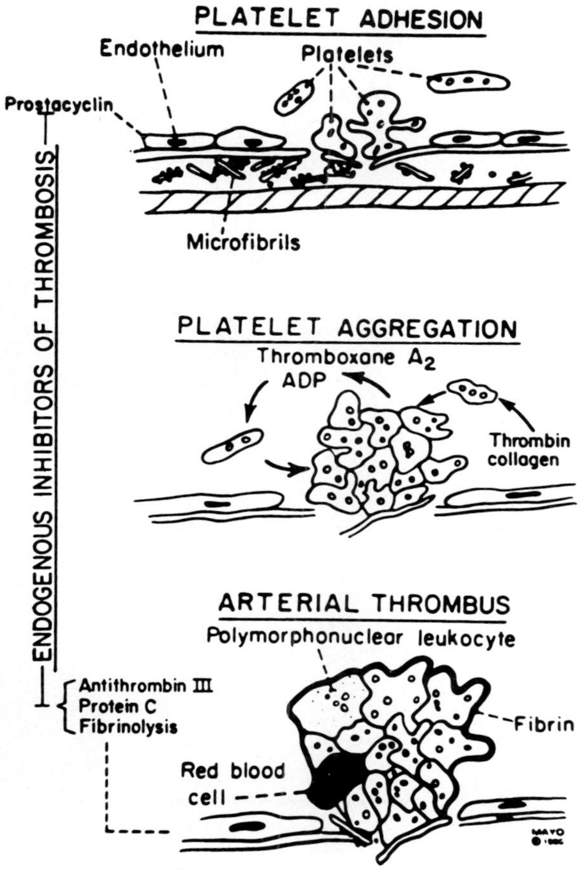

Figure 4–3. Schematic representation of four phases of arterial thrombus formation: platelet adhesion and spreading, secretion of granule contents and platelet aggregation, activation of the coagulation system, and activation of endogenous inhibitors of thrombosis.

aggregation, and activation of the coagulation system (see Fig. 4–3). Not all of these reactions necessarily occur. As described earlier, following mild vessel wall injury, only platelet adhesion occurs which may lead to platelet-dependent intimal hyperplasia. After deep vessel injury, platelet aggregation and activation of the clotting system take place, which may result in thrombus formation.[20]

Platelet Adhesion and Spreading (Figs. 4–3 and 4–4)

Platelet-vessel wall interaction occurs after the endothelial barrier has been injured or removed. Platelet adhesion to the subendothelium is not only important in the hemostatic process but also plays an important role in thrombosis and in atherogenesis (see below). Subendothelial collagen and fibronectin are the most reactive elements that trigger platelet adhesion. Platelets adhere more avidly to collagen that lies deep within the vascular wall than to that found beneath the endothelium.[21,22]

Platelet membrane receptors are essential in the process of adhesion (see Fig. 4–4). The glycoprotein Ib (GPIb) functions as the platelet-binding site for von Willebrand factor (vWF), which seems to play a critical role in platelet adhesion, especially at high shear rates.[23,24] Patients with Bernard-Soulier syndrome lack the platelet receptor GPIb, which results in defective platelet adhesion[25] and

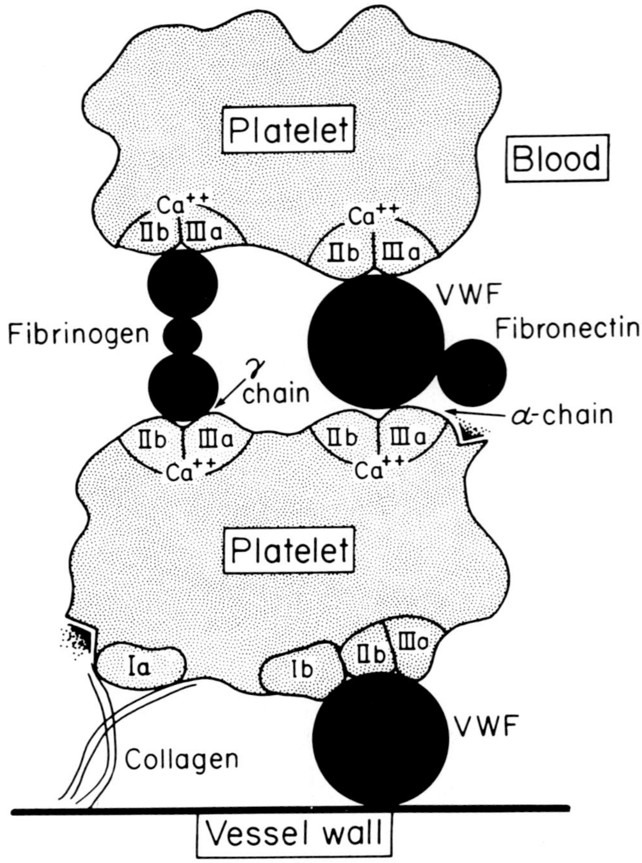

Figure 4–4. Schematic of the binding of adhesive macromolecules to platelet membrane glycoproteins (GP). Fibrinogen binds to GPIIb-IIIa-Ca^{++} complex (γ-chain), constituting an essential process in platelet aggregation. Von Willebrand factor (VWF) can either bind to GPIb or to the GPIIb-IIIa-Ca^{++} complex (α-chain) in association with fibronectin, thus contributing to both platelet adhesion and aggregation. Collagen may bind to GPIa and thus may participate in the process of adhesion.

increased hemorrhagic tendency. Another platelet receptor, the glycoprotein IIb-IIIa (GPIIb-IIIa), not only plays an essential role in platelet aggregation by binding fibrinogen but it also has been shown to interact with vWF and fibronectin in the process of adhesion.[23–26] Studies in patients with Glanzmann's thrombasthenia (who lack the receptor GPIIb-IIIa) or experiments using monoclonal antibodies against GPIIb-IIIa have demonstrated the importance of this receptor in both platelet adhesion and aggregation. The receptor GPIa binds collagen at low shear rates [26] and may have an additional role in the process of adhesion.

The high shear stress found in stenotic areas or at branching points results in increased platelet deposition and thrombus growth. This may be, in part, due to increased arrival and cohesion of platelets at the vicinity of the affected surface caused by a higher shear rate.[27] In addition, red blood cells, by pushing platelets to the periphery of the circulating mass, facilitate their interaction with the vessel wall.[18] In fact, studies have shown that both the red cell concentration and the

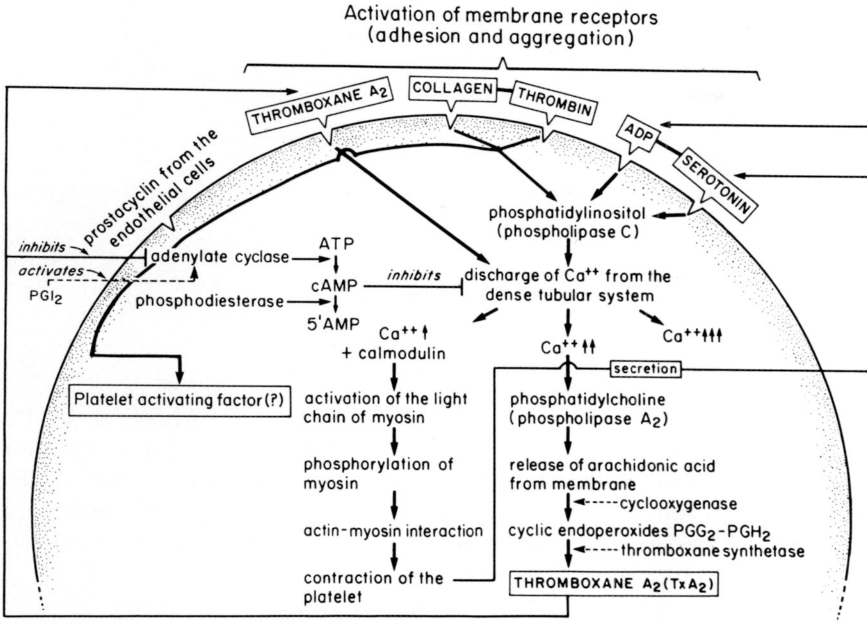

Figure 4–5. Mechanisms of platelet activation. Platelet membrane activators lead to the mobilization of calcium, which functions as a mediator of platet activation via three metabolic pathways: (a) Platelet contraction and secretion of its granule contents (i.e., ADP, serotonin). (b) Activation of the arachidonate pathway with generation of thromboxane A_2. (c) Activation via powerful extrinsic activators (thrombin, collagen). Cyclic AMP inhibits calcium mobilization from the dense tubular system. Note that thrombin and collagen can independently activate platelets via platelet activating factor. Upright arrows indicate increased availability of calcium. Broken line denotes inhibition of a metabolic pathway.

local shear rate are important determinants of thrombus growth on subendothelium.[27] Moreover, the blood turbulence that takes place at stenotic areas may result in red blood cell lysis with release of adenosine diphosphate (ADP), which in turn may stimulate both platelet adhesion and aggregation.

For hemostasis to occur, platelets need not only to adhere to the injured area but to spread across it. Following adhesion, platelets lose their discoid shape, form pseudopods, and spread out on the injured surface. Parallel assembly of actin filaments are essential for the following processes: pseudopod extension, platelet stabilization on an irregular surface, and platelet contraction which helps to seal the hemostatic plug.[28,29]

Platelet Secretion and Aggregation (Figs. 4–3 through 4–5)

Platelets have different organelles including mitochondria, dense granules, alpha granules, lysosomes, and peroxisomes. When platelets are activated by a number of agonists (i.e., collagen, thrombin, epinephrine, TXA_2), they undergo a change in shape from discs to spiny spheres. An increase in cytoplasmic calcium results in the activation of the actin-myosin system, which leads to platelet contraction. Platelet granules are forced to the center of the cell by a centripetal movement of the circumferential band of microtubules, in a preparatory stage for the secretion of their contents.

Table 4–1. Content of Platelet Granules

Dense granules	
	Serotonin, ADP, calcium
Alpha granules	
	Proteins present in plasma: fibrinogen, fibronectin, von Willebrand factor, factor V, thrombospondin, albumin
	Proteins not present in plasma: platelet factor 4, beta-thromboglobulin, platelet-derived growth factor
Lysosomes	
	Acid hydrolases, cathepsin D,E
Peroxisomes	
	Catalase

Platelets contain different types of secretory granules (Table 4–1). Dense granules contain serotonin, ADP, calcium, and inorganic phosphate. Serotonin is a vasoconstrictor, but its role in human hemostasis is probably small. ADP is a powerful proaggregating compound that stimulates a change in platelet shape, resulting in the exposure of platelet binding sites for fibrinogen, which are important in the process of aggregation (see below).

Alpha granules contain a number of substances with diverse physiologic activities. Fibrinogen is a critical mediator of platelet aggregation. As mentioned above, vWF and fibronectin are important in platelet adhesion. The role of thrombospondin in platelet adhesion remains to be defined.[30] Fibrinogen, vWF, and fibronectin are not only secreted by platelets but are also found in plasma. Whether the intraplatelet or the plasmatic compounds are physiologically more important in the process of aggregation remains to be elucidated.

Other products of alpha granules include platelet-derived growth factor (PDGF) and platelet factor 4. PDGF is a potent mitogen for smooth muscle cells,[31] a vasoconstrictor,[32] and has chemotactic activity on neutrophils and smooth muscle cells.[33] Platelet factor 4 (antiheparin factor) attracts monocytes and neutrophils[34] and is found in the subendothelium after endothelial injury,[35] perhaps serving as stimulus to leukocyte accumulation in areas of platelet deposition.

The process whereby platelets attach to each other is called aggregation. The degree of platelet aggregation and thrombus formation within the vascular system is dependent on a number of different factors including: the functional status of platelets, the extent of vessel wall injury, the presence or absence of underlying vascular disease, hemorrheologic factors, the size of the circulating mass of platelets and erythrocytes, the balance between PGI_2 and TXA_2 production, and the activity of the coagulation system.[29,36]

Most platelet agonists seem to act via the hydrolysis of platelet membrane phosphatidylinositol by phospholipase C, which leads to the mobilization of calcium from the dense tubular system.[37] Calcium is an important mediator of platelet activation which can occur via three metabolic pathways: ADP-dependent, arachidonate-dependent, and thrombin-collagen-dependent.[38]

ADP-Dependent Pathway (Fig. 4–5). ADP is released during platelet activation and is a potent inducer of platelet aggregation in the presence of calcium and fibrinogen. ADP binds to its receptor in the platelet membrane in a calcium-independent reaction, and induces a change in the platelet shape, which is calcium-dependent. This change in shape exposes the binding sites for fibrinogen and vWF on the platelet. Fibrinogen and vWF bind to their receptor (GPIIb-IIIa) on adjacent platelets and form stable platelet aggregates.[23,26,39] The fibrinogen bridges between platelets constitute the critical reaction in the process of aggregation. The fibrinogen receptor is located in the C-terminal end of the gamma-chain of the GPIIb-IIIa complex.[20] In addition, a different sequence of amino acids in the gamma-chain binds vWF and fibronectin. During platelet aggregation, the gamma-chain binding site of fibrinogen competes successfully, whereas during adhesion, the alpha-chain site of wWF and fibronectin may predominate (see Fig. 4–4).[40]

ARACHIDONATE-DEPENDENT PATHWAY AND CYCLIC AMP (FIG. 4–5). Platelet activation by diverse stimuli (i.e., collagen, thrombin, and epinephrine) leads to the synthesis and release of TXA_2. Calcium activates phospholipase A_2, which by hydrolysis of platelet membrane phosphatidylcholine, catalyzes the release of arachidonic acid.[37] Cyclooxygenase oxydizes arachidonic acid to form the unstable prostaglandin PGG_2, which is converted to PGH_2. Thromboxane synthetase converts PGH_2 to TXA_2, which is the most important product of platelet prostaglandin metabolism. TXA_2 is not only a powerful platelet-aggregating substance but is also a potent vasoconstrictor.

PGI_2 is, on the other hand, the main product of prostaglandin metabolism in endothelial cells.[2,41] Furthermore, PGG_2 and PGH_2 derived from platelet arachidonic acid can be utilized by endothelial cells to synthesize PGI_2.[42] PGI_2 stimulates adenylate cyclase, which leads to an increase in cyclic AMP (cAMP) levels and a reduction in calcium mobilization from intracellular storage sites. It is probably through this mechanism that PGI_2 inhibits platelet aggregation induced by a number of agonists including thrombin, collagen, epinephrine, ADP, and arachidonate.[43]

The basal level of cytoplasmic cAMP seems to determine platelet activation by controlling calcium mobilization from intracellular storage sites. The level of cAMP is regulated by the activity of two enzymes, adenylate cyclase and phosphodiesterase. PGI_2 probably exerts its platelet-inhibitory effects by stimulating adenylate cyclase and increasing the concentration of cAMP.[43] On the other hand, TXA_2 may stimulate platelets through its ability to mobilize calcium from storage sites through a direct or indirect inhibitory action on adenylate cyclase.[44]

THROMBIN-COLLAGEN-DEPENDENT PATHWAY (FIG. 4–5). When an atherosclerotic plaque ruptures, a number of extrinsic factors are more important in releasing calcium and promoting platelet aggregation than the physiological low concentrations of ADP and TXA_2.[45–47] The most important of these factors is probably thrombin, which is generated during activation of the coagulation cascade and may independently activate platelets via a platelet-activating factor. Other factors include collagen from the vessel wall, large amounts of ADP released during erythrocyte lysis, and platelet-activating factor, released from leukocytes and macrophages.

Currently used platelet inhibitor drugs (namely, aspirin) are capable of interfering with only one of the aforementioned pathways of platelet activation. Aspirin blocks the generation of TXA_2 but has no activity on the processes dependent on ADP or thrombin and collagen. This may explain why conventional platelet inhibitors are inefficient in preventing arterial thrombosis in certain clinical situations.[47,48]

Platelet Procoagulant Activity (Fig. 4–6)

In addition to adhesion and aggregation, which contribute to the hemostatic process, platelets markedly accelerate the generation of thrombin.[49–51] Activated platelets, perhaps by rearranging their surface lipoproteins during contraction, promote the interaction of clotting factors (Figure 4–6).[52] It is on the platelet surface where interaction between activated factors IX and VIII occurs, which results in the activation of factor X. Additionally, the interaction between activated factors X and V, which leads to prothrombin activation, also takes place on the platelet surface,[49] where specific receptors for several clotting factors have been identified.[49–51] Furthermore, the binding of certain activated clotting factors (including thrombin) to platelets may protect them from inhibition.[53,54]

Studies by Weiss and coworkers[55] on fibrin deposition at different shear rates in patients with quantitative and qualitative platelet defects have demonstrated that a complex interrelation exists among specific platelet properties, the clotting system, and rheologic factors. The foregoing observations support the presence of a strong link between platelets and the coagulation system in the development of thrombosis.

The Coagulation System (Fig. 4–6)

During vessel wall injury, not only platelet adhesion and aggregation occur, but the coagulation system is activated via the exposure of blood components to the negatively charged injured vessel surface (intrinsic pathway) or via the release

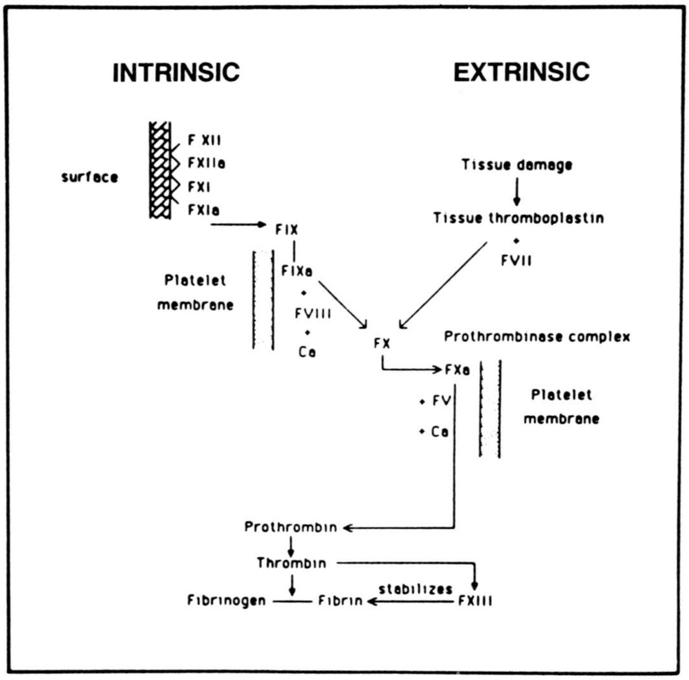

Figure 4–6. The coagulation mechanism. Note the interaction between activated clotting factors and the platelet membrane.

of tissue thromboplastin (extrinsic pathway). The result of these series of complex reactions is the activation of thrombin, which not only promotes further platelet aggregation but also leads to the generation of fibrin. Fibrin stabilizes the platelet mass and allows the arterial thrombus to resist removal by the high shear forces of blood flow.

The clotting factors circulate as inactive precursors or zymogenes (except for factors V and VIII). The coagulation sequence consists of a chain of enzymatic reactions, in which a zymogen is converted to an enzyme, which in turn activates another zymogen (see Fig. 4–6).[56] As already mentioned, the interaction between clotting factors is markedly increased by their being adsorbed and concentrated on surfaces, predominantly that of platelets, but probably also that of endothelial cells[57] and monocytes.[58] With each step, the coagulation system is amplified to produce increasing numbers of activated factors, which ultimately lead to the massive generation of thrombin, the enzyme that converts fibrinogen to fibrin.[56]

Although the clotting system is traditionally divided into intrinsic and extrinsic, there is clear evidence that both pathways are interrelated.[52] The intrinsic pathway, in which all necessary factors are present in plasma, is initiated when blood comes in contact with the deendothelialized vascular surface. Activated factor XII is generated with the participation of two plasma proteins, kallikrein and high molecular weight kininogen. In a sequential reaction, factor XIIa activates factor XI, which in turn activates factor IX. Factor IXa activates factor X in the presence of factor VIII, calcium, and negatively charged phospholipids.

In the extrinsic pathway, it is not a plasma factor but a tissue component—a phospholipoprotein called tissue thromboplastin—which activates factor VII. Factor VIIa, in the presence of factor V, calcium, and phospholipids, activates factor X, and the two pathways merge into a common one.

Platelets provide a phospholipid surface for the assembly of the prothrombinase complex, formed by factors Xa and V and calcium. Thrombin converts soluble fibrinogen into fibrin monomers, which polymerize into a insoluble network. Thrombin also activates factor XIII which catalyzes a transamidation reaction that results in the covalent crosslinking and stabilization of fibrin molecules.[52] Finally, as mentioned previously, thrombin is a powerful platelet activator.

Inhibition of Thrombus Formation (Fig. 4–3)

During the process of platelet activation and fibrin generation, several endogenous inhibitory mechanisms are activated, which tend to limit thrombus formation. The most important of these are prostacyclin, antithrombin III, protein C, protein S, and the fibrinolytic system.

Prostacyclin

As previously mentioned, prostacyclin (PGI_2) is the main product of prostaglandin metabolism by the vascular tissue. Its concentration is highest in the endothelium and decreases toward the adventitia of the vessel. PGI_2 inhibits platelet aggregation by increasing platelet cAMP and thus reducing calcium mobilization from its storage sites.[43] PGI_2 is also a powerful systemic vasodilator. It is synthesized from arachidonic acid by the action of cyclooxygenase and prostacyclin synthetase and its production is stimulated in two ways: by thrombin and in response to vessel wall injury.[20] In addition, platelet PGG_2 and PGH_2, produced as intermediate steps in the synthesis of TXA_2, can be converted to PGI_2 by endothelial cells, thus limiting platelet aggregation and thrombosis. An imbalance between platelet proaggregating and antiaggregating activity of both prostaglandin systems—TXA_2 and PGI_2—may be an important factor in thrombogenesis.[43,59]

Diets rich in eicosapentaenoic acid may affect prostaglandin metabolism by altering the substrate (eicosapentaenoic acid instead of arachidonic acid) and the product of prostaglandin metabolism (TXA_3 and PGI_3 instead of TXA_2 and PGI_2, respectively). Both TXA_3 and PGI_3 have platelet-inhibitory activity.[44,60] Some of the risk factors of atherosclerosis and thrombosis possibly exert their effects by altering the TXA_2–PGI_2 equilibrium.[21,61]

Antithrombin III

Antithrombin III is an important endogenous coagulation inhibitor. It inhibits thrombin and activated factors X, IX, XI, and XII; its inhibitory action is markedly increased by heparin.[62,63] Thrombin is inactivated by antithrombin III after it binds to heparan sulfate and other glycosaminoglycans found on the endothelial cell surface.[64] In addition, antithrombin III inhibits thrombin bound to thrombomodulin.[65]

The importance of antithrombin III as a modulator of the coagulation system is suggested by the increased incidence of deep vein thrombosis and pulmonary embolism in patients with antithrombin III deficiency.[66]

Protein C and Protein S

Protein C is a vitamin K-dependent serine protease that is rapidly activated following the association of thrombin with its endothelial cofactor thrombomodulin.[8] Activated protein C is a potent anticoagulant; it inactivates factors VIIIa and Va[67] and initiates fibrinolysis by releasing tissue plasminogen activator from endothelial cells.[68] Protein C deficiency is an autosomal-dominant disease, and its clinical manifestations usually consist of venous thromboembolism.[69] Although there are isolated reports of stroke and myocardial infarction in young patients with protein C deficiency, there is no convincing evidence that arterial thrombosis results from alterations in this protein.[52]

Activated protein C requires a cofactor—protein S—for maximal anticoagulant activity.[70] Protein S deficiency has been described in families with recurrent venous thromboembolic disease, which usually occurs at a young age.[71–73] Patients with protein C or protein S deficiency may be treated effectively with long-term warfarin therapy.

Fibrinolytic System

Plasminogen is converted into plasmin by activated protein C and other plasminogen activators. Recent work suggests that activated protein C increases plasminogen activator activity by neutralizing a circulating inhibitor of tissue-type plasminogen activator (t-PA).[74] Plasmin hydrolyzes fibrin into soluble fragments and degrades fibrinogen, prothrombin, and factors VIII and V.[56]

During fibrin formation, plasminogen bound to fibrin is incorporated into the thrombus. Intact endothelial cells produce t-PA, which specifically binds to fibrin[75] and activates fibrin-bound plasminogen, with the subsequent generation of plasmin.[76]

Like the coagulation system, the fibrinolytic system has its natural inhibitors. The most important of these is alpha$_2$-antiplasmin. Other inhibitors include alpha$_1$-proteinase inhibitor, antithrombin III, and alpha$_2$-macroglobulin. Recurrent thrombosis has been described in patients with elevated titers of plasminogen inhibitors,[77] defective plasminogen,[78] or low fibrinolytic response.[79]

PATHOPHYSIOLOGY OF ACUTE CORONARY SYNDROMES

The pathophysiology, clinical presentation, and consequences of acute coronary occlusion have interested and challenged cardiologists for many years. In 1912, James Herrick[80] proposed that coronary thrombosis was the cause of myocardial infarction. Autopsy studies done in the last two decades[81–83] suggested that coronary thrombosis was secondary to myocardial infarction and not the cuase of it. More recently, pathologic,[84–87] angiographic,[88,89] and angioscopic[90] studies have clearly demonstrated the role of coronary thrombosis in the development of unstable angina, myocardial infarction, and ischemic sudden death.

We will review the pathophysiology of acute coronary syndromes, with a particular emphasis on the roles of plaque rupture and platelet activation in the development of coronary thrombosis.

Unstable Angina (Table 4–2)

During the evolution of coronary artery disease, the surface of an atherosclerotic plaque may fracture or rupture,[91] with subsequent exposure of the constituents of the plaque and subendothelial tissue to the circulating blood. This sequence may lead to the development of an intraintimal or luminal thrombus. Careful pathologic studies by Falk[87] in patients dying within 24 hours of the onset of unstable angina revealed the presence of thrombi with layered appearence overlying areas of plaque rupture, which suggested that repeated episodes of mural thrombosis occurred, and these, in turn, led to progressive narrowing of the vascular lumen. Furthermore, small fragments of thrombus material were found in the intramyocardial arteries supplied by the affected vessel, which suggested that peripheral embolization occurred distal to the evolving coronary thrombosis. These observations gave rise to the concept of "dynamic coronary stenosis" in which recurrent episodes of thrombus formation and thrombus fragmentation with peripheral embolization take place.[85]

Table 4–2. Hypothesis of the Pathogenesis of the Acute Coronary Syndromes

		Thrombus	
Syndrome	**Plaque Damage**	**Fixed**	**Labile**
Unstable angina	+	+*	+++
Non-Q-wave infarct	++	++†	++
Q-wave infarct	+++	+++†	+

Relative significance: (+) low, (++) moderate, (+++) high.
*Vasoconstriction may contribute to coronary occlusion.
†Collaterals may decrease the extension of infarction.

Hemodynamic studies[92,93] have supported the concept whereby reductions in coronary blood flow, rather than increases in myocardial oxygen demand play a predominant role in episodes of angina at rest. Transient reductions in blood flow can be associated with focal vasospasm[94] or with platelet aggregation and labile thrombus formation—both processes usually occurring in areas of fixed coronary atherosclerosis. Numerous angiographic studies have demonstrated the presence of intracoronary thrombi in patients with unstable angina.[89,95–100] A recent study by Gotoh and associates[96] revealed the presence of an intracoronary thrombus in 57 percent of patients with unstable angina. Ambrose and colleagues[101] found an eccentric stenosis with scalloped or overhanging edges in the ischemia-producing vessel in 71 percent of patients with unstable angina but in only 16 percent of stable angina patients. Postmortem angiographic studies have shown that eccentric and irregular lesions frequently represent plaque rupture or superimposed partially occlusive or recanalyzed thrombus.[102]

On the other hand, increased myocardial oxygen demand plays a role in unstable angina in a certain number of patients. Gotoh and associates showed[96] that 38 percent of patients with unstable angina had fixed, obstructive coronary stenosis without evidence of thrombus; in this group, transient increases in myocardial oxygen demand probably accounted for the symptoms of unstable angina.

Patients with stable or crescendo angina, but without rest pain, studied at angioscopy,[90] revealed the presence of endothelial ulceration without macroscopic evidence of intracoronary thrombus. In this context, atherosclerotic plaque rupture can cause an abrupt change in the geometric configuration of the stenotic lesion, which may result in a significant reduction in coronary blood flow and crescendo anginal symptoms. This reduction in coronary flow may occur even in the absence of superimposed thrombosis. There is strong clinical and pathologic evidence that supports the role of plaque rupture with or without superimposed thrombosis or vasospasm as the essential pathogenetic process in unstable angina.

On the other hand, when patients with angina at rest were studied angioscopically during bypass surgery,[90] an occlusive or partially occlusive thrombus at the site of plaque rupture was frequently found. Plaque damage in unstable angina is probably not as severe as in patients with myocardial infarction and, therefore, the resulting thrombosis is more transient or labile. The future development of anterograde coronary angioscopy done at the time of chest pain may elucidate the relative contributions of spasm and persistent or recurrent thrombosis in the pathogenesis of unstable angina.[103]

Phasic increases in metabolites of TXA_2 (11-dehydro-thromboxane B_2 in plasma and 2,3-dinor-thromboxane B_2 in urine) and of PGI_2 (urinary 2,3-dinor-6-keto prostaglandin $F_1\alpha$) have been found in patients with rest angina.[104] These findings support the role of platelet activation in the pathophysiology of unstable coronary disease.[103] Furthermore, increased TXA_2 metabolites may reflect the amount and extent of angiographically visible coronary thrombus formation in patients with unstable angina refractory to aggressive medical therapy.[105]

Fibrinopeptide A, which is a product of fibrinogen cleavage by thrombin and a reliable marker of blood clotting activation, has been found to be elevated in patients with unstable angina.[106,107] Moreover, a reduction in the plasma level of fibrinopeptide A during streptokinase therapy has been associated with successful vessel recanalization.[108] Thus, biochemical markers for the activation of platelets or the clotting system may be useful predictors of the severity of the clinical situation (i.e., patients with ongoing coronary thrombosis) and the response to therapy.[109] Owing to the fact that, in addition to TXA_2, there are other pathways of platelet activation and other platelet products released, additional biochemical markers are needed.[109]

As mentioned previously, vasoconstriction may contribute to the development of unstable angina. Platelet deposition and activation occur in areas of injured endothelium[14] or ulcerated atherosclerotic plaques, with the subsequent release of vasoactive substances (TXA_2, serotonin, PDGF) that may contribute to subsequent vasoconstriction. There is experimental evidence that supports a correlation between quantitative platelet deposition and localized vasoconstriction at the site of angioplasty-induced arterial injury, as well as reduction in vasoconstriction by platelet inhibition with aspirin.[110] Furthermore, atherosclerotic arteries may be deficient in endothelial-derived relaxing factor production and, thus, be more prone to spasm. Abnormalities of endothelial vasodilator function in atherosclerotic coronary arteries have been demonstrated angiographically by intracoronary injection of acetylcholine.[111]

Based on the previous experimental and clinical observations, a pathophysiologic concept of unstable angina has been developed. Minor injury to a midly stenotic atherosclerotic plaque may occur, which changes the geometric configuration of the plaque and leads to a reduction in coronary flow, with subsequent exacerbation of angina. Transient and labile thrombosis overlying the disrupted plaque may ensue, which results in angina at rest. During these transient episodes, coronary flow is markedly impaired, but is not of sufficient duration to cause clinically detectable myocardial necrosis. Vasoconstriction may play an additional role, triggered by a combination of platelet activation with release of vasoactive substances, and endothelial-derived relaxing factor deficiency in areas of atherosclerosis. Additionally, transient increases in myocardial oxygen demand may play a significant role in some cases of unstable angina.

Non-Q-Wave Myocardial Infarction (Table 4–2)

The pathophysiologic mechanisms associated with non-Q-wave infarction are not entirely clear. Pathologic studies in patients dying soon after a non-Q-wave infarct found a lower incidence of complete vessel occlusion as compared with patients with Q-wave infarcts.[82,112,113] Angiographic studies have indicated a lower incidence of complete occlusion of the infarct-related artery in non-Q-wave infarct.[114–117] DeWood and coworkers[114] found that patients studied within the first 24 hours of presentation had a 26 percent complete occlusion rate, which increased to 37 percent and 42 percent in the groups studied 1 to 3 and 3 to 7 days after presentation, respectively. Collaterals to the infarct area were seen in 85 percent of cases with total occlusion. Ambrose and colleagues[117] studied the morphology of the ischemia-related vessel and found that an eccentric lesion with narrow neck and overhanging edges was commonly present in both unstable angina and non-Q-wave infarct. As mentioned previously, these angiograpic findings correlate with the presence of ulcerated plaques with or without overlying thrombus at autopsy.[102]

Recent clinical and arteriographic studies by Gibson[115] and Timmis and coworkers[116] showed an increase in the patency rate of the infarct-related artery in cases of non-Q-wave infarct; this finding may suggest that, at the time of coronary angiography, the intracoronary thrombus had lysed spontaneously. Furthermore, these patients—with patent infarct-related arteries—had a higher ejection fraction and creatine kinase time curves that were undistinguishable from patients with thrombotic coronary occlusion who underwent successful reperfusion with thrombolytic drugs. This finding suggests that acute coronary thrombotic occlusion with subsequent spontaneous thrombolysis plays an important role in the pathogenesis of non-Q-wave infarct.

Based on the aforementioned observations we propose a common pathophysiologic link between unstable angina and non-Q-wave infarct.[117,118] Plaque disruption with thrombus formation is probably the common denominator among all acute coronary syndromes (Fig. 4–7). A greater degree of atherosclerotic plaque damage in infarction as compared with unstable angina results in the formation of a more fixed and persistent arterial thrombus. As a consequence, coronary blood flow is markedly impaired and leads to some degree of myocardial necrosis. In addition, superimposed vasoconstriction in the area of plaque injury may contribute to ischemia. After approximately 1 hour of vessel occlusion, some degree of myocardial reperfusion develops as a result of intrinsic lysis of the occluding thrombus or resolution of vasospasm. The shorter duration of total coronary occlusion in non-Q-wave infarct or the functional adequacy of collateral blood flow may explain the difference in the amount of myocardial necrosis in non-Q-wave versus Q-wave infarcts.[118] If coronary occlusion persists for a longer interval and collateral flow is inadequate, Q wave infarct may develop.

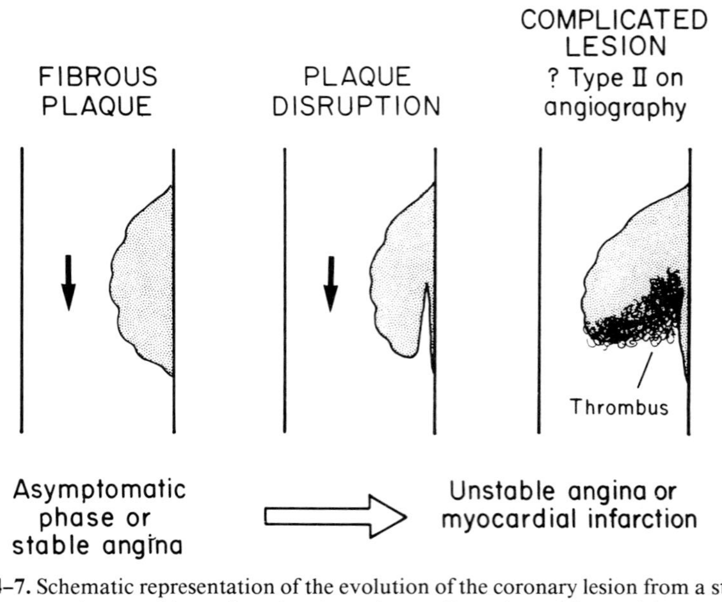

Figure 4–7. Schematic representation of the evolution of the coronary lesion from a stable fibrous plaque (asymptomatic or stable angina phase) to plaque disruption with or without superimposed thrombus formation (unstable angina, acute myocardial infarction, or sudden ischemic death). Angiographic type II lesion represents an eccentric stenosis with scalloped or overhanging edges frequently seen in unstable angina and non-Q-wave infarct.[101]

Q-Wave Myocardial Infarction (Table 4–2)

At present, there is no doubt that coronary thrombosis is the most important pathogenetic mechanism in the development of myocardial infarction. Pathologic studies have shown fissuring of an atherosclerotic plaque or rupture of its fibrous cap associated with overlying thrombus formation in the majority of fatal cases of unstable angina, myocardial infarction, and sudden ischemic death.[84,85,87,91] Falk[85] demonstrated the presence of plaque rupture underlying the coronary thrombus, with plaque contents dispersed deeply in the thrombus, which indicated that plaque rupture preceded, rather than resulted from, thrombus formation. In addition, at the site of rupture the thrombus consisted mostly of aggregated platelets, which supports the concept that plaque rupture is a powerful stimulus for platelet activation and thrombus formation. Necropsy studies by Davies and Thomas[91] have increased our knowledge regarding the pathophysiologic process associated with myocardial infarction. Atherosclerotic plaques consist of a crescentic mass of extracellular lipid (mainly cholesterol and its esters) encapsulated within the thickened intima and separated from the circulating blood by a fibrous cap.[119] Rupture of the fibrous cap leads to free communication between flowing blood from the vessel lumen and exposed collagen and lipids, which are powerful platelet activators. Dissection of blood from the lumen into the plaque results in the formation of a platelet-rich intraintimal thrombus, which is in continuity with a large luminal thrombus. Over the fissured plaque, the thrombus is formed mainly by platelets and fibrin, whereas the thrombus that extends into the lumen and distally in the vessel, consists predominantly of red blood cells and fibrin.[91]

Why do atherosclerotic plaques rupture? Advanced atherosclerotic plaques are relatively soft due to the accumulation of fat beneath their fibrous cap, particularly at the margin of the plaque. In addition, there is fragmentation of the elastic plaque elements. Increased wall shear stress in areas of focal arterial narrowing, changes in vascular tone, and even the normal bending and twisiting of the arteries with each cardiac contraction may lead to plaque rupture or ulceration, which exposes underlying collagen and promotes thrombus formation.[47]

Angiographic studies by DeWood and coworkers[88] demonstrated an 87 percent incidence of total coronary occlusion in patients with Q-wave infarction studied within the first 4 hours of presentation. This incidence decreased to 65 percent when angiography was done 12 to 24 hours after the onset of symptoms, which suggests that spontaneous thrombolysis with recanalization or resolution of vasospasm, or both, occur in a number of patients with Q-wave infarct. In a subgroup of patients who underwent emergency bypass surgery, a thrombus was retrieved by Fogarty catheter in 88 percent of cases.[88]

Careful angiographic observations of coronary morphology by Brown and colleagues[120] in patients undergoing thrombolysis for acute myocardial infarction revealed the presence of luminal thrombosis in the majority. Moreover, the stenotic lesion responsible for the infarct was less than 50 percent of the vessel diameter in one-third of cases and less than 60 percent in two-thirds of them. The finding of mild to moderate stenosis underlying an area of coronary occlusion suggests that plaque rupture with thrombus formation, with or without vasoconstriction, may be the primary determinant of acute occlusion, rather than the severity of the underlying stenosis. Although autopsy studies by Falk[85] and Davies and Thomas[86] have indicated that a severe preexisting stenosis was commonly associated with thrombosis in fatal cases of myocardial infarction and unstable angina, more recent studies suggest that the underlying stenotic lesion is less severe in a large number of patients.[120,121] In these cases, extensive thrombus formation overlies areas of plaque rupture that are only mild to moderately stenotic. These pathologic and angiographic findings are consistent with the frequent occurrence of acute myocardial infarction and ischemic sudden death in previously asymptomatic individuals.

The morphology of the infarct-related vessel in patients with acute infarction is similar to that in unstable angina,[122] which supports the concept of a common pathophysiologic process in both syndromes. In Q-wave infarction, there is probably a more severe degree of plaque damage or ulceration, which leads to the formation of a more fixed and persistent occlusive thrombus and, thus, a longer period of blood flow deprivation and greater myocardial damage.

In addition to vessel wall injury, there are other factors that predispose to the development of myocardial infarction. Epidemiologic studies have disclosed the strong association between high serum fibrinogen levels and cardiovascular disease.[123–125] The Framingham study[123] indicated that the fibrinogen level was a significant predictor of coronary heart disease in both men and women. In the Goteborg study,[124] an association between high fibrinogen levels in men and increased incidence of myocardial infarction and stroke was found. In addition, fibrinogen levels and smoking were strongly related to each other, which suggests that the importance of smoking as a coronary risk factor may be partially mediated through its effects on fibrinogen levels. The Northwick Park Heart Study[125] demonstrated a strong association between cardiovascular mortality and high levels of clotting factor VII activity and plasma fibrinogen. Furthermore, the relationship of coronary artery disease with fibrinogen and factor VII activity was even stronger than with the serum cholesterol level. Although these studies show a strong association between fibrinogen and ischemic heart disease, they do not prove causation. The independent contribution of a high fibrinogen level to atherosclerotic cardiovascular disease may be mediated through its effects on blood coagulability, viscosity, and hemorrheology, particularly in patients with compromised arterial circulation due to hyperlipidemia, hypertension, or impaired glucose tolerance.[123]

Recent biochemical studies suggest that a relationship between myocardial infarction and enhanced platelet activation exists.[104,126] Moreover, increased plasma concentration of cross-linked fibrin polymers[127] and fibrin-related antigens,[128] which reflects the activation of the clotting system with thrombin generation and fibrin formation, has been found in patients with acute myocardial infarction. In addition, decreased activity of endogenous t-PA and increased concentrations of an inhibitor of t-PA were found in young survivors of myocardial infarctions,[129] in patients with acute infarction and angiographically normal coronary arteries,[130] and in patients with coronary artery disease as compared with controls.[131] These studies further support the roles of platelet activation, thrombin and fibrin formation, and impaired fibrinolysis in the pathogenesis of myocardial infarction.

Ischemic Sudden Death

Sudden death can be defined as unexpected death of a patient within 6 hours of the onset of symptoms. Davies and Thomas[86] studied 100 patients who died suddenly and in whom the diagnosis of ischemic death was based on the presence of at least a 50 percent diameter narrowing of one or more coronary arteries, in the absence of other discernible causes of death. They found intraluminal thrombi in 74 percent of the specimens; the majority of the thrombi had a coexisting intraintimal thrombus that resulted from plaque fissuring. Of the remaining 26 percent, the majority had an intraintimal thrombus usually in areas of plaque fissuring, and in only 5 percent of the cases was there no evidence of an acute arterial lesion.

Postmortem angiograms have revealed that only about 25 percent of sudden death victims have a large, occlusive or near-occlusive intraluminal thrombus.[119] Most of the remaining 75 percent of cases show an eccentric, irregular coronary lesion that correlates with the histologic finding of plaque fissure with intraintimal or intraluminal thrombus but without luminal occlusion.[91] Interestingly, this arterial morphology is similar to that of unstable angina, suggesting a common pathophysiologic mechanism.[118] Moreover, platelet aggregates in the distal small intramyocardial vessels supplied by the affected coronary artery were found in one-third of sudden death victims.[87] These platelet emboli result in multiple microscopic areas of myocardial necrosis and may lead to electrical instability, which can result in ventricular fibrillation and sudden death. Nevertheless, the most important preciptating factor for sudden death in these patients is the plaque rupture (with or without thrombosis) that occurs proximally in the coronary arteries.

SUMMARY

We support the concept of a common anatomic and physiologic link between the acute coronary syndromes, which consists of plaque fissuring or rupture, leading to exposure of the circulating blood to collagen, lipids, and smooth muscle cells. This, in turn, results in marked platelet activation and the initiation of the coagulation sequence, both of which lead to thrombus formation. What determines the clinical outcome in these patients is the suddenness of coronary occlusion, the completeness of blood flow deprivation, and most importantly, its duration.

In unstable angina, either plaque disruption resulting in an abrupt change in its morphologic configuration with reduction of coronary blood flow or increased myocardial oxygen demand are associated with increased exertional symptoms. In rest angina, two events may take place: formation of a transient and labile thrombus due to platelet and clotting activation, or vasospasm associated with the release of platelet-derived vasoconstrictive substances or loss of endothelial relaxing properties. As a result, transient myocardial ischemia occurs, which may be intermittent and recurrent and may progress to myocardial infarction or sudden death.

In myocardial infarction, plaque rupture is usually more severe, leading to the formation of an occlusive or near-occlusive thrombus which may be more persistent and fixed to the arterial wall. The duration of coronary blood flow deprivation needs to be sufficiently long in order to produce myocardial cell death. Moreover, the difference between Q-wave and non-Q-wave infarction is probably determined by the duration of blood flow obstruction, being longer in the former. The presence of a functionally adequate collateral circulation will, in part, determine the survival of the area of myocardium at jeopardy.

The coronary events that take place in ischemic sudden death are probably similar to those in unstable angina, namely plaque rupture with thrombus formation. In sudden death, the resulting myocardial ischemia may precipitate fatal ventricular arrhythmias. Alternatively, platelet microemboli from ulcerated arterial plaques may produce multiple areas of myocardial necrosis which can result in electrical instability and ventricular fibrillation.

REFERENCES

1. Gimbrone, MA: Vascular endothelium: Nature's blood-compatible container. In Leonard, EF, Turitto, VT, and Vroman, L (eds): Blood in Contact with Natural and Artificial Surfaces. Ann NY Acad Sci 516:5, 1987.
2. Moncada, A and Vane, JR: Arachidonic acid metabolites and the interactions between platelets and blood-vessel walls. N Engl J Med 300:1142, 1979.
3. Weksler, BB and Jaffe, EA: Prostacyclin and the endothlium. In Gimbrone, MA (ed): Vascular Endothelium in Hemostasis and Thrombosis. Churchill Livingstone, Edinburgh, 1986, p 40.
4. Hoak, JC, Brotherton, AA, Czervionke, RL, et al: Role of prostacyclin in inhibiting platelet adherence to cells of the vessel wall. In Oates, JA, Hawiger, J, and Ross, R (eds): Interaction of Platelets with the Vessel Wall. American Physiologic Society, Bethesda, 1985, p 117.
5. Rosenberg, RD and Rosenberg, JS: Natural anticoagulant mechanisms. J Clin Invest 74:1, 1984.
6. Busch, CW and Owen, WG: Identification in vitro of an endothelial cell surface cofactor for antithrombin III. J Clin Invest 69:726, 1982.
7. Mustard, JF, Groves, HM, Kinlough-Rathbone, RL, et al: Thrombogenic and nonthrombogenic biological surfaces. In Leonard, EF, Turitto, VT, and Vroman, L (eds): Blood in Contact with Natural and Artificial Surfaces. Ann NY Acad Sci 516:12, 1987.
8. Esmon, NL, Owen, WG, and Esmon, CT: Isolation of a membrane-bound cofactor for thrombin-catalyzed activation of protein C. J Biol Chem 257:859, 1982.
9. Lollar, P, McIntosh, SC, and Owen, WG: Reaction of antithrombin III with thrombin bound to the vascular endothelium. J Biol Chem 259:4535, 1984.
10. Buchanan, MR, Butt, RW, Magas, Z, et al: Endothelial cells produce a lipoxygenase derived chemo-repellent which influences platelet-endothelial cell interactions. Effect of aspirin and salicylate. Thromb Haemost 53:306, 1985.
11. Sawyer, PN and Srinivasan, S: The role of electrochemical surface properties in thrombosis at vascular surfaces: Cumulative experience of studies in animals and man. Bull NY Acad Med 48:235, 1972.
12. Hawiger, J: Formation and regulation of platelet and fibrin hemostatic plug. Human Pathol 18:111, 1987.
13. Goldsmith, HL and Turitto, VT: Rheological aspects of thrombosis and haemostasis: Basic principles and applications. Thromb Haemost 55:415, 1986.
14. Badimon, L, Badimon, JJ, Galvez, A, et al: Influence of arterial wall damage and wall shear rate on platelet deposition: Ex vivo study in a swine model. Arteriosclerosis 6:312, 1986.
15. Turitto, V: Blood viscosity, mass transport and thrombogenesis. In Spaet, TH (ed): Progress in Hemostasis and Thrombosis, Vol 6. Grune & Stratton, New York, 1982, p 139.
16. Davies, MJ and Thomas, T: The pathological basis and microanatomy of occlusive thrombus formation in human coronary arteries. Philos Trans R Soc Lond (Biol) 294:225, 1981.
17. Adams, PC, Fuster, V, Badimon, L, et al: Platelet/vessel wall interactions, rheologic factors and thrombogenic substrate in acute coronary syndromes: Preventive strategies. Am J Cardiol 60 (Suppl):9G, 1987.
18. Stemerman, MB: Vascular injury: Platelets and smooth muscle cell response. Philos Trans R Soc Lond (Biol) 294:217, 1981.
19. Groves, HM, Kinlough-Rathbone, RL, Richardson, M, et al: Thrombin generation and fibrin formation following injury to the rabbit neointima. Studies of vessel wall reactivity and platelet survival. Lab Invest 46:605, 1982.
20. Fuster, V, Badimon, L, Badimon, J, et al: Drugs interfering with platelet functions: Mechanisms and clinical relevance. In Verstraete, M, Vermylen, J, Linjen, HR, and Arnout, J (eds.): Throm-

bosis and Haemostasis 1987. International Society on Thrombosis and Haemostasis and Leuven University Press, Leuven, 1987, p 349.

21. Fuster, V, Adams, PC, Badimon, JJ, et al: Current concepts of thrombogenesis: Platelet inhibitor drugs' role in coronary artery disease. Prog Cardiovasc Dis 5:325, 1987.
22. Crowley, JG and Pierce, RA: The affinity of platelets for subendothelium. Am J Surg 47:529, 1981.
23. Hawiger, J, Kloczewiak, H, and Timmons, S: Platelet receptor mechanisms for adhesive macromolecules. In Oates, J, Hawiger, J, and Ross, R (eds): Interaction of Platelets with the Vessel Wall. American Physiological Society, Bethesda, 1985, p 1.
24. Turitto, VT, Weiss, HJ, and Baumgartner, HR: Platelet interaction with rabbit subendothelium in von Willebrand's disease. Altered thrombus formation distinct from defective platelet adhesion. J Clin Invest 74:1730, 1984.
25. Weiss, HJ, Tschopp, TB, Baumgartner, HR, et al: Decreased adhesion of giant (Bernard-Soulier) platelets to subendothelium. Am J Med 57:920, 1974.
26. Niewenhuis, HK and Sixma, JJ: Platelet receptors. In Born, GVR and Neri Serneri, GG (eds): Antiplatelet Therapy: Twenty Years' Experience. Proceedings of a European Conference. Excerpta Medica, Amsterdam, 1987, p 28.
27. Turitto, VT, Weiss, HJ, Baumgartner, HR, et al: Cells and aggregates at surfaces. In Leonard EF, Turitto, VT, Vroman, L (eds): Blood in Contact with Natural and Artificial Surfaces. Ann NY Acad Sci 516:453, 1987.
28. Escolar, G, Krumwiede, M, and White, JG: Organization of the actin cytoskeleton of resting and activated platelets in suspension. Am J Pathol 123:86, 1986.
29. White, JG: Platelet structural physiology: The ultrastructure of adhesion, secretion, and aggregation in arterial thrombosis. In Mehta, JL, Conti, RC, and Brest, AN (eds): Thrombosis and Platelets in Myocardial Ischemia. FA Davis, Philadelphia, 1987, p 13.
30. Coller, BD: Blood elements at surfaces: Platelets. In Leonard, EF, Turitto, VT, and Vroman, L (eds): Blood in Contact with Natural and Artificial Surfaces. Ann NY Acad Sci 516:362, 1987.
31. Antoniades, HN and Hunkapiller, MW: Human platelet-derived growth factor (PDGF): Aminoterminal amino acid sequence. Science 20:963, 1983.
32. Berk, BC, Alexander, RW, Brock, TA, et al: Vasoconstriction: A new activity for platelet-derived growth factor. Science 232:87, 1986.
33. Grotendorst, GR, Seppa, EJ, Kleinman, HK, et al: Attachment of smooth muscle cells to collagen and their migration toward platelet-derived growth factor. Proc Natl Acad Sci USA 78:3669, 1981.
34. Deuel, TF, Senior, RM, Chang, D, et al: Platelet factor 4 is chemotactic for neutrophils and monocytes. Proc Natl Acad Sci USA 78:4584, 1981.
35. Goldberg, ID, Stemerman, MB, and Handin, RI: Vascular permeation of platelet factor 4 after endothelial injury. Science 209:611, 1980.
36. Packham, MH and Mustard, JF: The role of platelets in the development of atherosclerosis. Semin Hematol 23:8, 1986.
37. Lagarde, M: Control mechanisms of platelet aggregation with special reference to eicosanoids and related components. In Born, GVR and Neri Serneri, GG (eds): Antiplatelet Therapy: Twenty Years' Experience. Proceedings of a European Conference. Excerpta Medica, Amsterdam, 1987, p 18.
38. Vermylen, J, Verstraete, M, and Fuster, V: Role of platelet activation and fibrin formation in thrombogenesis. J Am Coll Cardiol 8 (Suppl):2B, 1986.
39. Peerschke, EIB: The platelet fibrinogen receptor. Semin Hematol 22:241, 1985.
40. Luscher, EF: Mechanisms of platelet aggregation. In Born, GVR and Neri Serneri, GG (eds): Antiplatelet Therapy: Twenty Years' Experience. Proceedings of a European Conference. Excerpta Medica, Amsterdam, 1987, p 9.
41. Eldor, A, Falcone, DJ, Hajjar, DP, et al: Recovery of prostacycline production by de-endothelialized rabbit aorta: Critical role of neointimal smooth muscle cells. J Clin Invest 67:735, 1981.
42. Marcus, AJ, Weksler, BB, Jaffe, EA, et al: Synthesis of prostacyclin from platelet-derived endoperoxides by cultured human endothelial cells. J Clin Invest 66:979, 1980.
43. Moncada, S: Prostacyclin—discovery and biological importance. In Longenecker, GL and Schaffer, SW (eds): Prostaglandins: Research and Clinical Update. Alpha Editions, Minneapolis, 1985, p 1.
44. Cliveden, PB and Salzman, EW: Platelet metabolism and the effect of drugs. In Bowie, EJW and

Sharp, AA (eds): Hemostasis and Thrombosis. Butterworth and Company Publishers, Ltd, London, 1985, p 1.
45. Zucker, MB and Nachmias, VT: Platelet activation. Arteriosclerosis 5:2, 1985.
46. Verstraete, M, Dejana, E, Fuster, V, et al: An overview of antiplatelet and antithrombotic drugs. Haemostasis 15:89, 1985.
47. Fuster, V, Steele, PM, and Chesebro, JH: Role of platelets and thrombosis in coronary atherosclerotic disease and sudden death. J Am Coll Cardiol 5 (Suppl):175B, 1985.
48. Harker, LA and Fuster, V: Pharmacology of platelet inhibitors. J Am Coll Cardiol 8 (Suppl):21B, 1986.
49. Majerus, PW, Miletich, JP, Kane, WH, et al: The formation of thrombin on the platelet surface. In Mann, KG and Taylor, FB (eds): The Regulation of Coagulation. Elsevier, New York, 1980, p 215.
50. Hemeker, HC, van Rijn, JLML, Rosing, J, et al: Platelet membrane involvement in blood coagulation. Blood Cells 9:303, 1983.
51. Walsh, PN and Schmaier, AH. Platelet–coagulation protein interactions. In Colman, RW, Hirsh, J, Marder, J, and Salzman, EW (eds): Hemostasis and Thrombosis. JB Lippincott, Philadelphia, 1985, p 689.
52. Hirsh, J, Buchanan, MR, Ofosu, FA, et al: Evolution of thrombosis. In Leonard, EF, Turitto, VT, and Vroman, L (eds): Blood in Contact with Natural and Artificial Surfaces. Ann NY Acad Sci 516:586, 1987.
53. Ofosu, FA, Cerskus, AL, Hirsh, J, et al: The inhibition of the anticoagulant activity of heparin by platelets, brain phospholipids and tissue factor. Br J Haematol 57:229, 1984.
54. Rick, ME and Krizek, DM: Platelets modulate the proteolysis of factor VIII:C protein by plasmin. Blood 67:1649, 1986.
55. Weiss, HJ, Baumgartner, HR, and Turitto, VT: Regulation of platelet-fibrin thrombi on subendothelium. In Leonard, EF, Turitto, VT, and Vroman, L (eds): Blood in Contact with Natural and Artificial Surfaces. Ann NY Acad Sci 516:380, 1987.
56. Wessler, S and Gitel, SN: Pharmacology of heparin and warfarin. J Am Coll Cardiol 8 (Suppl):10B, 1986.
57. Stern, DM, Nawroth, PP, Kisiel, W, et al: A coagulation pathway or bovine aortic segment leading to generation of factor Xa and thrombin. J Clin Invest 74:1910, 1984.
58. Tracy, PB, Rohrbach, MS, and Mann KG. Functional prothrombinase complex assembly on isolated monocytes and lymphocytes. J Biol Chem 258:7264, 1983.
59. Chierchia, S and Patrono, C: Role of platelets and vascular eicosanoids in the pathology of ischemic heart disease. Fed Proc 46:81, 1987.
60. Kromhout, D, Bosschieter, EB, and Coulander, CDL: The inverse relation between fish consumption and 20-year mortality from coronary heart disease. N Engl J Med 312:1205, 1985.
61. Moncada, S, Palmer, RMJ, and Higgins, EA: Prostacyclin and endothelium-derived relaxing factor: Biological interactions and significance. In Verstraete, M, Vermylen, J, Lijnen, HR, and Arnout, J (eds): Thrombosis and Haemostasis 1987. International Society on Thrombosis and Haemostasis and Leuven University Press, Leuven, 1987, p 597.
62. McNeely, TB and Griffith, MJ: The anticoagulant mechanism of action of heparin in contact-activated plasma: Inhibition of factor X activation. Blood 65:1226, 1985.
63. Hemker, HC: The mode of action of heparin in plasma. In Verstraete, M, Vermylen, J, Lijnen, HR, and Arnout, J (eds): Thrombosis and Haemostasis 1987. International Socieity on Thrombosis and Haemostasis and the Leuven University Press, Leuven, 1987, p 17.
64. Colburn, P and Buonassisi, V: Anti-clotting activity of endothelial cell cultures and heparin sulfate proteoglycans. Biochem Biophys Res Commun 104:220, 1982.
65. Lollar, P and Owen, WG: Clearance of thrombin from circulation in rabbits by high affinity binding sites on endothelium: Possible role in the inactivation of thrombin by antithrombin III. J Clin Invest 66:1222, 1980.
66. Marciniak, E, Farley, CH, and De Simone, PA: Familial thrombosis due to antithrombin III deficiency. Blood 43:219, 1974.
67. Marlar, RA, Kleiss, AJ, and Griffin, JG: Human protein C: Inactivation of factor V and VIII in plasma by the activated molecule. Ann NY Acad Sci 370:303, 1981.
68. Comp, PC and Esmon, CT: Evidence for multiple roles for activated protein C in fibrinolysis. In Mann, KG and Taylor FB (eds): Regulation of Coagulation. Elsevier, New York, 1980, p 583.
69. Clouse, LH and Comp, PC: The regulation of hemostasis: The protein C system. N Engl J Med 314:1298, 1986.

70. Walker, FJ: Regulation of activated protein C by a new protein: A possible role for bovine protein S. J Biol Chem 255:5521, 1980.
71. Comp, PC, Nixon, RR, Cooper, MR, et al: Familial protein S deficiency is associated with recurrent thrombosis. J Clin Invest 74:2082, 1984.
72. Schwartz, HP, Fisher, M, Hopmeier, P, et al: Plasma protein S deficiency in familial thrombotic disease. Blood 64:1297, 1984.
73. Comp, PC, Nixon, RR, Cooper, MR, et al: Recurrent venous thromboembolism in patients with partial deficiency of protein S. N Engl J Med 311:1525, 1984.
74. Van Hinsbergh, VWM, Bertina, RM, van Wijngaarden, A, et al: Activated protein C decreases plasminogen activator–inhibitor activity in endothelial cell-conditioned medium. Blood 65:444, 1985.
75. Matsuo, O, Rijken, DC, and Collen, D: Comparison of the relative fibrinogenolytic, fibrinolytic and thrombolytic properties of tissue plasminogen activator and urokinase in vivo. Thromb Haemost 45:225, 1981.
76. Hoylaerts, M, Rijken, DC, Lijnen, MR, et al: Kinetics of the activation of plasminogen by human tissue plasminogen activator. Role of fibrin. J Biol Chem 257:2912, 1982.
77. Alexandre, P, Larcan, A, and Briqul, ME: Recurring thromboembolic accidents caused by family-related deficiency of the fibrinolysis system. Blut 41:437, 1980.
78. Aoki, N, Moroi, M, Saketa, Y, et al: Abnormal plasminogen: A hereditary molecular abnormality found in a patient with recurrent thrombosis. J Clin Invest 61:1186, 1978.
79. Dreyer, NA and Pizzo, SV: Blood coagulation and idiopathic thromboembolism among fertile women. Contraception 22:123, 1980.
80. Herrick, JB: Clinical features of sudden obstruction of the coronary arteries. JAMA 59:2015, 1912.
81. Ehrlich, JC and Shinohara, Y: Low incidence of coronary thrombosis in myocardial infarction. A restudy of serial block technique. Arch Pathol 78:432, 1964.
82. Roberts, WC and Buja, LM: The frequency and significance of coronary arterial thrombi and other observations in fatal acute myocardial infarction: A study of 107 necropsy patients. Am J Med 52:425, 1972.
83. Silver, MD, Baroldi, G, and Mariani, F: The relationship between acute occlusive coronary thrombi and myocardial infarction studied in100 consecutive patients. Circulation 61:219, 1980.
84. Horie, T, Sekiguchi, M, and Hirosawam, K: Coronary thrombosis in pathogenesis of acute myocardial infarction. Histopathological study of coronary arteries in 108 necropsied cases. Br Heart J 40:153, 1978.
85. Falk, E: Plaque rupture with severe pre-existing stenosis precipitating coronary thrombosis. Characteristics of coronary atherosclerotic plaques underlying fatal occlusive thrombi. Br Heart J 50:127, 1983.
86. Davies, MJ and Thomas, A: Thrombosis and acute coronary artery lesions in sudden cardiac ischemic death. N Engl J Med 310:1137, 1984.
87. Falk, E: Unstable angina with fatal outcome: Dynamic coronary thrombosis leading to infarction and/or sudden death. Circulation 71:699, 1985.
88. DeWood, MA, Spores, J, Notske, R, et al: Prevalence of total coronary occlusion during the early hours of transmural myocardial infarction. N Engl J Med 303:897, 1980.
89. Capone, G, Wolf, NM, Meyer, B, et al: Frequency of intracoronary filling defects by angiography in angina pectoris at rest. Am J Cardiol 56:403, 1985.
90. Sherman, CT, Litvack, F Grundfest, W, et al: Coronary angioscopy in patients with unstable angina pectoris, N Engl J Med 315:913, 1986.
91. Davies, MJ and Thomas, AC: Plaque fissuring—the cause of myocardial infarction, sudden ischemic death, and crescendo angina. Br Heart J 53:363,1985.
92. Ganz, P, Abben, RP, and Barry, WH: Dynamic variations in resistance of coronary arterial narrowings in angina pectoris at rest. Am J Cardiol 59:66, 1987.
93. Chierchia, S, Brunelli, C, Simonette, I, et al: Sequence of events in angina at rest: Primary reduction in coronary flow. Circulation 61:759, 1980.
94. Maseri, A: Role of coronary artery spasm in symptomatic and silent myocardial ischemia. J Am Coll Cardiol 9:249, 1987.
95. Holmes, DR, Harzler, GO, Smith, HC, et al: Coronary artery thrombosis in patients with unstable angina. Br Heart J 45:411, 1981.
96. Gotoh, K, Minamino, T, Katoh, O, et al: The role of intracoronary thrombus in unstable angina:

Angiographic assessment and thrombolytic therapy during ongoing anginal attacks. Circulation 77:526, 1988.
97. Vetrovec, GW, Cowley, MJ, Overton, H, et al: Intracoronary thrombus in syndromes of unstable myocardial ischemia. Am Heart J 102:1202, 1981.
98. Mandelkorn, JB, Wolf, NM, Singh, S, et al: Intracoronary thrombus in nontransmural myocardial infarction and in unstable angina pectoris. Am J Cardiol 52:1, 1983.
99. Zack PM, Ischinger, T, Aker, UT, et al: The occurrence of angiographically detected intracoronary thrombus in patients with unstable angina pectoris. Am Heart J 108:1408, 1984.
100. Ambrose, JA, Hjemdahl-Monsen, C, Borrico, S, et al: Quantitative and qualitative effects of intracoronary streptokinase in unstable angina and non-Q wave infarction. J Am Coll Cardiol 9:1156, 1987.
101. Ambrose, JA, Winters, SL, Stern, A, et al: Angiographic morphology and the pathogenesis of unstable angina pectoris. J Am Coll Cardiol 5:609, 1985.
102. Levin, DC and Fallon, JT: Significance of the angiographic morphology of localized coronary stenoses. Histophathologic correlates. Circulation 66:316, 1982.
103. Fuster, V and Chesebro, JA: Mechanisms of unstable angina. N Engl J Med 315:1023, 1986.
104. Fitzgerald, DJ, Catella, F, and FitzGerald, GA: Platelet activation in unstable coronary disease. N Engl J Med 315:983, 1986.
105. Hamm, CW, Lorenz, RL, Bleifeld, W, et al: Biochemical evidence of platelet activation in patients with persistent unstable angina. J Am Coll Cardiol 10:998, 1987.
106. Neri Serneri, GG, Gensisni, GF, Carnovali, M, et al: Association between time of increased fibrinopeptide A levels in plasma and episodes of spontaneous angina: A controlled prospective study. Am Heart J 113:672, 1987.
107. Theroux, P, Latour, JG, Leger-Gauthier, C, et al: Fibrinopeptide A and platelet factor levels in unstable angina pectoris. Circulation 75:156, 1987.
108. Eisenberg, PR, Sherman, L, Rich, M, et al: Importance of continued activation of thrombin reflected by fibrinopeptide A to the efficacy of thrombolysis. J Am Coll Cardiol 7:1255, 1986.
109. Chesebro, JH and Fuster, V: The therapeutic challenge of plaque rupture: Value of biochemical markers. J Am Coll Cardiol 10:1005, 1987.
110. Lam, JYT, Chesebro, JH, Steele, PM, et al: Is vasospasm related to platelet deposition? In vivo relationship in a pig model of arterial injury. Circulation 75:243, 1987.
111. Ludmer, PL, Selwyn, AP, and Shook, TL: Paradoxical vasoconstriction induced by acetylcholine in atherosclerotic coronary arteries. N Engl J Med 315:1046, 1986.
112. Levine, HD: Subendocardial infarction in retrospect: Pathologic, cardiographic and ancillary features. Circulation 72:790, 1985.
113. Erhardt, LR: Clinical and pathological observations in different types of acute myocardial infarction. A study of 84 patients deceased after treatment in coronary care unit. Acta Med Scand 560 (Suppl):1, 1974.
114. DeWood, MA, Stifter, WF, Simpson, CS, et al: Coronary arteriographic findings soon after non-Q-wave myocardial infarction. N Engl J Med 315:417, 1986.
115. Gibson, RS: Clinical, functional, and angiographic distinctions between Q wave and non-Q wave myocardial infarction: Evidence of spontaneous reperfusion and implications for intervention trials. Circulation 75 (Suppl):V128, 1987.
116. Timmis, AD, Griffin, B, Crick, JCP, et al: The effects of early coronary patency on the evolution of myocardial infarction: A prospective arteriographic study. Br Heart J 58:345, 1987.
117. Ambrose, JA, Hjemdahl-Monsen, CE, Borrico, S, et al: Angiographic demonstration of a common link between unstable angina pectoris and non-Q wave acute myocardial infarction. Am J Cardiol 61:244, 1988.
118. Fuster, V, Badimon, L, Cohen, M, et al: Insights into the pathogenesis of acute ischemic syndromes. Circulation 77:1213, 1988.
119. Davies, MJ: Thrombosis in acute myocardial infarction and sudden death. In Mehta, JL, Conti, RC, and Brest, AN (eds): Thrombosis and Platelets in Myocardial Ischemia. FA Davis, Philadelphia, 1987, p 151.
120. Brown, BG, Gallery, CA, Badger, RS, et al: Incomplete lysis of thrombus in the moderate underlying atherosclerotic lesion during intracoronary infusion of streptokinase for acute myocardial infarction: Quantitative angiographic observations. Circulation 73:653, 1986.
121. Ambrose, JA, Tannenbaum, M, Alexopoulos, D, et al: Angiographic progression of coronary artery disease and the development of myocardial infarction. J Am Coll Cardiol 12:56, 1988.
122. Ambrose, JA, Winters, SL, Arora, RR, et al: Coronary angiographic morphology in myocardial

infarction: A link between pathogenesis of unstable angina and myocardial infarction. J Am Coll Cardiol 6:1233, 1985.

123. Kannel, WB, Wolf, PA, Castelli, WP, et al: Fibrinogen and risk of cardiovascular disease. JAMA 258:1183, 1987.
124. Wilhelmsen, L, Svardsudd, K, Korsan-Berngtsen, K, et al: Fibrinogen as a risk factor for stroke and myocardial infarction. N Engl J Med 311:501, 1984.
125. Meade, TW, Brozovic, M, Chakrabarti, RR, et al: Haemostatic function and ischaemic heart disease: Principal results of the Northwick Park Heart Study. Lancet 2:533, 1986.
126. Tofler, GH, Brezinski, D, Schafer, AI, et al: Concurrent morning increase in platelet aggregability and the risk of myocardial infarction and sudden cardiac death. N Engl J Med 316:1514, 1987.
127. Francis, CW, Connaghan, DG, Scott, WL, et al: Increased plasma concentration of cross-linked fibrin polymers in acute myocardial infarction. Circulation 75:1170, 1987.
128. Kruskal, JB, Commerford, PJ, Franks, JJ, et al: Fibrin and fibrinogen-related antigens in patients with stable and unstable coronary artery disease. N Engl J Med 317:1361, 1987.
129. Hamsten, A, Wiman, B, de Faire U, et al: Increased plasma levels of a rapid inhibitor of tissue plasminogen activator in young survivors of myocardial infarction. N Engl J Med 313:1557, 1985.
130. Verheugt, FWA, Wouter ten Cate, J, Sturk, A, et al: Tissue plasminogen activator activity and inhibition in acute myocardial infarction and angiographically normal coronary arteries. Am J Cardiol 59:1075, 1987.
131. Francis, RB, Kwanishi, D, Baruch, T, et al: Impaired fibrinolysis in coronary artery disease. Am Heart J 115:776, 1988.

CHAPTER 5

Coronary Artery Spasm and Acute Myocardial Infarction

Charles R. Lambert Jr., M.D., Ph.D.
Carl J. Pepine, M.D.

In recent years the importance of thrombosis and changing atherosclerotic plaque morphology in setting the stage for acute myocardial infarction has become clear. Evidence in this regard has accumulated from both the research laboratory and, probably more importantly, from multiple large-scale clinical trials with early coronary angiography after or concurrent with systemic or intracoronary administration of thrombolytic agents. Despite the clearcut association of most myocardial infarctions with thrombosis, there remains a subset of patients who have myocardial infarction in association with exaggerated coronary vasomotion and angiographically normal coronary arteries once spasm is relieved pharmacologically. Beyond this group of patients, however, is a much larger group comprising perhaps the majority of those with ischemic heart disease who have some degree of "fixed" atherosclerosis and superimposed coronary vasomotion. The latter substrate allows for pathophysiologic reductions in coronary flow with changes in myocardial oxygen demand and supply, and also acts to promote thrombosis, platelet activation, and a possible cascade of summated vasoconstrictor responses within the labile local environment of the "dynamic coronary artery stenosis." Thus a current concept of coronary artery spasm in acute myocardial infarction must address the spectrum of vascular smooth muscle activation ranging from the near-maximal response associated with cessation of flow in a hypersensitive smooth-walled coronary artery with a relaxed cross-sectional area of 10 mm^2 to the minimal vasoconstriction required to stop flow in a coronary artery with an eccentric stenosis limiting cross-sectional area to 2 mm^2. Both of these responses involve coronary artery constriction, which, if left unchecked, might result in prolonged ischemia and myocardial infarction. Both situations fall under the heading of coronary artery spasm. However, it is important to realize that the degree of vasomotion involved is greatly different in these two situations. Coronary artery spasm in vivo should be thought of in terms of a continuum between these two extremes.

Recent experimental reports, pertinent in this context, provide strong evidence suggesting that focal arterial constriction, not of sufficient magnitude to reduce resting blood flow, may damage the arterial wall and possibly promote further vasospasm.[1-3] In one such study, vasoconstriction that reduced the rabbit carotid artery diameter 42 percent, without changing blood flow, produced marked longitudinal folding of the luminal surface.[3] Endothelial desquamation with extensive platelet deposition occurred on the exposed subendothelium. After 15 minutes, attached thrombus developed. Calcium deposits were seen on the luminal side of the internal elastic lamina. After 24 hours, marked leukocyte deposition occurred. With this substrate, platelet generation of thromboxane A_2 and leukocyte-triggered release of vasoactive arachidonic acid metabolites might initiate further vasoconstriction. Such a sequence of events, with an atherosclerotic substrate, nonobstructive coronary constriction, endothelial changes described above, promulgation of platelet deposition, leukocyte infiltration, and release of vasoconstrictive substances may play a role in the clinical association of coronary artery spasm and acute myocardial infarction to be discussed below.

These principles are illustrated by a case illustrated in Figures 5–1 and 5–2. A 68-year-old male presented initially with both rest and exertional angina poorly controlled by beta blockers and nitrates. The admission electrocardiogram showed anterior precordial T wave inversions; cardiac enzymes indicated necrosis; and the diagnosis of a non-Q-wave myocardial infarction was made. Despite intensive medical therapy, chest pain recurred several days later and coronary arteriography demonstrated only moderately severe coronary atherosclerotic obstruction involving principally the left anterior descending coronary artery.

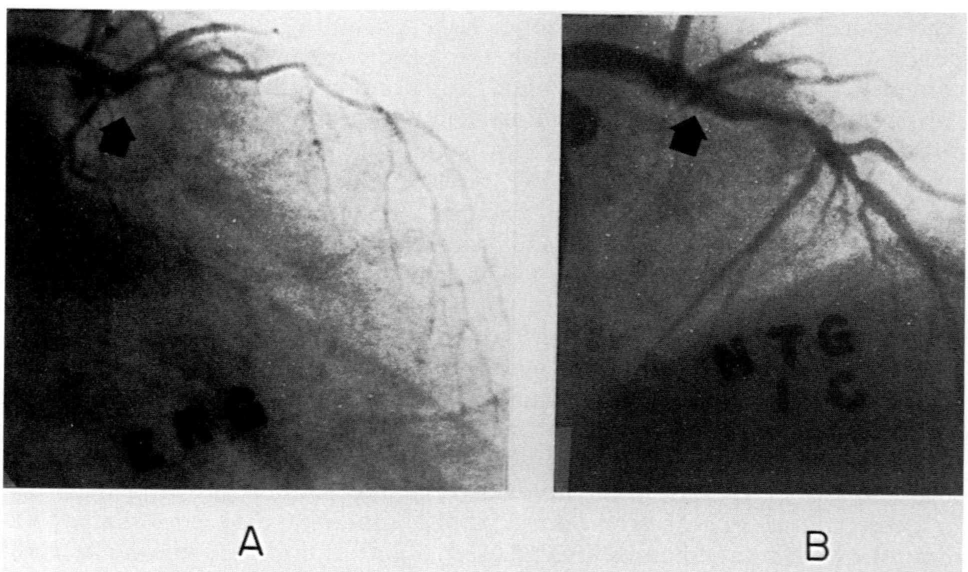

Figure 5–1. As described in the text, *panel A* is a left coronary artery angiogram (RAO) showing total occlusion of the left anterior descending coronary artery at the arrow after administration of intravenous ergonovine. Repeat arteriography *(panel B)* following administration of 0.1 mg intracoronary nitroglycerin reveals a patent vessel with moderate atherosclerosis involving the region of spasm.

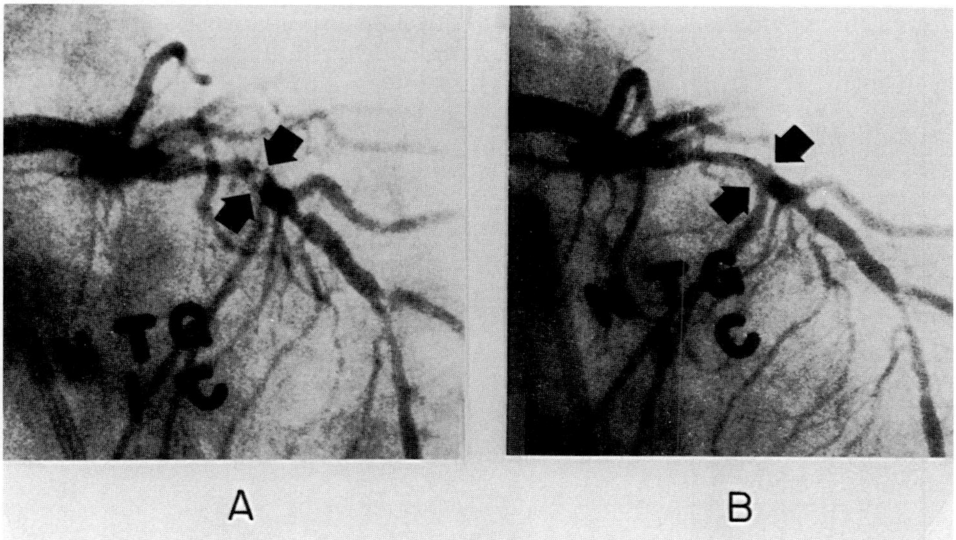

Figure 5–2. *Panel A* reveals an intraluminal filling defect, characteristic of thombus, in the proximal portion of the left anterior descending coronary artery where spasm had been demonstrated previously. *Panel B* shows resolution of the thrombus after administration of intracoronary streptokinase.

Ergonovine (0.1 mg) administered intravenously provoked total occlusion of the proximal left anterior descending artery (see Fig. 5–1*A*), which was promptly relieved with intracoronary nitroglycerin (see Fig. 5–1*B*). The patient subsequently did well taking diltiazem and long-acting nitrates and was discharged. However, he was admitted 1 week later during an episode of prolonged chest pain at rest. His ECG now showed ST segment elevation in the anterior precordial leads consistent with evolving anterior ischemic injury. Coronary arteriography performed approximately 6 hours after the onset of pain showed a non-occlusive intraluminal filling defect within the proximal left anterior descending artery in the region of previously documented spasm (see Figure 5–2*A*). Intracoronary steptokinase infusion caused resolution of the filling defect, confirming intraluminal thrombus (see Figure 5–2*B*). The patient subsequently did well with combination aspirin, nifedipine, diltiazem, and nitrate therapy. This case demonstrates not only coronary artery spasm, which was relatively refractory to conventional therapy, but also the manifestations of the complex pathophysiological mechanisms, mentioned above, which are involved in this disease.

CLININICAL ASSOCIATIONS OF CORONARY SPASM WITH MYOCARDIAL INFARCTION

Nitrate Withdrawal

Probably the first firm association between myocardial infarction and coronary spasm was made by Lange and coworkers[4] who described four patients developing acute myocardial infarction within 3 days after withdrawal from industrial nitroglycerin exposure. Subsequent coronary arteriography revealed normal-appearing vessels without evidence of important atherosclerotic obstruction in three patients. The fourth patient developed spontaneous spasm of both right and left coronary arteries during cardiac catheterization, which was relieved by nitroglycerin. An interesting animal model that may have clinical relevance in this regard has been described by Reeves and coworkers.[5] Using a rabbit model, these investigators described myocardial infarction, ventricular arrhythmia, and sudden death believed due to coronary spasm developing after abrupt withdrawal of nitroglycerin. Their observations were similar to those described in the aforementioned patients. Other investigators have noted development of acute myocardial infarction[6] and/or sudden death[7] soon after withdrawal of either nitroglycerin or oral isosorbide dinitrate. Although not documented angiographically, these observations are suggestive of coronary artery spasm as a possible etiology. Thus, it appears that sudden withdrawal of occupational exposure to aliphatic nitrates can definitely result in myocardial infarction due to coronary spasm.[8] Whether or not there is an absolute causal role for coronary spasm in the ischemic events sometimes observed after withdrawal of nitrates administered clinically remains to be established.

Catheter-Related Coronary Artery Spasm

Several episodes of catheter-related spasm resulting in myocardial infarction have been reported.[9,10] It may be difficult in such cases, however, to determine whether coronary artery dissection or thrombo-embolus caused the infarction. Likewise, the possible coexistence of variant angina is usually open to question. Considering the fact that catheter-related coronary spasm is not uncommon, there are very few cases of associated infarction reported. In general, myocardial infarction is not frequently caused by non-interventional catheter procedures; even during coronary angioplasty, coronary spasm is not a major problem.

Patients With Variant Angina

In 1976 Wiener and coworkers[11] described six patients with variant angina (rest angina and ST segment elevation) who eventually developed myocardial infarction. These patients later underwent coronary arteriography, which revealed spontaneous spasm of arteries supplying regions of myocardium involved in infarction. These observations provided a retrospective association between spontaneous coronary artery spasm, variant angina, and myocardial infarction. In1978 Maseri and coworkers[12] reported a systematic study of 187 patients with recurrent rest angina and ST segment shifts. Of these patients, 37 evolved a myocardial infarction in the myocardial areas localized to the region reflecting the transient ST segment shifts during episodes of rest angina. Of the 187 patients, 76 also underwent hemodynamic monitoring together with thallium 201 scintigraphy or coronary angiography during angina episodes. Evidence for coronary spasm (e.g., reversible perfusion defect or coronary artery narrowing) was seen in all of these patients during angina. Of these 76 patients, 8 developed acute myocardial infarction with, during, or shortly after the hemodynamic studies. Hemodynamic changes observed during angina due to spasm were indistinguishable from those seen at the onset of myocardial infarction. After infarction, occlusion of the coronary artery previously shown to undergo spasm was documented angiographically in two patients. One patient who died 6 hours after the onset of infarction had freshly formed thrombus at autopsy at the site of the previously noted spasm. These observations offer strong support to the role of coronary spasm as a primary event in myocardial infarction in some patients with variant or unstable angina pectoris and demonstrate the association which may be evident with thrombosis.

Walling and coworkers[13] recently reported results of long-term followup (mean 65 months) in a group of 217 patients hospitalized with variant angina. Of these patients, 87 had no coronary narrowings greater than 70 percent at cardiac catheterization. Overall, cardiac death occurred in 30 patients, and another 54 suffered a nonfatal myocardial infarction. In the group without severe coronary artery disease, only 15 patients suffered a myocardial infarction (17 percent). These data again point out the association of variant angina and presumed coronary artery spasm in myocardial infarction.

Nakamura and coworkers[14] reported followup data from a multicenter Japanese study of 349 patients with variant angina and coronary spasm. Only 101 of these patients had severe coronary artery disease, and the myocardial infarction rate in this group (mean followup 3.4 years) was only 5 percent. Thus, although these data represent a relatively good prognosis, an association of coronary artery spasm with myocardial infarction was documented again.

Beyond these series, numerous case reports exist in which coronary spasm, variant angina, and myocardial infarction are associated. For example, Zellinger and coworkers[15] reported a patient with variant angina and persistent inferior T wave abnormalities. After a symptom-free period, the patient developed recurrent rest angina with marked inferior lead ST segment elevation. Both symptomatic and asymptomatic periods with ST elevation continued despite intravenous nitroglycerin. At cardiac catheterization, a right coronary artery thrombus was found which fragmented during streptokinase infusion. Subsequent serum CK and electrocardiographic changes documented myocardial infarction. The authors speculated that during the period of unstable angina, coronary spasm produced intermittent ischemia. They suggested that timing of the angiographic study in such cases may lead to false conclusions regarding relative roles for thrombotic versus vasospastic events.

Tanimoto and coworkers[16] recently reported a patient with atherosclerotic left main coronary artery obstruction, who developed an acute inferior infarction in the perioperative period that was thought clinically to be related to right coronary artery spasm. At subsequent arteriography, ergonovine-induced spasm of the right coronary was confirmed. Egashira and coworkers[17] described a patient thought to have coronary spasm, who evolved an acute myocardial infarction during treatment with diltiazem. In this case, spasm was not confirmed angiographically. Halper and Factor[18] recently described a patient who died during acute myocardial infarction that was thought to be secondary to coronary spasm associated with neurofibromatosis. At autopsy, abnormal perivascular coronary innervation was found. The authors speculated that this abnormal innervation in association with right stellate ganglion blockade, provoked coronary spasm and acute transmural myocardial infarction. Topol and Fortuin[19] described a patient with carcinoid heart disease thought to have coronary artery spasm as the etiology for exercise-related cardiac arrest.

From all of the aforementioned evidence, it seems reasonable to conclude that coronary spasm, which is definitely associated with variant angina, plays a role in the evolution of myocardial infarction in certain patients.

Patients With Unstable Angina

Coronary spasm is thought to be present in a substantial number of unselected patients with unstable angina, based upon the frequency of recurrent ST segment elevation. However, obviously there is considerable overlap of these patients with those described under variant angina. In a systematic study by Bertrand and associates[20] of patients with chest pain undergoing cardiac catheterization, spasm was found in approximately 14 percent of patients (19 of 138) with both rest and effort angina and 38 percent of patients with only rest angina (77 of 203). They subdivided these patients according to their electrocardiographic responses. Eighty-five percent of those with ST segment elevation during rest angina had spasm, whereas 45 percent and 65 percent of those with ST depression and T wave changes, respectively, had coronary spasm. The latter two subsets are those most commonly encountered in the unstable angina population. Unstable angina patients are recognized to be at relatively high risk for development of acute myocardial infarction compared with patients with more stable effort angina. Whether or not those patients with spasm constitute an even higher risk for myocardial infarction is unknown. Supportive data were reported by Neill and coworkers[21] who prospectively studied 70 patients with unstable angina and reversible ST abnormalities. Coronary arteriography was performed acutely and after 4 months. These studies revealed a high incidence of complete coronary occlusion at 4 months in coronary arteries that had been patent but with high-grade atherosclerotic obstructions at the earlier study. The occlusions were associated with myocardial infarction in the region supplied and suggested that the unstable angina period represented intermittent coronary occlusion. Whether intermittent occlusion was due to rapid progression of atherosclerosis with thrombotic occlusion, or secondary to spasm could not be determined. The clinical similarity of this patient population, however, to that with rest angina and spasm reported by Maseri and colleagues[12] suggests a common mechanism for both transient ischemia and infarction.

From the foregoing, it seems reasonable to conclude that coronary spasm may be responsible for acute myocardial infarction in a subset of patients with unstable angina.

Patients Presenting With Acute Myocardial Infarction

Oliva and Breckinridge[22] reported results of coronary arteriography in 15 patients within 12 hours of acute myocardial infarction. Coronary spasm, defined as total or subtotal occlusion with subsequent opening after nitroglycerin, was found in 6 (40 percent) of these patients. In each instance, spasm occurred at the site of an atherosclerotic obstruction. These observations were interpreted as suggesting that coronary spasm preceded the formation of an occlusive thrombus, which leads to myocardial infarction in some patients.

Experience with thrombolytic therapy in acute myocardial infarction has offered support to proponents of thrombosis as the primary mediator of most myocardial infarctions. These data, however, consistently show a small number of patients with nitroglycerin-responsive coronary occlusion when angiography is performed early. The primary problem in delineating the precise etiology of acute myocardial infarction in these patients is the timing of arteriographic study and the acutal onset of the event ("time zero"). Difficulties with timing the onset of the event from the onset of symptoms and the lack of data at "time zero" prohibit solving this problem at present. Ganz and coworkers[23] studied 20 patients within 3 hours of the onset of chest pain. Eighteen were found to have complete coronary artery occlusion, and only two occlusions opened with intracoronary nitroglycerin. Mathey and coworkers[24] studied 39 patients with complete coronary occlusion in a similar time frame, and only one nitroglycerin response was seen. Markis and coworkers[25] reported on nine patients within 2 to 4 hours of the onset of chest pain, and none responded to intracoronary nitroglycerin. Rentrop and coworkers[26] studied 29 patients within 1.5 to 16 hours after the onset of chest pain, and 5 responded to intracoronary nitroglycerin. Reduto and coworkers[27] found, within a similar time frame, 1 of 26 coronary occlusions to be nitroglycerin-responsive.

Mandelkorn and coworkers[28] reported their experience with intracoronary streptokinase and nitroglycerin in patients with unstable angina, transmural infarction, and nontransmural infarction. Only one patient with unstable angina responded to intracoronary nitroglycerin. After 1.5 to 3 hours, the majority of patients with nontransmural infarction and about half of those with unstable angina responded to streptokinase, but not nitroglycerin, with either opening of an occluded vessel, an increase in stenosis diameter, or dissolution of an intracoronary filling defect. These findings are consistent with a thrombotic role for coronary artery diameter reduction in both unstable angina and myocardial infarction after 1.5 to 3 hours.

Cipriano and coworkers[29] reported 11 patients with documented coronary artery spasm either before or after myocardial infarction. Arteriographic study of the vessels supplying infarcted regions showed six that had minimal or no visible atherosclerotic disease. The coincidence of the location of the infarction and that of spasm was interpreted as evidence that the latter was probably causally related to the former. Benacerraf and coworkers[30] described a 37-year-old man with an evolving inferior myocardial infarction who underwent coronary arteriography approximately 2.5 hours after the onset of chest pain. Angiography initially revealed complete occlusion of the proximal right coronary artery, which responded to intracoronary nitroglycerin, revealing a discrete stenosis and associated intraluminal filling defect suggestive of thrombus. No streptokinase was administered because of previous cardiopulmonary resuscitation. Later coronary arteriography revealed resolution of the intraluminal filling defect and slight outline irregularity in the area. An ergonovine provocation test was positive, and later negative after treatment with diltiazem. These authors postulated that coronary artery spasm initiated the thrombotic process as suggested by the circumstantial evidence presented. Additional evidence that lends support to the coronary artery spasm–myocardial infarction connection is supplied by Bertrand and coworkers.[20] The high frequency (21 percent) of ergonovine-provoked coronary artery spasm after myocardial infarction in their study establishes a temporal if not causal relationship between the two phenomena. Additional data in patients presenting with acute myocardial infarction were reported recently by Bory and coworkers.[31] Using methylergometrine testing in the cardiac catheterization laboratory, 6 of 23 patients with acute myocardial infarction had coronary artery spasm demonstrated after autonomic blockade with atropine and labetalol. Before blockade, none of the patients exhibited spasm. Although the frequency of coronary artery spasm in these myocardial infarction patients before autonomic blockade was not as high as in the study cited above, an association between infarction and spasm was demonstrated again. The exact role of the autonomic nervous system in mediation of spasm in this setting deserves further investigation. A recent review[32] of findings with early coronary arteriography indicates that an average of 8 percent of patients demonstrate a nitroglycerin-responsive occlusion when studied early in the course of acute myocardial infarction. Thus, even without data at "time zero," a small but definite role is seen for coronary artery spasm in the pathogenesis of acute myocardial infarction. Additional evidence supporting coronary vasoconstriction as an important mediator of ischemia in the setting of acute myocardial infarction was recently supplied by Hackett and coworkers.[33] Using continuous ECG monitoring and serial coronary arteriography, 28 episodes of coronary reopening and closure were documented in 45 patients receiving intracoronary streptokinase for acute myocardial infarction. During reocclusion, nitrate reopened the coronary artery in 14 of 28 episodes demonstrating the importance of vasoconstriction in this response.

That such peri-infarction coronary artery spasm may not be of primary importance in the evolving infarction, however, is suggested by both the Norwegian[34] and U.S.[35] multicenter nifedipine–myocardial infarction trials. Nifedipine did not prevent progression of threatened infarction or limit infarct size in these trials. If it is assumed that nifedipine treatment abolishes or attenuates coronary artery spasm, then the role of spasm in the patient with evolving myocardial infarction might be minimal. A possible explanation of this observation is that nifedipine treatment was administred too late in the course of a spasm-mediated event to affect a beneficial response.

Myocardial Infarction in Patients Receiving Antispasm Agents

In a 1-year followup study of 45 patients with rest angina due to coronary spasm who were receiving calcium blockers alone or in combination with nitrates,[36] we observed 5 patients who developed acute myocardial infarction and 3 others with sudden death. In controlled trials of patients with unstable angina assigned to either nifedipine or placebo therapy for periods ranging from 2 weeks to over 1 year, the frequency of myocardial infarction and sudden death was the same regardless of nifedipine therapy.[35,37] Thus, although spasm may have a role in development of acute myocardial infarction in patients with unstable angina, one must speculate about additional mechanisms. For example, each of the eight events observed in our followup study occurred in the 18-patient subgroup who had spasm superimposed upon important coronary atherosclerosis[36] similar to the case presented in the introduction. Another possibility is that spasm became refractory or unresponsive to calcium blocker treatment. Such an event could occur if, for example, the endothelium became damaged or platelet aggregation, plaque disruption, hemorrhages, and so on occurred. Evidence that spasm leads to intimal injury, thrombus formation, and/or plaque disruption is present in reports of unstable angina patients who later develop myocardial infarction.[38,39]

SUMMARY

From the studies and observations reviewed in this chapter, it can be appreciated that there is considerable direct and circumstantial evidence to implicate coronary artery spasm as a primary phenomenon in some patients with myocardial infarction. Although currently available data indicate that the number of acute myocardial infarctions due primarily to "pure" coronary artery spasm is relatively small, it should be emphasized that essentially very little if any data exist at "time zero" or at the actual onset of infarction. Most myocardial infarctions are probably multifactorial in etiology. To what extent coronary artery spasm, atherosclerosis, platelets, in situ thrombosis, endothelial mediators, and passive influences on vascular caliber interact in the pathogenesis of acute myocardial infarction remains incompletely understood.

REFERENCES

1. Gertz, SD, Uretsky, G, Wajnberg, RS, et al: Endothelial cell damage and thrombus formation after partial arterial constriction: Relevance to the role of coronary artery spasm in the pathogenesis of myocardial infarction. Circulation 63:476, 1981.
2. Joris, I and Majno, G: Endothelial changes induced by arterial spasm. Am J Pathol 102:346, 1981.
3. Kurgan, A, Gertz, SD, and Wajnberg RS: Intimal changes associated with arterial spasm induced by periarterial application of calcium chloride. Exp Mol Pathol 39:176, 1983.
4. Lange, RL, Reid, MD, Tresch, DD, et al: Nonatheromatous ischemic heart disease following withdrawal from chronic idustrial nitroglycerin exposure. Circulation 46:666–678, 1972.
5. Reeves, WC, Cook, L, Wood, MA, and Whitesell, L: Coronary artery spasm after abrupt withdrawal of nitroglycerin in rabbits. Am J Cardiol 55:1066–1069, 1985.
6. Muller, JE and Gunther, SJ: Nifedipine therapy for Prinzmetal's angina. Circulation 57:137–139, 1978.
7. Franciosa, JA, Nordstrom, LA, and Cohn, JN: Nitrate therapy for congestive heart failure. JAMA 240:443–446, 1978.
8. Morton, WE: Occupational habituation to aliphatic nitrates and the withdrawal hazards of coronary disease and hypertension. J Occup Med 19:197–200, 1977.
9. Cheng, TD, Bashour, T, Singh, BK, and Kelser, GA: Myocardial infarction in the absence of coronary atherosclerosis. Am J Cardiol 30:680–682, 1972.
10. Engel, HJ, Page, HL, and Campbell, WB: Coronary artery spasm as the cause of myocardial infarction during coronary arteriography. Am Heart J 91:501–506, 1976.
11. Wiener, L, Kasparian, H, Duca, PR, et al: Spectrum of coronary arterial spasm—clinical, angiographic and myocardial metabolic experience in 29 cases. Am J Cardiol 38:945–955, 1976.
12. Maseri, A, L'Abbate, A, Biroldi, G, et al: Coronary vasospasm as a possible cause of myocardial infarction. N. Engl J Med 299:1271–1277, 1978.
13. Walling, A, Waters, DD, Miller, DD, et al: Long-term prognosis in patients with variant angina. Circulation 76:990–997, 1987.
14. Nakamura, M, Takeshita, A, and Nose, Y: Clinical characteristics associated with myocardial infarction, arrhythmias, and sudden death in patients with vasospastic angina. Circulation 75:1110–1116, 1987.
15. Zellinger, AB, Abramowitz, BM, Schick, EC, and Ryan, TJ: Variant angina culminating in coronary thrombosis and myocardial infarction. Chest 82:188–192, 1982.
16. Tanimoto, Y, Matsuda, Y, Kobayashi, Y, et al: Coronary spasm as a cause of perioperative myocardial infarction. Jap Heart J 25:275–281, 1984.
17. Egashira, K, Araki, H, Koiwaya, Y, et al: Acute myocardial infarction following asymptomatic ST elevation despite diltiazem therapy. Am Heart J 109:379–380, 1985.
18. Halper, J and Factor, SM: Coronary lesions in neurofibromatosis associated with vasospasm and myocardial infarction. Am Heart J 108:420–422, 1984.
19. Topol, EJ and Fortuin, NJ: Coronary artery spasm and cardiac arrest in carcinoid heart disease. Am J Med 77:950–952, 1984.
20. Bertrand, ME, Lablanche, JM, Tilmant, PY, et al: The provocation of coronary arterial spasm in patients with recent transmural myocardial infarction. Eur Heart J 4:1532–1535, 1983.
21. Neill, WA, Wharton, TP, Fluri-Lundeen, J, and Cohen, IS: Acute coronary insufficiency—coronary occlusion after intermittent ischemic attacks. N Engl J Med 302:1157–1162, 1980.
22. Oliva, PB and Breckinridge, JC: Arteriographic evidence of coronary arterial spasm in acute myocardial infarction. Circulation 56:366–374, 1977.

23. Ganz, W, Buchbinder, N, Marcus, H, et al: Intracoronary thrombolysis in evolving myocardial infarction. Am Heart J 101:4–13, 1981.
24. Mathey, DG, Kuck, K, Tilsmer, V, et al: Nonsurgical coronary artery recanalization in acute transmural myocardial infarction. Circulation 63:489–497, 1981.
25. Markis, JE, Malagold, M, Parker, JA, et al: Myocardial salvage after intracoronary thrombolysis with streptokinase in acute myocardial infarction. N Engl J Med 305:777–782, 1981.
26. Rentrop, P, Blanke, H, Karsch, KR, et al: Selective intracoronary thrombolysis in acute myocardial infarction and unstable angina pectoris. Circulation 63:307–317, 1981.
27. Reduto, LA, Smalling, RW, Freund, GC, and Gould KL: Intracoronary infusion of streptokinase in patients with acute myocardial infarction: Effects of reperfusion on left ventricular performance. Am J Cardiol 48:403–309, 1981.
28. Mandelkorn, JB, Wolf, NM, Singh, S, et al: Intracoronary thrombus in nontransmural myocardial infarction and in unstable angina pectoris. Am J Cardiol 53:1–6, 1983.
29. Cipriano, PR, Koch, FH, Rosenthal, SJ, et al: Myocardial infarction in patients with coronary artery spasm demonstrated by angiography. Am Heart J 105:542–547, 1983.
30. Benacerraf, A, Scholl, JM, Achard, F, et al: Coronary spasm and thrombosis associated with myocardial infarction in a patient with nearly normal coronary arteries. Circulation 67:1147–1150, 1983.
31. Bory, M, Joly, P, Bonnet, J, et al: Methergin testing with angiographically normal coronary arteries. Am J Cardiol 61:298–302, 1088.
32. Conti, CR: Myocardial infarction: Thoughts about pathogenesis and the role of coronary artery spasm. Am Heart J 110:187–193, 1985.
33. Hackett, D, Davies, G, Chierchia, S, and Maseri, A: Intermittent coronary occlusion in acute myocardial infarction. N Engl J Med 317:1055–1059, 1987.
34. Sirnes, PA, Overskeid, K, Pedersen, TR, et al: Evolution of infarct size during the early use of nifedipine in patients with acute myocardial infarction: The Norwegian nifedipine multicenter trial. Circulation 70:638–644, 1984.
35. Muller, JE, Morrison, J, Stone, PH, et al: Nifedipine therapy for patients with threatened and acute myocardial infarction: A randomized double-blind, placebo-controlled comparison. Circulation 69:740–747, 1984.
36. Pepine, CJ, Feldman, RL, Hill, JA, et al: Clinical outcome after treatment of rest angina with calcium blockers: Comparative experience during the initial year of therapy with diltiazem, nifedipine, and verapamil. Am Heart J 106:1341–1347, 1983.
37. Ouyang, P, Brinker, JA, Mellits, ED, et al: Variables predictive of successful medical therapy in patients with unstable angina: Selection by multivariate analysis from clinical, electrocardiographic and angiographic evaluations. Circulation 70:367, 1984.
38. Ambrose, JA, Winters, SL, Stern, A, et al: Angiographic morphology and the pathogenesis of unstable angina pectoris. J Am Coll Cardiol 5:509–516, 1985.
39. Mandelkorn, JB, Wolf, NM, and Singh, S: Intracoronary thrombus in nontransmural myocardial infarction and in unstable angina pectoris. Am J Cardiol 52:1, 1983.

PART 3

Diagnosis/New Methods—New Concepts

CHAPTER 6

Early Biochemical Markers of Myocardial Necrosis

Peter Puleo, M.D.
Robert Roberts, M.D.

The biochemical diagnosis of acute myocardial infarction (AMI) has improved dramatically since the first description of aspartate transaminase elevation (AST; formerly designated SGOT) by LaDue and coworkers in 1954.[1,2] Plasma enzymes now provide the most accurate means of diagnosing acute myocardial necrosis and allow for reliable estimates of infarct size. However, the recent demonstrations that thrombolytic intervention in the first hours of AMI can result in myocardial salvage have created the need for biochemical indicators of myocardial necrosis that are diagnostic within 3 hours of the onset of symptoms. The availability of such markers would be useful also in the appropriate triage of emergency room patients having chest pain. Unfortunately, the diagnostic enzymes currently in widespread use are not reliable within this time frame. Consequently, recent work has been focused on the subforms of the MM and MB creatine kinase (CK) isoenzymes.

BIOCHEMICAL MARKERS OF AMI

Biochemical markers of AMI have in common the property of being present within cardiac myocytes, with release into the blood following the onset of myocardial infarction. Release is presumably a result of the cell membrane breakdown that accompanies irreversible ischemia. Elevations of blood enzyme levels usually do not occur with reversible ischemia in the dog[3,4] or in humans.[5] Transport from the necrotic myocardium to the blood occurs via the cardiac lymphatics.[6]

The most important factors that affect the timing of marker appearance in the blood are molecular size and solubility. Small molecules such as myoglobin (molecular weight: 17,800) diffuse rapidly and appear in the blood in the first hours of AMI; large molecules such as lactate dehydrogenase (LDH; molecular weight 135,000) have a delayed appearance in the blood. In addition, poorly soluble molecules, such as those constituting the contractile apparatus, exhibit a very delayed rise in plasma levels. An important practical consideration for early molecular markers of AMI is the reliability and speed with which an assay for the molecule can be performed; assays requiring an hour to perform or highly trained personnel are unlikely to be useful. Finally, the utility of any molecular diagnostic marker for AMI is critically dependent on the extent to which it is present in myocardium but not in other tissues, so that a rise in blood levels is specific for myocardial injury.

CREATINE KINASE

CK catalyzes the reversible transfer of a high-energy phosphate group from adenosine triphosphate (ATP) to creatine:

$$\text{Cr} + \text{ATP} \overset{\text{CK}}{\rightleftharpoons} \text{Cr-P} + \text{ADP}$$

(Cr = creatine; Cr-P = creatine phosphate; ADP = adenosine diphosphate)

Creatine phosphate (Cr-P) is believed to function as an energy carrier in a "shuttle" system wherein ATP formed in the mitochondria transfers its high-energy phosphate bond to the smaller, more rapidly diffusing molecule Cr-P, in a reaction catalyzed by the mitochondrial CK isoenzyme. Cr-P then diffuses out of the mitochondria to cytosol where, in the presence of cytosolic CK and ADP, ATP can be regenerated for energy utilization.[7,8]

Molecular Properties of CK

CK is a dimer of molecular weight 86,000. The three cytosolic CK isoenzymes are formed by dimeric association of the CK polypeptide subunits M and B in one of three possible combinations: MM, MB, and BB CK (also designated CK-3, CK-2, and CK-1, respectively). MM CK, the predominant cytosolic form present in skeletal muscle, is isoelectric at physiologic pH; BB CK, the only cytosolic isoenzyme present in the brain, has a net negative charge; MB CK has a charge intermediate between the two. Mitochondrial CK has a net positive charge at pH 7.4; it is a homodimer that differs antigenically,[9] biochemically,[10] and in charge[11] from the three cytosolic enzymes. The isoenzymes also differ in stability: MM is stable for several days at room temperature; MB CK is stable for several days if refrigerated; BB and mitochondrial CK are very labile molecules, even with optimum storage. The M, B, and mitochondrial chains are encoded by different genes.[12]

CK Assays

Total CK activity is assayed by the three-step, coupled enzyme system of Rosalki,[13] in which nicotinamide adenine dinucleotide phosphate-H^+ (NADPH) is generated as a final product and measured by ultraviolet light absorption at 340 nm. Artifactual elevation may occur in hemolyzed specimens owing to release of the enzyme adenylate kinase from erythrocytes.

Assay of the CK isoenzymes has been achieved by a wide variety of techniques; the most commonly employed technique in clinical laboratories is electrophoresis on agarose or cellulose acetate. This method physically separates the isoenzymes on the basis of their charge differences; after electrophoresis the gel is incubated with "Rosalki reagent" and NADPH is produced in situ at the location of the CK isoenzymes. The relative percentage of each isoenzyme is determined by scanning densitometry. The normal range for MB CK is defined (somewhat arbitrarily) as less than 3 percent, 4 percent, or 5 percent (depending on the investigator) of total CK activity.[14] Application of samples having high activity to the gel without dilution can result in falsely elevated MB CK values. Albumin-bound bilirubin may also produce false-positive results. A major limitation of electrophoresis is the need for individual sample handling by experienced personnel and the relatively long assay time (30 to 45 minutes); consequently, this assay is unavailable in most "stat" labs.

A more convenient and rapid method of isoenzyme assay is the batch adsorption assay of Henry and associates,[15] which employs glass beads coated with a positively charged ion-exchange resin. Negatively charged MB CK binds the resin while MM remains unbound and is washed away; subsequent rinses using high ionic strength buffer elute MB CK, which is then quantitated by the Rosalki assay. This technique is highly sensitive, precise, reproducible, and can be completed in 5 minutes by personnel with minimal training. This allows for easy handling of "stat" specimens so that isoenzyme results are available within minutes of blood sampling. Furthermore, MB CK determinations obtained at 4-hour intervals facilitate movement of patients with serial negative assays out of the coronary care unit (CCU) to less expensive, nonintensive care beds. A disadvantage of the batch adsorption assay is that BB CK binds the resin and is assayed with MB CK. However, BB CK is rarely present in the blood at clinically meaningful concentrations.[16]

A number of immune assays have been developed; none is in widespread use. Radioimmunoassay (RIA) affords high sensitivity and precision[17] at the expense of long assay time; these tests are performed only once daily in most laboratories. This limitation and the need for handling radiopharmaceuticals have made the RIA unpopular among both cardiologists and clinical pathologists. Similarly, nonradioactive immunoprecipitation, immunoinhibition, and enzyme-linked immunoadsorption assays are used in only a minority of clinical laboratories[18] because they are cumbersome and time consuming, and may be unreliable.[19] However, a recently developed colorimetric assay based on an MB-specific monoclonal antibody[20] appears to be reliable and has been partially automated[21]; nevertheless, the assay requires approximately 1 hour for accurate results.

CK Tissue Distribution

The quantity and isoenzyme distribution of the cytosolic CK isoenzymes are shown in Figure 6–1. Skeletal muscle contains the highest CK activity per gram of tissue. Although the vast majority of CK in adult skeletal muscle is MM CK, up to 40 percent of normal muscles biopsied also contain small (1 percent to 3 percent) quantities of MB CK.[22] More importantly, disease or injury (including acute or chronic exercise) may induce skeletal muscle MB CK synthesis and release,[23–28] repeating a pattern characteristic of fetal muscle.[29]

Myocardium is the only tissue that harbors substantial quantities of MB CK:

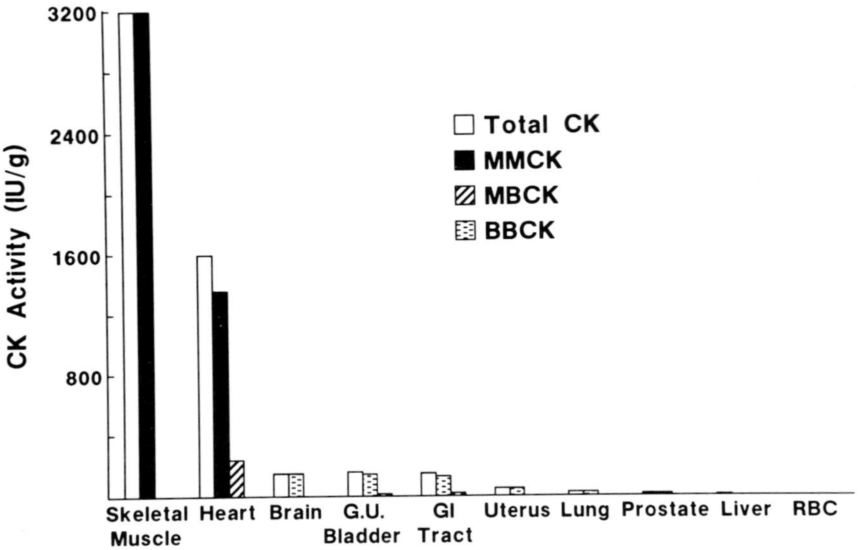

Figure 6–1. Tissue distribution of the CK cytosolic isoenzymes.

approximately 15 percent to 20 percent of myocardial cytosolic CK is MB CK; the remainder is MM CK. A recent report contending that nondiseased human myocardium is free of MB CK, with induction of MB CK synthesis by ischemia or hypertrophy,[30] has not been confirmed by others and conflicts with other published data from studies of healthy humans[31,32] and nonhuman primates.[33]

Organs other than heart and skeletal muscle, particularly organs containing smooth muscle, such as the uterus, GI tract, prostate, and urinary tract, contain CK activity in low levels per gram of tissue; most CK present in this tissue is the BB isoenzyme. BB CK is also the only isoenzyme present in brain. None of these tissues contains significant levels of MB CK. Rarely, malignant tumors may synthesize and release CK, usually BB CK.[34]

CK Isoenzymes in the Diagnosis of AMI

Blood levels of total and MB CK remain within the normal range for the first 4 to 6 hours after the onset of AMI; these markers subsequently exhibit a steady rise until peak values are attained an average of 24 hours after the onset of symptoms. Peak plasma levels are reached earlier in non-Q-wave (15 hours) than in Q-wave AMI (28 hours).[35] Levels then return to normal by 48 to 72 hours after AMI onset. The MB/MM ratio in the blood reflects that of the myocardium (i.e., 15/85).

The specificity of the MB CK molecule for myocardium distinguishes it from other biochemical markers of AMI. In addition, the high levels of MB CK activity present in myocardial tissue, combined with the low concentration present in the serum of healthy individuals, make this determination a very sensitive indicator of myocardial necrosis. Consequently, overall precision of MB CK assay for the diagnosis of AMI exceeds 95 percent for the commonly used assays.[19,36] False-negative results are very rare if blood samples are available within an appropriate time frame. False-positive results, although uncommon, may occur in a variety of circumstances:

1. *Release of nonmyocardial MB CK from injured or diseased skeletal muscle.* This is encountered most commonly in association with rhabdomyolysis,[26] but also occurs with electric injury,[26,27] inflammatory myopathies,[25] muscular dystrophy,[28] chronic high levels of exercise,[23,24] and following DC countershock.[37] A nonmyocardial source of elevated plasma MB CK should be suspected if skeletal muscle injury is likely, especially if: (a) clinical and ECG data are atypical of AMI, (b) plasma MB CK activity elevation is delayed and/or sustained rather than following a time course typical of AMI, (c) total CK activity is elevated to very high levels with a relative percentage rise of MB CK below that usually found in AMI (i.e., 3 percent to 10 percent of total CK activity rather than 15 percent to 20 percent).
2. *Laboratory error or artifact.* This occurs most commonly with electrophoretic assays. Artifactual bands may be present because of renal failure[38] or because of albumin-bound drugs, including diazepam, chlordiazepoxide, and tricyclic antidepressants. The so-called macro-CK complexes, which consist of BB or mitochondrial CK polymers formed in the blood after release of dimeric CK from tissue, may cause diagnostic confusion in immunoassays.[39] Injury to tissue rich in BB CK, such as the prostate or uterus, may result in misdiagnosis if a method that measures MB and BB CK together is employed. BB CK may be released also following blunt trauma to the brain or diffuse cerebral injury but is generally not detectable after bland cerebral infarction.[40]
3. Hypothyroidism may be associated with sustained elevation of total and MB CK activity, presumably on the basis of impaired enzyme clearance from the blood.[41]

In our institution, plasma samples for total and MB CK activity are obtained on admission to the CCU and every 4 hours for 24 hours. The glass bead method is used, and assays are performed in the laboratory within 30 minutes of specimen withdrawal. The diagnosis of AMI is made if serial samples exhibit MB CK above the upper normal limit (14 IU per liter), with a time-activity curve and percent MB (of total CK) typical of AMI. If only one sample is available from within the appropriate time frame, the diagnosis of AMI is made only if plasma MB CK activity exceeds the upper normal limit by 100 percent, and returns to the normal range in the expected time period. Frequent plasma sampling permits accurate estimation of infarct size[42] and allows for early transfer out of the CCU of the 65 percent to 70 percent of patients in whom the diagnosis of AMI is ruled out.

As already noted, MB CK plasma concentration usually remains within the normal range for 4 to 6 hours after the onset of AMI. The introduction of sensitive and quantitative MB CK assays, such as the glass bead assay and the RIA, have not significantly changed the time at which AMI can be detected biochemically. To avoid high rates of false-positive results, the upper limit of the normal reference range for plasma MB CK must be significantly higher than the mean value in a normal population. Consequently, an individual with a baseline plasma MB CK of 3 to 5 IU per liter must have sufficient MB release from AMI to at least triple preinfarction plasma CK levels before AMI can be detected biochemically. If a lower value were selected for the upper reference limit, AMI might be detectable at an earlier time, but a substantial proportion of a normally distributed population without AMI would exhibit levels outside the normal range, and thus "early diagnosis" would come at the expense of lower assay specificity. Inasmuch as these constraints apply to all MB CK isoenzyme assays, "early diagnosis" within the time frame required for decision making in the thrombolysis era (i.e., in the first 3 hours of AMI) does not appear to be possible using MB isoenzyme activity values alone. Indeed, the sensitivity of MB CK for the diagnosis of AMI is only 25 percent within 4 hours of onset, and 54 percent in the first 12 hours.[43]

SERUM MYOGLOBIN

Myoglobin is a heme-containing protein of molecular weight 17,800; like hemoglobin, it has a high affinity for molecular oxygen. Myoglobin is thought to function as a "reservoir" for oxygen in striated muscle. Because this molecule is abundant in both cardiac and skeletal muscle and has no known tissue-specific isoenzymes, its release into the blood is not a specific marker for myocardial injury; skeletal muscle trauma is associated with marked myoglobinemia. Inasmuch as myoglobin functions as a carrier molecule and not as an enzyme, it is assayed immunologically by RIA rather than by a catalytic activity. Following AMI, myoglobin rapidly appears in the blood with detectable elevation as early as 1½ hours after the onset of symptoms.[44] This early rise is probably a result of its low molecular weight and rapid diffusing capacity. Its small molecular size also results in myoglobin clearance through the glomerular filtration apparatus, hence the danger of myoglobin precipitation in the renal tubules and acute renal failure following massive skeletal muscle injury. As a result of rapid renal clearance, plasma myoglobin levels return to the normal range within 34 hours after onset of symptoms of AMI.[44] In small infarctions, the marker may be falsely negative if the assay is performed after 24 hours of AMI onset. The poor specificity of myoglobin for cardiac muscle injury is the major drawback for the use of this molecule as a diagnostic marker of AMI.[45]

The early rise of plasma myoglobin following acute myocardial necrosis would suggest that this marker might serve as an early diagnostic marker of AMI. However, the currently available immunoassays for myoglobin require much more time for completion than the glass bead or electrophoretic MB CK assays, thus eliminating the 3- to 4-hour time advantage for plasma myoglobin elevation as compared with MB CK.[45] These disadvantages, combined with the lack of tissue specificity, make this marker unacceptable as a reliable guide for early diagnosis of AMI and for the utilization of thrombolytic therapy.

MM AND MB CK SUBFORMS

In the late 1970s, Wevers and his coworkers[46,47] in the Netherlands observed that serum from patients who had suffered an AMI, upon prolonged gel electrophoresis, demonstrated three CK bands in the MM region rather than the expected single band. Similarly, MB CK could be resolved into two component bands. These bands have subsequently been designated sub-bands, and the CK molecules corresponding to each band have been termed subforms or subisoenzymes. Wevers also demonstrated a shift in relative sub-band intensity with time after AMI: the less mobile MM and MB bands were most intense in the early hours after AMI; with increasing time after infarction the faster migrating forms become dominant. The same group showed that only the slow migrating MM subform, or MM3, is present in tissue. The faster migrating subforms, MM2 and MM1, are produced sequentially by a modification of MM3 after release into the blood. (Note that, like the three CK isoenzymes, the subisoenzymes can be designated by speed of electrophoretic migration toward the anode: MM3 and MB2 are the slow migrating forms, MM1 and MB1 the fast migrating forms, and MM2 is intermediate between MM3 and MM1. This convention has been a source of some confusion, inasmuch as the numeric designation is the reverse of the order of temporal appearance following AMI.) Finally, Wevers reproduced the conversion of MM3 to MM1 in vitro by incubating purified tissue MM3 with serum.[47] Similarly, conversion of MB2 to MB1 can be demonstrated in vitro.

In 1981, we isolated and purified the three MM subforms by chromatofocusing.[48] We also showed that the conversion reaction in the blood was mediated by the plasma enzyme carboxypeptidase-N (CP-N), and reproduced the conversion in vitro in the absence of serum by incubating purified tissue MM3 with CP-N.[49,50] The mechanism of MM3 modification was demonstrated to be via cleavage of the positively charged amino acid lysine from the carboxy terminal of the M subunit(s); the result is a polypeptide chain having a slightly greater net charge (by one unit) and, therefore, a faster rate of migration toward the positive electrode.[50,51] The conversion reaction has been shown to progress rapidly, both in vivo and in vitro.

Therefore, the sequential predominance of the three MM subforms can be explained as follows: cleavage of the terminal lysine from one of the two M polypeptides of MM3 by CP-N yields the heterodimer MM2; removal of the remaining terminal lysine for the second M-chain produces MM1 (Fig. 6–2). Preliminary work in our laboratory has indicated that a similar mechanism is involved in the conversion of MB2 to MB1.

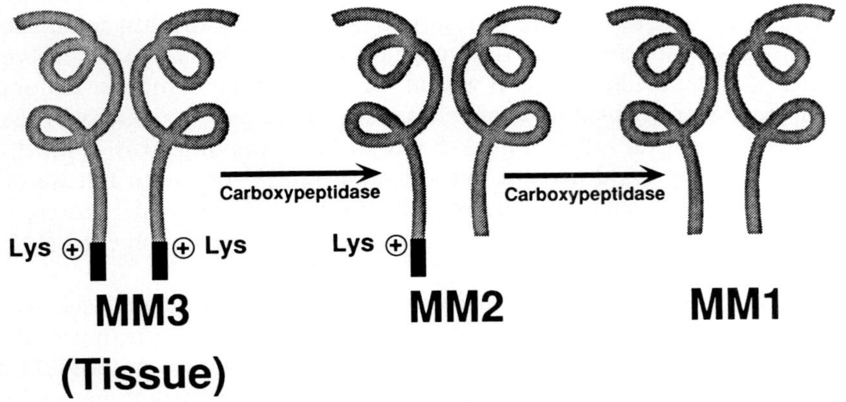

Figure 6–2. Schematic representation of the modification of MM3 CK after release from tissue, to the sequential forms MM2 and MM1. The same mechanism governs the conversion of the M chain of MB2 CK after release from the myocardium, so that MB1 is formed in the blood.

Early Diagnosis of AMI

Because thrombolytic therapy is most efficacious when administered within the first 4 hours, the decision to initiate treatment is, of necessity, based on symptoms and ECG findings, which are of low sensitivity and specificity.[52] Given the risk, albeit small, of severe hemorrhage accompanying thrombolysis, an early diagnostic marker with a low rate of false positives (i.e., a high specificity) would be a valuable aid in avoiding treatment of patients without AMI. The problem of diagnostic uncertainty in the early hours of AMI will be further compounded if the indications for thrombolysis are extended to include non-Q-wave infarction; in this setting, ECG changes are completely nonspecific.

CK subform analysis shows promise as an early indicator of AMI. At steady state in a normal individual, small amounts of MM CK (and MB CK from cardiac tissue) are continuously released into the blood, and then converted to the modified subforms. Inasmuch as the conversion reaction is rapid, the tissue form MM3 contributes only a relatively small percentage of the total MM CK isoenzyme activity (30 percent to 35 percent). With the onset of AMI, the rate of myocardial MM3 release quickly exceeds the rate of conversion of MM3 to MM2 and MM1, and MM3 as a percentage of total MM activity rises. Thus, rapid release of relatively small quantities of MM3 will be sufficient to raise the percent MM3 before the values for total CK activity is increased sufficiently to exceed the upper limit of normal. For example, if the MM CK activity in a patient at baseline is 60 IU per liter, with the upper limit of normal at 120 IU per liter, the baseline MM3 percent would approximate 20 IU per liter—33 percent of MM activity. An initial rapid release of MM3 CK early in AMI would raise the MM3 to 60 IU per liter but the total only to 100, a value within normal limits; however, the MM3 CK will now consitute 60 percent of MM CK activity. In effect, each patient's plasma MM activity serves as its own control, with perturbations in steady-state activity readily detectable as changes in subisoenzyme distribution even when CK activity is in the normal reference range.

Initial studies using this technique have been promising in animal studies[53] and were successful in detecting AMI 3.9 hours after the onset of symptoms in one study involving a small number of human subjects.[54] Unfortunately, assays for CK subforms are not applicable for clinical use. The methods employed in the above studies required 36 to 48 hours to obtain data. Currently available electrophoretic assays are more rapid, but are insufficiently sensitive to resolve MM subforms when total CK activity is within the normal range. Another major drawback for the use of MM subform analysis is the problem of specificity of the MM subforms. Use of total rather than MB CK to make the diagnosis of AMI introduces a 20 percent to 30 percent false-positive rate[43,55] owing to release of MM CK from noncardiac sources, usually skeletal muscle. Noncardiac sources of elevated total CK plasma activity are accompanied by a rise in percent MM3, thus reducing the specificity of this finding.[56–58]

Because of the lack of specificity of MM CK subform analysis, we have recently evaluated the use of MB CK subforms in the early diagnosis of AMI. Unlike previous systems used for subform separation, which required 1½ hours of electrophoresis at 90 volts for adequate resolution, the prototype instrument we tested (Rep, Helena Laboratories, Beaumont, TX) performs electrophoresis at 1800 volts on a dynamically cooled gel to separate the tissue subform, MB2, from the plasma-modified subform, MB1, in 5 minutes. We validated the system using purified MB2 and MB1 reconstituted in heat-inactivated serum. The assay is linear for both MB subforms even at very low levels (r = 0.99 between 2.5 and 10.0 IU per liter; n = 70, upper normal limit = 14 IU per liter), is highly reproducible, and generates the expected MB2/MB1 ratio when both subforms are present in serum (r = 0.95, n = 144). Sensitivity is 1.0 IU per liter; total assay time is 20 minutes.

MB subform assay was applied to 24 normal subjects and to 11 patients with AMI in whom an initial plasma sample, obtained within 3 hours of the onset of symptoms, was still within the normal range for MB CK (Fig. 6–3). The mean percentage of MB2 was 64.1 percent among the normal individuals and 81.4 percent among the early infarct patients. Eight of 11 patients with AMI had a percent MB2 greater than 80 percent; samples were positive as early as 1 hour after the onset of symptoms. In contrast, among the 24 normal individuals, only one had more than 80 percent of MB CK present as the MB2 subform. Thus, these preliminary data suggest that MB subform analysis is rapid and specific and provides early diagnosis in the first 3 hours of AMI.

CK subform analysis has also been shown to be of value in the noninvasive assessment of reperfusion success by ourselves[59] and others.[60]

The role of early diagnostic methods in conjunction with thrombolysis remains to be defined. As currently practiced, thrombolytic therapy is initiated in the emergency room after physician evaluation. An assay with a 15-minute "turnaround time" might allow for obtaining objective data prior to the initiation of therapy. An alternative protocol would be initiation of treatment in all patients with suspected AMI, with termination of drug infusion within minutes of initiating thrombolytic therapy in patients shown not to have AMI by MB subform analysis. The latter course would maximize the potential for myocardial salvage while awaiting subform results, and potentially limit the risk associated with a full course of thrombolytic therapy to a patient without AMI. A similar protocol could be employed if thrombolytic therapy were initiated by paramedics at the site of initial patient contact "in the field."

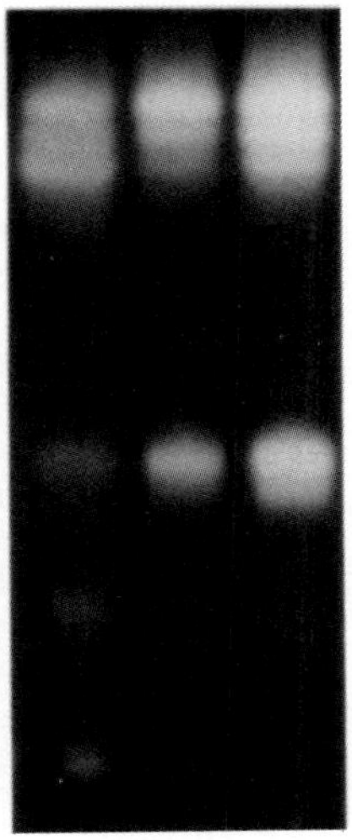

Figure 6–3. MM and MB subforms in the early hours of AMI. MM subforms are visible at the top and MB subforms in the center of each lane. *(Left Lane)* Two hours after AMI onset; total and MB CK activity are 85 and 6 IU per liter, respectively (upper normal = 120 and 14 IU per liter). MM3/MM1 ratio is normal. The faint MB band is exclusively MB2, indicating new release of MB from tissue. The faint bands visible below MB are albumin and BB CK. *(Center Lane)* Same patient, 6 hours after AMI onset; total and MB CK activity are 250 and 43 IU per liter. The MB2 band is now more prominent; no MB1 is yet visible. *(Right Lane)* 10 hours after AMI; total and MB CK 900 and 150 IU per liter (specimen diluted). MB1 band now present due to conversion of released MB2.

REFERENCES

1. LaDue, JS, Wroblewski, F, and Karmen, A: Serum glutamic oxaloacetic transaminase activity in human acute transmural myocardial infarction. Science 120:497, 1954.
2. Karmen, A, Wroblewski, F, and LaDue, J: Transaminase activity in human blood. J Clin Invest 34:126, 1954.
3. Ahmed, SA, Williamson, JR, Roberts, R, et al: The association of increaed plasma MB CPK activity and irreversible ischemic myocardial injury in the dog. Circulation 54:187, 1976.
4. Siegel, RJ, Said, JW, Shell, WE, et al: Identification and localization of creatine kinase B and M in normal, ischemic and necrotic myocardium. An immunohistochemical study. J Mol Cell Cardiol 16:95, 1984.
5. Roberts, R: Diagnostic assessment of myocardial infarction based on lactate dehydrogenase and creatine kinase isoenzymes. Heart Lung 10:486, 1981.
6. Michael, LH: Cardiac lymph: Monitor of myocardial membrane and vascular alterations. Life Sciences 29:1495, 1981.
7. Bessman, S and Carpenter, C: The creatine–creatine phosphate energy shuttle. Annu Rev Biochem 54:831, 1985.
8. Mahler, M: First-order kinetics of muscle oxygen consumption, and an equivalent proportionality between Qo_2 and phosphorylcreatine level. J Gen Physiol 86:135, 1985.
9. Roberts, R and Grace, AM: Purification of mitochondrial creatine kinase. J Biol Chem 255:2870, 1980.
10. Basson, CT, Grace, AM, and Roberts, R: Enzyme kinetics of a highly purified mitochondrial creatine kinase in comparison with cytosolic forms. Mol Cell Biochem 67:151, 1985.
11. Jacobus, WE and Lehninger, AL: Creatine kinase of rat heart mitochondria. J Biol Chem 248:4803, 1973.
12. Villareal-Levy, G, Ma, TS, Kerner, SA, et al: Human creatine kinase: Isolation and sequence analysis of cDNA clones for the B subunit, development of subunit specific probes and determination of gene copy number. Biochem Biophys Res Comm 144:1116, 1987.
13. Rosalki, SB: An improved procedure for creatine phosphokinase determination. J Lab Clin Med 69:696, 1967.
14. Lott, JA and Stang, JM: Serum enzymes and isoenzymes in the diagnosis and differential diagnosis of myocardial ischemia and necrosis. Clin Chem 26:1241, 1980.
15. Henry, PD, Roberts, R, and Sobel BE: Rapid separation of plasma creatine kinase isoenzymes by batch absorption on glass beads. Clin Chem 21:844, 1975.
16. Apple, FS, Greenspan, NS, and Dietzler, DN: Elevation of creatine kinase BB CK in hospitalized patients. Ann Clin Lab Sci 12:398, 1982.
17. Ritter, CS, Mumm, SR, and Roberts, R: Improved radioimmunoassay for creatine kinase isoenzymes in plasma. Clin Chem 27:1878, 1981.
18. Boone, DJ, Duncan, PH, MacNeil, ML, et al: Results of a nationwide survey of analyses for creatine kinase and creatine kinase isoenzymes. Clin Chem 30:33, 1984.
19. Lott, JA: Serum enzyme determinations in the diagnosis of acute myocardial infarction. Human Pathol 15:706, 1984.
20. Vaidya, HD, Maynard Y, Dietzler DN, et al: Direct measurement of creatine kinase MB activity in serum after extraction with a monoclonal antibody specific to the MB isoenzyme. Clin Chem 32:657, 1986.
21. Landt, Y, Vaidya, HC, Porter, SE, et al: Semi-automated direct colorimetric measurement of creatine kinase isoenzyme MB activity after extraction from serum by use of a CK MB-specific monoclonal antibody. Clin Chem 34:575, 1988.
22. Tsung, JS and Tsung, SS: Creatine kinase isoenzymes in extracts of various human skeletal muscles. Clin Chem 32:1568, 1986.
23. Siegel, AJ, Silverman, LM, and Evans, WJ: Elevated skeletal muscle creatine kinase MB isoenzyme levels in marathon runners. JAMA 250:2835, 1983.
24. Apple, FS, Rogers, MA, Sherman, WM, et al: Profile of creatine kinase isoenzymes in skeletal muscles of marathon runners. Clin Chem 30:413, 1984.
25. Keshgegian, AA and Feinberg, NV: Serum creatine kinase MB isoenzyme in chronic muscle disease. Clin Chem 30:575, 1984.
26. Shahanglan, S, Ash, OW, Wahlstrom, NO, et al: Creatine kinase and lactate dehydrogenase isoenzymes in serum of patients suffering burns, blunt trauma, or myocardial infarction. Clin Chem 30:1332, 1984.

27. McBride, JW, Labrosse, KR, McCoy, HG, et al: Is serum creatine kinase-MB in electrically injured patients predictive of myocardial injury? JAMA 255:764, 1986.
28. Somer, H, Dubowitz, V, and Donner, M: Creatine kinase isoenzymes in neuromuscular diseases. J Neurol Sci 29:129, 1976.
29. Tzvetanova, E: Creatine kinase isoenzymes in muscle tissue of patients with neuromuscular diseases and human fetuses. Enzyme 12:279, 1971.
30. Ingwall, JS, Kramer, MF, Fifer, MA, et al: The creatine kinase system in normal and diseased human myocardium. N Engl J Med 313:1050, 1985.
31. Marmor, A, Margolis, T, Alpan, G, et al: Regional distribution of the MB isoenzyme of creatine kinase in the human heart. Arch Pathol Lab Med 104:425, 1980.
32. Baraka, M, Deveaux, N, Frank, R, et al: Creatine kinase MB isoenzyme activity after endocardial catheter fulguration (abstr). Circulation 76:IV-174, 1987.
33. Yasmineh, WG, Pyle, RB, and Nicoloff, DM: Rate of decay and distribution volume of MB isoenzyme of creatine kinase, intravenously injected into the baboon. Clin Chem 22:1095, 1976.
34. Tsung, SH: Creatine kinase activity and isoenzyme pattern in various normal tissues and neoplasms. Clin Chem 29:2040, 1983.
35. Roberts, R: Recognition, pathogenesis, and management of non-Q wave infarction. Mod Concepts Cardiovasc Dis 56:17, 1987.
36. Lee, RH and Goldman, L: Serum enzyme assays in the diagnosis of acute myocardial infarction. Ann Intern Med 105:221, 1986.
37. Puleo, P: Unpublished data.
38. Jaffe, AS, Ritter, C, Meltzer, V, et al: Unmasking artifactual increases in creatine kinase isoenzymes in patients with renal failure. J Lab Clin Med 104:193, 1984.
39. Lang, H and Wurzburg, U: Creatine kinase, an enzyme of many forms. Clin Chem 28:1439, 1982.
40. Kaste, M, Somer, H, and Konttinen, A: Brain-type creatine kinase isoenzyme. Arch Neurol 34:142, 1977.
41. Goldman, J, Matz R, Montimer, R, et al: High elevations of creatine phosphokinase in hypothyroidism: An isoenzyme analysis. JAMA 238:325, 1977.
42. Roberts, R, Henry, PD, and Sobel, BE: An improved basis for enzymatic estimation of infarct size. Circulation 52:743, 1975.
43. Lee, TH, Weisberg, MC, Cook, EF, et al: Evaluation of creatine kinase and creatine kinase-MB for diagnosing myocardial infarction. Arch Intern Med 147:115, 1987.
44. Grenadier, E, Keidar, S, Kahana, L, et al: The roles of serum myoglobin, total CPK, and CK-MB isoenzyme in the acute phase of myocardial infarction. Am Heart J 105:408, 1983.
45. Nørregaard-Hansen, K, Petersen, PH, Hangaard, J, et al: Early observations of S-myoglobin in the diagnosis of acute myocardial infarction. The influence of discrimination limit, analytical quality, patient's sex and prevalence of disease. Scand J Clin Lab Invest 46:561, 1986.
46. Wevers, RA, Olthuis, HP, Van Neil, JCC, et al: A study on the dimeric structure of creatine kinase. Clin Chim Acta 75:377, 1977.
47. Wevers, RA, Delsing, M, Klein Gebbink, JAG, et al: Postsynthetic changes in creatine kinase isoenzymes. Clin Chem Acta 86:323, 1978.
48. Sims, HS, Ritter, CS, Fukayama, T, and Roberts, R: Characterization of the modification of creatine kinase following its release into plasma after infarction (abstr). Clin Res 29:242A, 1981.
49. George, S, Ishikawa, Y, and Roberts, R: Molecular basis for multiple forms of MM creatine kinase in plasma (abstr). Circulation 66:II-203, 1982.
50. George, S, Ishikawa, Y, Perryman, MB, et al: Purification and characterization of naturally occurring and in vitro induced multiple forms of MM creatine kinase. J Biol Chem 259:2667, 1984.
51. Perryman, MB, Knell, JD, and Roberts, R: Carboxypeptidase-catalyzed hydrolysis of C-terminal lysine: Mechanism for in vivo production of multiple forms of creatine kinase in plasma. Clin Chem 30:662, 1984.
52. Lee, TH, Gregory WR, Weisberg, MC, et al: Sensitivity of routine clinical criteria for diagnosing myocardial infarction within 24 hours of hospitalization. Ann Intern Med 106:181, 1987.
53. Hashimoto, H, Abendschein, DR, Strauss, AW, et al: Early detection of myocardial infarction in conscious dogs by analysis of plasma MM creatine kinase isoforms. Circulation 71:363, 1985.
54. Jaffe, AS, Serota, H, Grace, A, et al: Diagnostic changes in plasma creatine kinase isoforms early after the onset of acute myocardial infarction. Circulation 74:105, 1986.
55. Klein, MD, Shell, WE, and Sobel, BE: Serum creatine phosphokinase (CPK) isoenzymes after intramuscular injections, surgery, and myocardial infarction. Cardiovasc Res 7:412, 1973.

56. Annesley, TM, Strongwater, SL, and Schnitzer, TJ: MM subisoenzymes of creatine kinase as an index of disease activity in polymyositis. Clin Chem 31:402, 1985.
57. Apple, FS, Rogers, MA, and Ivy, JL: Creatine kinase isoenzyme MM variants in skeletal muscle and plasma from marathon runners. Clin Chem 32:41, 1986.
58. Clarkson, PM, Apple, FS, Byrnes, WC, et al: Creatine kinase isoforms following isometric exercise. Muscle Nerve 10:41, 1987.
59. Puleo, PR, Perryman, MB, Bresser, MA, et al: Creatine kinase isoform analysis in the detection and assessment of thrombolysis in man. Circulation 75:1162, 1987.
60. Tsukamoto, H, Hashimoto, H, Matsui, Y, et al: Detection of myocardial reperfusion by analysis of serum creatine kinase isoforms. Clin Cardiol 11:287, 1988.

CHAPTER 7

Radionuclide Diagnosis and Assessment of Acute Myocardial Infarction

Robert S. Gibson, M.D.

Radionuclide imaging procedures have been widely employed in the assessment of patients with acute myocardial infarction. In the acute phase, they may be used to identify, localize, and estimate the amount of myocardial necrosis. Radionuclide methods may also be used to evaluate myocardial perfusion, tissue metabolism and viability, and to determine the impact of infarction on both global and regional ventricular performance. At a later convalescent phase, radionuclide assessment provides valuable information concerning the degree of myocardial functional reserve and the presence and extent of stress-induced ischemia.

Because of advances in nuclear imaging techniques and the development of new radiotracers, it is appropriate to review currently or soon-to-be-available radionuclide methods that offer promise for providing diagnostic, prognostic, and pathophysiologic information in patients with acute myocardial infarction.

DETECTION OF ACUTE MYOCARDIAL INFARCTION WITH INFARCT-AVID IMAGING

Infarct-avid myocardial imaging refers to the accumulation of a radiopharmaceutical within a region of irreversibly damaged myocardium, allowing its visualization as a "hot spot" or positive area of increased uptake. Presently, the most commonly used imaging agent for detection of infarction is technetium-99m stannous pyrophosphate (^{99m}Tc PPi). Other infarct-avid imaging agents, which are promising but only in the preliminary stages of clinical investigation, include technetium- or indium-labeled antimyosin antibody.

Planar Imaging With ^{99m}Tc PPi

Since the pioneering work of Bonte and coworkers in 1974,[1] many studies have examined the ability of ^{99m}Tc PPi to identify acute myocardial infarction in

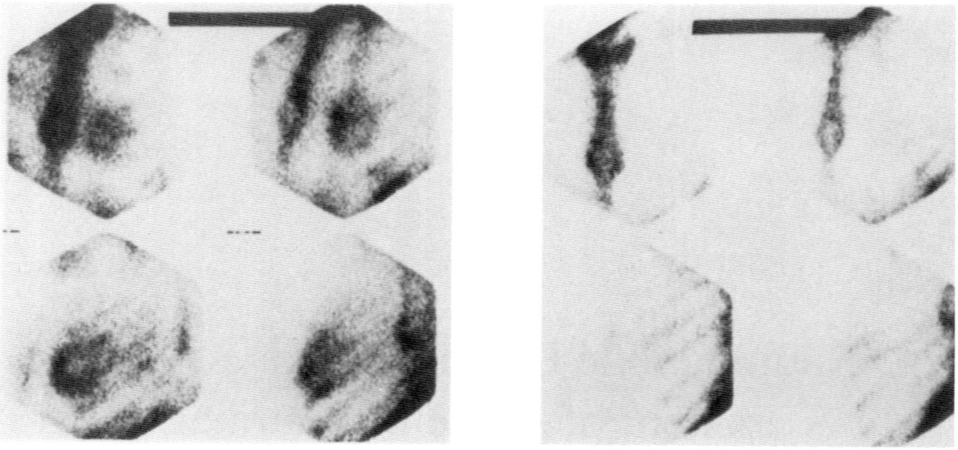

Figure 7–1. *(Left Panel)* Positive ^{99m}Tc PPi myocardial scintigram from a patient with anterolateral myocardial infarction showing abnormal radionuclide uptake in the anterior *(top left)*, 35-degree LAO *(top right)*, 70-degree LAO *(bottom left)*, and left lateral *(bottom right)* views. *(Right Panel)* For comparison, negative ^{99m}Tc PPi myocardial scintigram is shown in the same views. (From Willerson JT: How reliable is myocardial imaging in the diagnosis of acute myocardial infarction? In Rahimtoola, SH (ed): Controversies in Coronary Artery Disease. Cardiovascular Clinics 13/1, FA Davis, Philadelphia, 1983, p. 35, with permission.)

the clinical circumstance.[2–15] Data from these studies showed: (1) that ^{99m}Tc PPi scintiscans do not become positive until 24 to 48 hours after onset of infarction and have their maximal yield at 72 hours; (2) that discrete (as opposed to diffuse) myocardial uptake of ^{99m}Tc PPi is a relatively specific marker of acute necrosis (Fig. 7–1); and (3) that radiopharmaceutical accumulation, detected by an external gamma scintillation camera and planar imaging techniques, is dependent on, among other factors, the presence of a certain minimal amount of necrosis. In studies of patients with isoenzyme-confirmed acute myocardial infarction, ^{99m}Tc PPi has been found to be moderately sensitive in detecting transmural myocardial injury (i.e., Q-wave infarcts). However, as Table 7–1 illustrates, the sensitivity of ^{99m}Tc PPi imaging is suboptimal for clinical use in the diagnosis of non-Q-wave infarcts. When data from the 14 published studies are pooled, one finds that only 42 percent of patients with validated acute non-Q-wave myocardial infarctions had positive scans. In view of this collective, multi-institutional experience, it appears that two conclusions can be drawn: (1) the amount of ^{99m}Tc PPi accumulation in non-Q-wave infarcts is too small to be detected by conventional planar imaging techniques; and (2) planar ^{99m}Tc PPi myocardial scintigraphy offers little, if any, additional diagnostic information beyond that obtained from routine clinical evaluation and enzymatic studies of patients in the coronary care unit.[16]

SPECT Imaging With ^{99m}Tc PPi

The introduction of commercially available camera systems that permit tomographic imaging has rekindled interest in using ^{99m}Tc PPi for the detection and sizing of acute myocardial infarction. This is because tomographic slices of radio-

Table 7–1. Sensitivity of Planar Imaging with ^{99m}Tc PPi in Patients with Q-Wave and Non-Q-Wave Myocardial Infarction

Study	No. of Patients	Sensitivity* All Infarcts (%)	Q-Wave (%)	Non-Q-Wave (%)
Parkey et al[2]	15	87	87	
Willerson et al[3]	17	35		35
McLaughlin et al[4]	17	71	83	40
Cowley et al[5]	69	86	95	46
Berman et al[6]	99	84	94	39
Ahmad et al[7]	48	60	94	0
Henning et al[8]	35	86	90	50
Holman et al[9]	15	73	64	100†
Massie et al[10]	74	62	84	32
Codini et al[11]	134	68	78	41
Rude et al[12]	67	85	89	69
Lyons et al[13]	350	67	82	44
Olson et al[14]	107	63	80	39
Corbett et al[15]	36	69	88	53
Pooled data	1083	70	85	42

*Positive ^{99m}Tc PPi scan defined as discrete, localizable uptake with myocardial activity greater than or equal to costal activity.

†Scanning performed 4 to 8 hours after onset of symptoms.

pharmaceutical distribution in the heart provide three-dimensional information that effectively separates overlying and underlying radioactivity (e.g., in the chest wall, bone, cartilage, breast, and blood pool) and increases relative contrast between adjacent structures (i.e., enhances anatomic resolution and permits more precise localization of abnormal tracer uptake in a specific left ventricular region). Recently, Corbett and associates[15] from Dallas reported their experience with single-photon emission computed tomography (SPECT) in 19 patients with small subendocardial infarcts (mean peak CK 398 $\pm$ 268 IU/L). Comparative sensitivities were 95 percent by SPECT versus 63 percent by planar imaging ($p < 0.05$). Furthermore, this same group of investigators showed that SPECT imaging with ^{99m}Tc PPi can accurately estimate myocardial infarct size.[17,18]

Antimyosin Antibody Imaging

An alternative to ^{99m}Tc PPi myocardial scintigraphy for detection of infarction is utilization of radiolabeled antimyosin antibodies. Haber and associates[19] in Boston have developed monoclonal antibodies specific against myosin that enter dying myocardial cells and bind to myosin in the interior of these cells. These investigators, and others, have also shown that visualization, localization, and sizing of experimental infarction by external gamma scintiscanning is possible with antimyosin antibodies labeled with iodine, indium, and, more recently, technetium-99m.[19–23]

Extensive clinical studies of patients with routine infarcts or those who have undergone reperfusion have not yet been published with this imaging approach. Reports from two groups[24,25] in small selected patient samples are encouraging, but further work will be necessary before determining what advantages antimyosin antibody imaging has over ^{99m}Tc PPi imaging in the clinical setting. Also, it remains to be established whether serial imaging using the antimyosin antibody approach will be safe and feasible.

Indications for Infarct-Avid Myocardial Scintigraphy

When it is not clear from the history, serial ECGs, and cardiac enzyme studies that myocardial infarction has occurred, ^{99m}Tc PPi or possibly antimyosin antibody imaging with SPECT may be helpful in identifying and/or localizing new infarction. Patients with left bundle branch block, those who delay their hospital admission by more than 24 hours, and patients undergoing open heart surgery with suspected perioperative myocardial infarction[26–29] are potentially good candidates for infarct-avid scintigraphy.

Recently, ^{99m}Tc PPi has been used as a means to predict successful reperfusion in patients given thrombolytic agents.[30–32] In the absence of reperfusion, ^{99m}Tc PPi does not begin to accumulate in necrotic myocardium for at least 12 to 24 hours after onset of symptoms. Early restitution of nutritive blood flow appears to accelerate this process. In clinical studies of patients with Q-wave infarcts who were treated with intracoronary or intravenous thrombolytic agents, abnormal regional ^{99m}Tc PPi uptake has been detected in the zone of infarction at a time when ^{99m}Tc PPi would not have been detectable ordinarily. Patients with early positive ^{99m}Tc PPi scintiscans, compared with those with little or no accumulation of the tracer, show early peaking of serum creatine kinase isoenzyme levels, angiographically patent infarct vessels, and improvement in serial measures of global left ventricular function. Although these results are fascinating, it is still not clear that ^{99m}Tc PPi imaging will facilitate determination of whether tissue has been salvaged or whether blood flow has been restored to myocardium already irreversibly injured.[33,34]

PERFUSION IMAGING WITH SINGLE-PHOTON-EMITTING TRACERS

Thallium-201 Myocardial Imaging

The physiologic principles that determine myocardial uptake of thallium-201 (^{201}TL) are quite different than those of ^{99m}Tc PPi and other infarct-avid imaging agents. Whereas ^{99m}Tc PPi accumulates primarily in irreversibly injured myocardium, ^{201} TL is taken up by normal myocardial cells in proportion to regional blood flow.[35] The relative absence of ^{201}TL uptake (Fig. 7–2) in a region of myocardium during the very early phase of acute infarction indicates the presence of either acute necrosis, scar formation from previous infarction, or an area of ischemia that has not yet progressed to necrosis. Although ischemia can usually be differentiated from irreversible damage by comparing early with 3-hour rest images,[35,36] thallium scintigraphy cannot distinguish acute infarction from old myocardial scar. Because of this, perfusion imaging with ^{201}TL is of limited value in the early diagnosis of acute myocardial infarction.

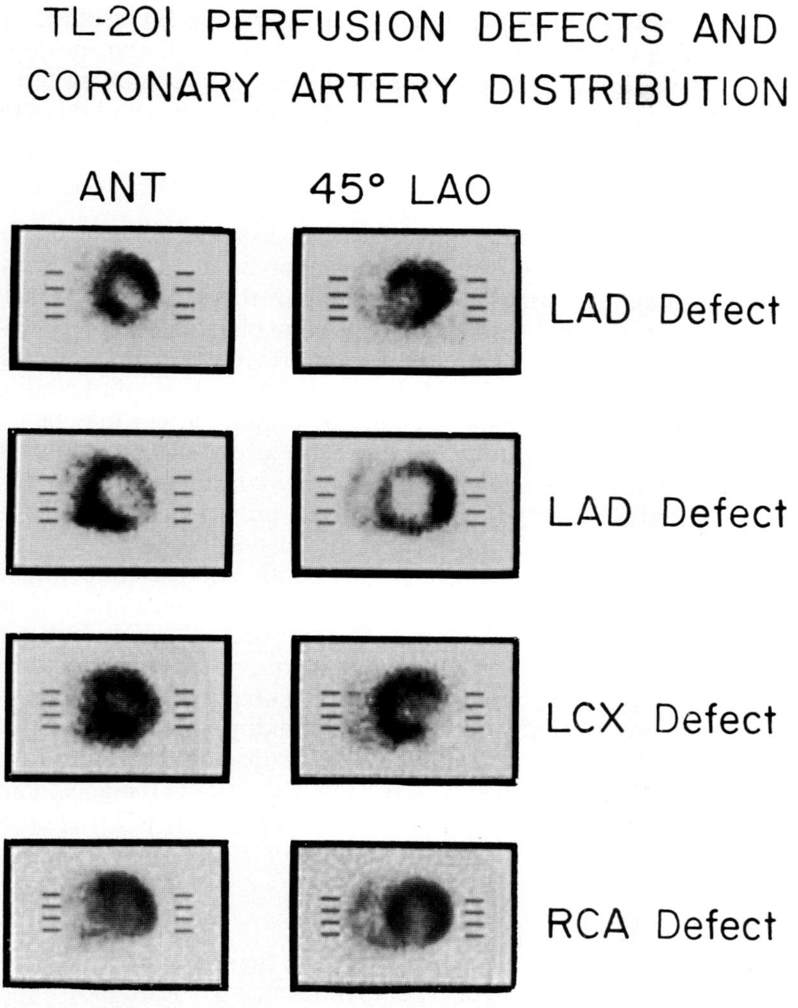

Figure 7–2. Anterior *(left)* and 45-degree LAO thallium-201 images *(right)* from four patients with perfusion defects involving myocardium subtended by the left anterior descending (LAD) artery, the left circumflex (LCx) artery, and the right coronary artery (RCA). Note the difference in defect size between a mid-LAD lesion *(top panel)* and a proximal LAD lesion *(second panel)*. (From Gibson and Watson,[35] with permission.)

In clinical studies of routine acute myocardial infarction, it has been reported that virtually all patients, including those with non-Q-wave infarcts, show ^{201}TL perfusion defects at rest if imaging is performed within 6 hours of the onset of symptoms.[37–42] With increase in time from onset of infarction, the sensitivity for detecting resting perfusion defects is diminished. This seems especially true in cases of non-Q-wave infarcts; in the series of Wackers and colleagues,[38] the sensitivity for detecting perfusion abnormablities at rest was 100 percent if imaging was carried out within 6 hours but only 52 percent if performed 24 hours or more after symptom onset. This tendency for ^{201}TL defects to decrease in size or disappear altogether over time suggests that: (1) peri-infarction ischemia contributes significantly to the size of the initial perfusion defect; and (2) resolution of ischemia, possibly as a result of improved collateral flow or spontaneous reopening of the infarct vessel, is largely responsible for the sometimes-found negative scans when rest imaging is performed late (i.e., ≥24 hours) after onset of infarction.[42–44]

Assessment of Coronary Thrombolysis with ^{201}TL Imaging

Myocardial perfusion scintigraphy with ^{201} TL has been advocated as a means of evaluating acutely the effectiveness of thrombolytic therapy. At present, however, there is a major question as to the ability of this technique to distinguish between changes in regional blood flow per se and changes caused by salvage of viable but jeopardized myocardium. In a recent review by Zaret and Wackers,[45] it was pointed out that improved ^{201}TL uptake during early postintervention scintigraphy in a region supplied by a recanalized coronary artery may be primarily a function of augmented flow despite the presence of significant necrosis and loss of myocardial viability. Because of this and other considerations (Table 7–2), it seems unlikely that ^{201}TL scintigraphy will play a prominent role in the immediate post-treatment assessment of reperfusion-related salvage.

Despite significant problems with preintervention and early postintervention imaging, ^{201}TL scintigraphy may still provide valuable information, if used at a time removed from the immediate reperfusion event. Clinical studies of post-thrombolytic patients have demonstrated that improvement in defect size on serial rest images predicts improvement in regional ventricular function and patency of the infarct-related vessel.[45–49] These findings, coupled with the observation that successfully reperfused patients have substantial amounts of exercise-induced peri-infarction ischemia,[49,50] suggest that additional therapeutic interventions (i.e., percutaneous transluminal coronary angioplasty [PTCA] or coronary bypass surgery) may be appropriate.

Table 7–2. Potential Limitations of Resting ^{201}TL Scintigraphy for Assessing Efficacy of Thrombolytic Therapy in Acute Myocardial Infarction

Practical Considerations

1. Acquisition of baseline (preintervention) imaging data interferes with initiation of time-dependent treatment regimen.
2. Long half-life of ^{201}TL (73 hours) precludes serial studies of myocardial perfusion.
3. Low energy of ^{201}TL (60–80 KeV) renders planar and even SPECT images highly vulnerable to external and self attenuation.
4. Quantitation of regional myocardial blood flow in ml/min/g of myocardium is not possible because of difficulties in correcting for attenuation.

Pathophysiologic Considerations in the Acute Reperfusion Phase

1. Early postintervention scintiscans may overestimate extent of myocardial salvage.
   - Animal studies indicate that pathologically defined infarct zones may have regional ^{201}TL activity as high as 50% of normal.
2. Smaller perfusion defect at rest after thrombolytic therapy may not represent myocardial salvage resulting from treatment-related reperfusion.
   - Size of ^{201}TL defect in patients receiving conventional treatment tends to decrease over time, possibly as a result of improved collateral flow or spontaneous reopening of infarct vessel.

PREDISCHARGE STRESS ^{201}TL IMAGING

Exercise myocardial perfusion scintigraphy with ^{201}TL has been used 3 to 10 days after onset of infarction for risk stratification and detection of residual ischemia.[51,52] Data from studies of patients not undergoing thrombolytic therapy indicate that: (1) ^{201}TL scintigraphy is more sensitive and specific in detecting ischemia than exercise testing alone[53–58]; (2) unlike stress electrocardiography, ^{201}TL scintigraphy can localize ischemia to a particular area or areas of myocardium subtended by a specific coronary artery[35]; and (3) ^{201}TL scintigraphy, compared with either angiographic anatomy or conventional exercise testing, is more reliable in risk stratification of postinfarction patients.[54,58,59] The more optimal prognostic efficiency of ^{201}TL scintigraphy is due, in part, to the fact that the error rate in falsely classifying patients as low risk is substantially and significantly smaller with ^{201}TL scintigraphy than with exercise testing or coronary arteriography.

Figure 7–3 illustrates the ability of quantitative ^{201}TL scintigraphy to detect prognostically important residual ischemia in patients recovering from acute uncomplicated myocardial infarction. Among 132 consecutive patients with negative submaximal exercise test responses (i.e., no angina or ST segment depression), ^{201}TL perfusion scintigraphy identified significant, albeit silent, ischemia in 72 (55 percent). As Figure 7–3 shows, the probability of survival without reinfarction during long-term followup was substantially lower in the 72 patients with ischemia versus the 60 without ischemia.

Until recently, most physicians have assumed that exercise-induced ST segment depression is a highly specific marker of residual ischemia in patients recovering from acute infarction. Although generally true for patients experiencing angina in conjunction with ST segment depression, this conclusion no longer seems appropriate for those who have ST segment depression alone. In our expe-

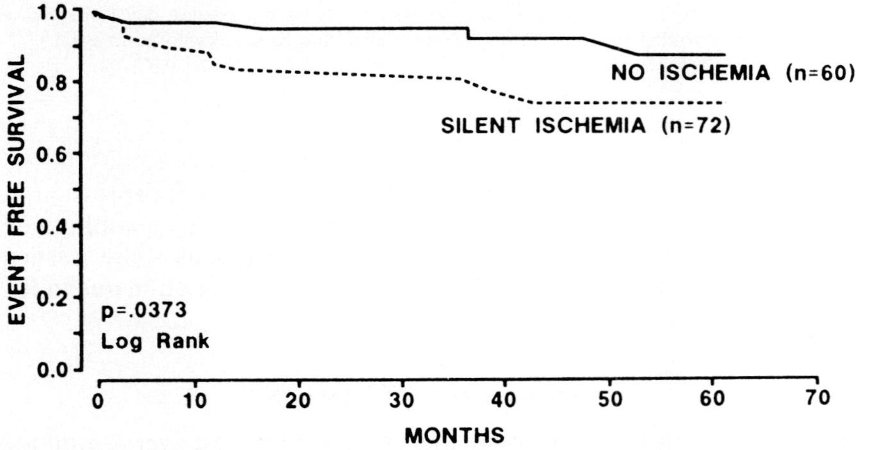

Figure 7–3. Kaplan-Meier survival curves for patients with no ischemia *(solid line)* and patients with ischemia *(broken line)* by exercise ^{201}TL scintigraphy. All 132 patients had negative submaximal exercise stress tests (target heart rate 120 bpm or workload 5 METs) 10 ± 3 days after onset of acute myocardial infarction. During long-term followup, the survival rate without reinfarction was significantly lower in patients with ischemia by ^{201}TL criteria ($p = 0.0373$ [log rank]). (From Gibson,[58] with permission.)

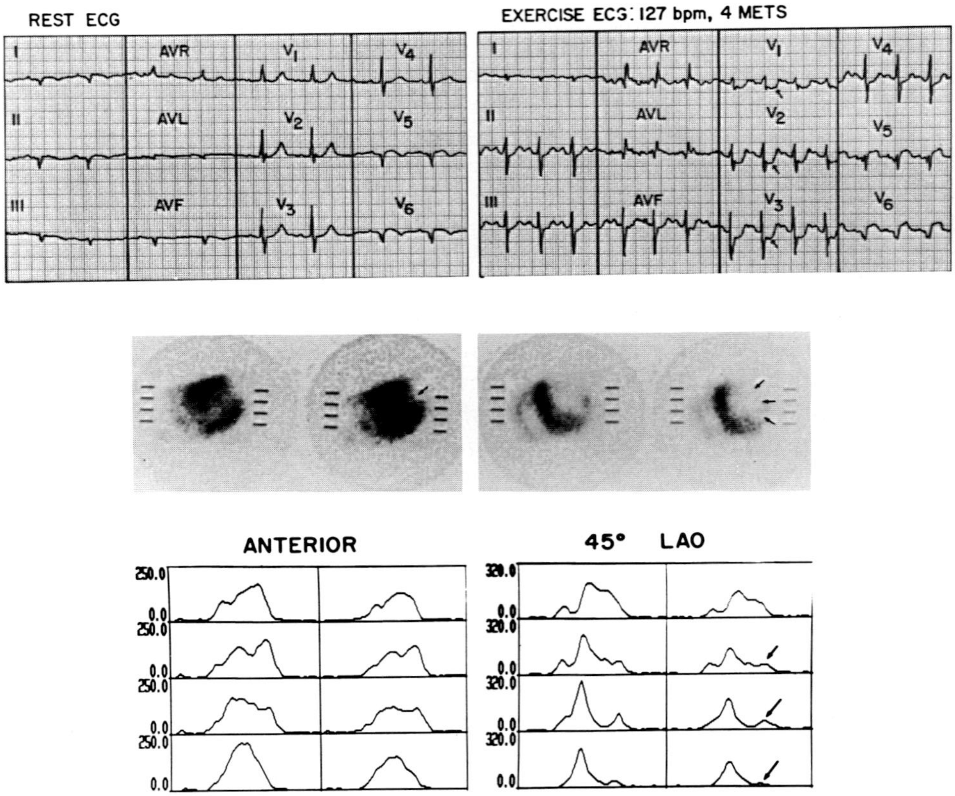

Figure 7–4. Rest and exercise ECG tracings *(top)* and ^{201}TL scintigram *(middle)* from a patient with inferoposterolateral Q-wave infarction owing to occlusion of the circumflex coronary artery. During submaximal exercise, painless ST segment depression in leads V_{1-4} occurred. The ^{201}TL scintigrams and corresponding time-activity curves *(bottom)* at 10 minutes *(left image of each pair)* and 2 hours after exercise *(right image of each pair)* shows an extensive persistent defect *(arrow)* without redistribution, compatible with scar. (From Gibson, Beller, and Kaiser,[56] with permission.)

rience, a sizable fraction of patients with painless ST segment depression during predischarge exercise testing show no evidence of ischemia by quantitative ^{201}TL criteria.[56] These false-positive electrocardiographic responses are particularly common among patients with moderately large Q wave infarction due to RCA or left circumflex occlusion (Fig. 7–4).

Dipyridamole ^{201}TL Imaging

Intravenous infusion of dipyridamole (i.e., 0.56 mg/kg over 4 minutes) has been suggested as an alternative to exercise for myocardial perfusion imaging with ^{201}TL. The powerful coronary vasodilating effects of dipyridamole increase regional blood flow in areas perfused by normal coronary vessels, but not in zones supplied by stenotic arteries. The resultant inhomogeneity of blood flow is detected by an abnormal ^{201}TL uptake pattern when the radiotracer is administered at peak vasodilatory effect. Because this pharmacologic approach to inducing myocardial ischemia may be comparable in efficacy to exercise stress, it should be considered in postinfarction patients who have claudication or orthopedic conditions preventing adequate exercise performance. In one study,[57] dipyridamole ^{201}TL scintigraphy before hospital discharge was found useful in predicting future prognosis, inasmuch as patients with reversible ^{201}TL perfusion defects had a significantly higher 1-year cardiac event rate (mortality and reinfarction) compared with patients showing a normal ^{201}TL uptake and washout pattern or merely a persistent defect. In agreement with other reports, this study also showed that ^{201}TL perfusion imaging was more sensitive than exercise testing for identifying high-risk postinfarction patients.

Qualitative Versus Quantitative ^{201}TL Scintigraphy

There is little doubt that the major clinical use of ^{201}TL scintigraphy is with exercise testing, or after maximal physiologic effect from intravenous dipyridamole, for purposes of identifying prognostic important residual ischemia. However, for stress-redistribution ^{201}TL scintigraphy to provide meaningful information, studies must be obtained with state-of-the-art, computer-assisted methods for quantitative analysis.

There are at least three important advantages in quantifying regional myocardial uptake and washout of ^{201}TL.[35,52] First, quantitative data analysis reduces reliance on visual interpretation (i.e., subjective analysis) and can be used to develop objective numerical standards. This, in turn, allows more accurate separation of normal and abnormal studies. Because interobserver and intraobserver variability is less when numerical standards are used, reproducibility is improved. Second, quantitative scintigraphic analysis enhances disease detection in individual coronary arteries and results in more optimal recognition of left mainstem or multivessel CAD. Lastly, by measuring ^{201}TL uptake on the initial set of postexercise images and characterizing washout kinetics from late images, quantitative scintigraphy offers the potential of more precisely estimating total ischemic burden, and for distinguishing scar from hypoperfused but still viable myocardium.

Technetium-99m Labeled Isonitriles

A new class of radiopharmaceuticals, the ^{99m}Tc-isonitriles, have shown considerable promise for routine use as myocardial perfusion imaging agents.[60,61] Such agents, when labeled with ^{99m}Tc, offer several potential advantages over ^{201}TL including: (1) lower radioisotope cost; (2) reduced radiation burden to the patient; and, most importantly, (3) more suitable photon energies for tomographic imaging with SPECT.

Unlike ^{201}TL, clearance of ^{99m}Tc-MIBI (^{99m}Tc-hexakis-2-methoxy-2-methylpropyl-isonitrile) from the myocardium in the initial few hours after injection is insignificant and there is no measurable redistribution into ischemic myocardium[62] (Fig. 7–5). This lack of redistribution over time represents a major difference when compared with ^{201}TL and suggests the potential for using ^{99m}Tc-MIBI for assessing reperfusion-related myocardial salvage. Although extensive clinical studies have not yet been performed, it seems possible to inject ^{99m}Tc-MIBI at the

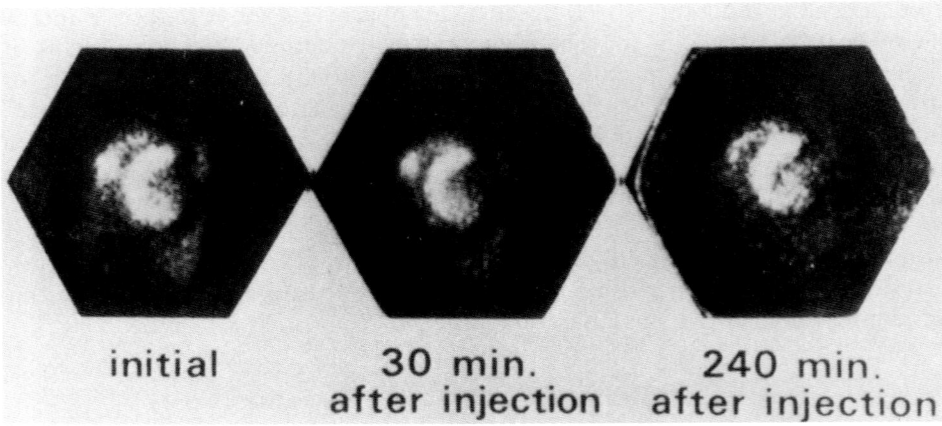

Figure 7–5. Myocardial gamma camera images from a dog with a left circumflex coronary artery stenosis. An initial posterior defect is readily apparent and persists for 4 hours. There is no evidence of redistribution. (From Okada, et al,[62] with permission.)

time of initiating of thrombolytic therapy but to image 2 to 3 hours later when the patient is already in the coronary care unit. Thus, as suggested by Zaret and Wackers,[45] imaging of the short-term flow deficit (i.e., risk zone) could be obtained without interfering with the time-dependent treatment regimen. A followup comparative imaging study, using a second injection at rest, could then be obtained several days later.

CLINICAL USES OF RADIONUCLIDE VENTRICULOGRAPHY

Either equilibrium or first-pass radionuclide ventriculography may be used to determine the functional impact of acute myocardial infarction on left and right ventricular ejection fraction, and regional wall motion. These assessments may be made relatively acutely after hospital admission and serially throughout the hospitalization. The initial measurements aid in the proper functional classification of patients and often identify a more severe degree of functional impairment than does clinical classification alone. Serial measurements of left ventricular performance may be used to document the effect of reperfusion-related salvage in a particular patient.[45] Furthermore, valvular regurgitation on one side of the heart may be identified, and left-to-right shunts (including ventricular septal defects developing acutely) can be detected and their size estimated. Thus, radionuclide ventriculograms may be used to identify alterations in global or segmental ventricular function occurring as a consequence of acute myocardial infarction. Although the general impact of acute myocardial infarction on ventricular function may be determined, these techniques do not allow one to distinguish old from new infarction or even myocardial ischemia from infarction. Thus, the information provided by radionuclide ventriculography should be viewed as complementary to that obtained with infarct-avid and myocardial perfusion assessments.

Radionuclide ventriculography at rest or with exercise may also be used at the time of hospital discharge to predict prognosis.[63–66] Patients demonstrating reductions in their left ventricular ejection fraction and/or increases in their end-systolic volumes at low levels of exercise have a higher risk of death, new myocardial infarction, unstable angina, and heart failure in the subsequent year.

POSITRON EMISSION TOMOGRAPHY

Historically, positron emission tomography (PET) of the heart has been a complicated, expensive imaging technology. Although its use and clinical application remain limited to a few major medical centers, PET clearly offers a new dimension to tissue characterization in normal and pathologic conditions. By combining quantitative tomographic imaging techniques with positron-emitting radiotracers of myocardial blood flow and tissue metabolism (Table 7–3), it is possible to obtain estimates of myocardial fuel uptake and utilization, thereby allowing identification of ischemically injured but viable myocardium. In this section, the principles of positron imaging and its application in patients with acute myocardial infarction will be discussed briefly.

PHYSICS OF POSITRON-EMITTING RADIOTRACERS

The fundamental physical property that makes positron-emitting radionuclides attractive for cardiac imaging is the annihilation radiation that results following emission of a positron. Positrons can be thought of as subatomic particles with the mass of an electron and a positive charge that are emitted with radionuclide decay. These particles travel only a short distance in biologic tissue (e.g., 1 to 2 mm) before encountering an electron. When a positron and electron interact, they both annihilate and the mass of each particle is transformed into energy in the form of two high-energy (511 KeV) gamma photons that travel in almost exactly opposite directions outward from the site of their production. This unique

Table 7–3. Commonly Used Positron Emitters for In-Vivo Cardiac PET Imaging of Myocardial Blood Flow and Tissue Metabolism

Isotope	Half-Life (Minutes)	Method of Production	Labeled Compound	Use
Nitrogen-13	10	Cyclotron	^{13}N ammonia ^{13}N glutamine	Perfusion Amino-acid metabolism
Oxygen-15	2	Cyclotron	^{15}O water	Perfusion
Carbon-11	20	Cyclotron	^{11}C palmitate ^{11}C pyruvate, glucose, acetate	Fatty-acid metabolism Carbohydrate metabolism
Flourine-18	108	Cyclotron	^{18}F 2-deoxyglucose	Carbohydrate metabolism
Rubidium-82	1.25	Generator	^{82}Rb Chloride	Perfusion

180-degree angular orientation of the annihilation photons permits electronic collimation by coincidence counting using one or more pairs of external radiation detectors aligned 180 degrees apart. Only counts that impinge on both detectors at virtually the same time are registered as true counts. Scintillation data collected in this manner can then be used to reconstruct mathematically the cross-sectional tissue concentration of the radiolabeled compound. Because the 511-KeV photons generated by positron annihilation are substantially more energetic than those of ^{201}TL (60 to 80 KeV) or ^{99m}Tc (140 KeV), attention correction is not a problem with positron-emitting radioisotopes.

All of the commonly used positron-emitting radioisotopes have short half-lives (see Table 7–3) and can be given repeatedly in relatively large quantities, yielding high count rates with minimal patient radiation burden.[67] A cyclotron, however, is usually necessary for their production and, because of their short half-lives, these facilities must be available at the imaging site. Because an on-site cyclotron currently costs from 1 to 2 million dollars, not including the cost of a dedicated PET camera, financial considerations presently limit the widespread availability of this technology. Possibly, the development of "baby" cyclotrons linked with automated chemical synthesizers may reduce cost and personnel requirements, enabling use of these unique radiotracers to become more widespread.

Clinical Applications of Cardiac PET

Results from several centers have demonstrated that PET provides unique information in patients with acute myocardial infarction.[68–71] These studies strongly suggest that the combined evaluation of regional blood flow and glucose utilization provides an accurate noninvasive determination of compromised but metabolically active myocardium, thereby allowing the differentiation of viable, potentially salvageable myocardium within an ischemic zone from irreversibly injured tissue. Such information is particularly useful in patients with major myocardial asynergy at rest.

Schelbert and colleagues[60,68,72] have demonstrated the ability of PET to identify metabolically active but ischemic tissue by demonstrating increased F-18 deoxyglucose (FDG) uptake in regions of diminished N-13 ammonia uptake in dogs (i.e., a metabolic/flow mismatch), and have subsequently shown the ability of this approach to detect reversible ischemic injury in patients (Fig. 7–6). More recently, this same group has demonstrated the presence of residual tissue viability in myocardial segments with markedly impaired contractility,[71] in electrocardiographic Q wave regions,[73] and in myocardial segments with fixed ^{201}TL perfusion defects,[74] using the FDG/N-13 ammonia PET technique. These observations, coupled with the finding that "PET viable" ischemic myocardium functionally benefits from therapeutic revascularization,[75] suggests that PET may identify acute infarct patients who are candidates for aggressive therapy to salvage endangered myocardium.

SUMMARY

The information presented in this review illustrates the different and potentially important clinical data that are obtainable from currently or soon-to-be-

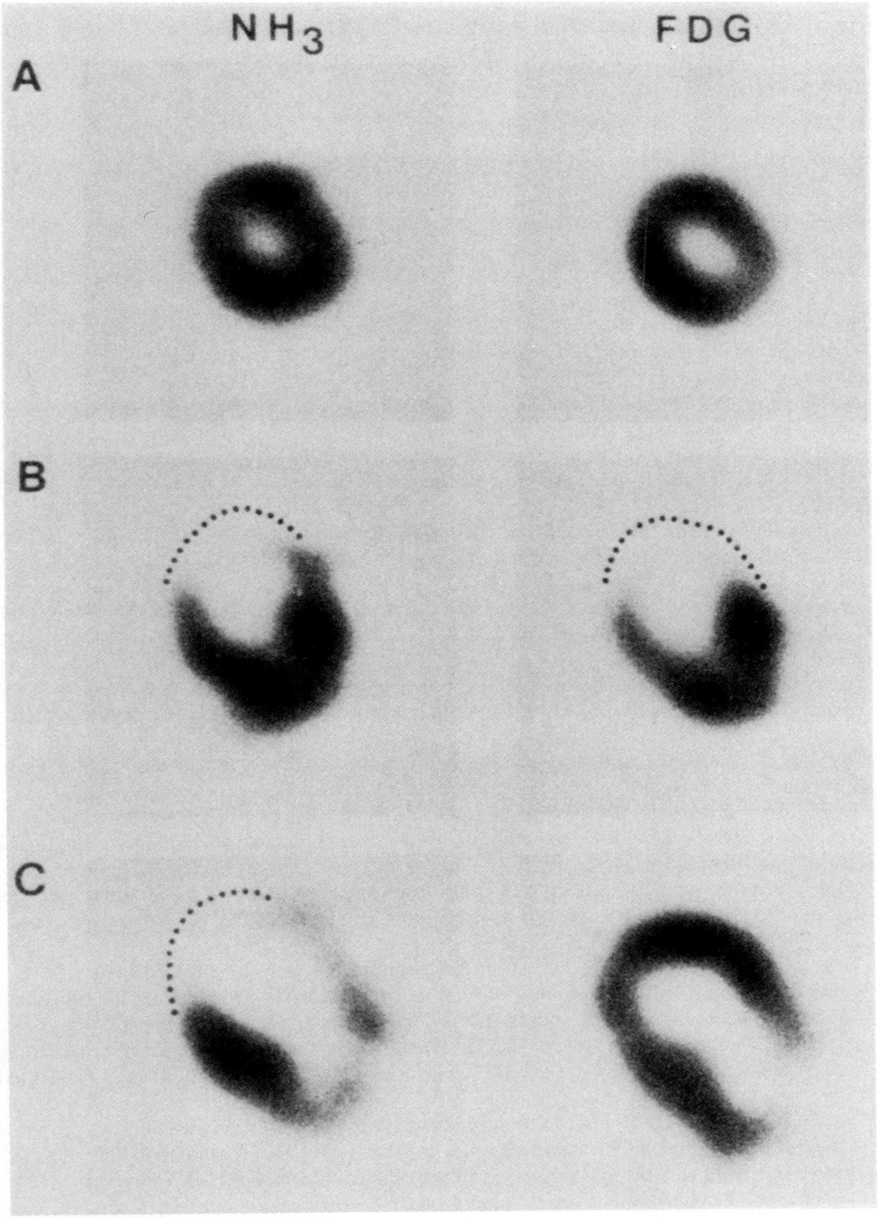

Figure 7–6. Regional myocardial blood flow and glucose utilization in a normal volunteer (*A*) and two patients with ischemic heart disease (*B* and *C*), evaluated with PET and N-13 ammonia (NH_3) and F-18 2 deoxyglucose (FDG), respectively. Only one mid-ventricular cross-sectional image per subject is shown. Note the homogeneous uptake of both tracers in the normal volunteer. In patient B, blood flow is decreased in the anterior wall *(broken line),* and this flow deficit is associated with a matched reduction in FDG uptake. This pattern reflects scar tissue. By comparison, in patient C, blood flow is decreased, while glucose utilization in the hypoperfused segment is markedly enhanced, reflecting tissue viability. (From Schelbert,[60] with permission.)

available radionuclide imaging procedures. Each modality has unavoidable intrinsic limitations. Nevertheless, in concert they have been useful in the clinical assessment of patients in the acute or convalescent phase of myocardial infarction.

REFERENCES

1. Bonte, FJ, Parkey, RW, Graham, KD, et al: A new method for radionuclide imaging of myocardial infarcts. Radiology 110:473, 1974.
2. Parkey, RW, Bonte, FJ, Meyer, SL, et al: A new method for radionuclide imaging of acute infarction in humans. Circulation 50:540, 1974.
3. Willerson, JT, Parkey, RW, Bonte, FJ, et al: Acute subendocardial myocardial in patients: Its detection by technetium 99-m stannous pyrophosphate myocardial scintigrams. Circulation 51:436, 1975.
4. McLaughlin, P, Coates, G, Wood, D, et al: Detection of acute myocardial infarction by technetium-99m pyrophosphate. Am J Cardiol 35:390, 1975.
5. Cowley, MJ, Mantle, JA, Rogers, WJ, et al: Technetium-99m stannous pyrophosphate myocardial scintigraphy: Reliability and limitation in assessment of acute myocardial infarction. Circulation 56:192, 1977.
6. Berman, DS, Amsterdam, EA, Hines, HH, et al: New approach to interpretation of technetium-99m pyrophosphate scintigraphy in detection of acute myocardial infarction. Am J Cardiol 39:341, 19777.
7. Ahmad, M, Dubiel, JP, Logan, KW, et al: Limited clinical diagnostic specificity of technetium-99m stannous pyrophosphate myocardial imaging in acute myocardial infarction. Am J Cardiol 39:50, 1977.
8. Henning, H, Schelbert, HR, Righetti, A, et al: Dual myocardial imaging with technetium-99m pyrophosphate and thallium-201 for detecting, localizing and sizing acute myocardial infarction. Am J Cardiol 40:147, 1977.
9. Holman, BL, Lesch, M, and Alpert, JS: Myocardial scintigraphy with technetium-99m pyrophosphate during the early phase of acute myocardial infarction. Am J Cardiol 41:39, 1978.
10. Massie, BM, Botvinick, EH, Werner, JA, et al: Myocardial scintigraphy with technetium-99m stannous pyrophosphate: An insensitive test for nontransmural myocardial infarction. Am J Cardiol 43:186, 1979.
11. Codini, MA, Turner, DA, Battle, WE, et al: Value and limitations of technetium-99m stannous pyrophosphate: An insensitive test for nontransmural myocardial infarction. Am J Cardiol 43:186, 1979.
12. Rude, RE, Rubin, HS, Stone, MJ, et al: Radioimmunoassay of serum creatine kinase B isoenzyme: Correlation with technetium-99m stannous pyrophosphate myocardial scintigraphy in the diagnosis of acute myocardial infarction. Am J Med 68:405, 1980.
13. Lyons, KP, Olson, HG, and Aronow, WS: Sensitivity and specificity of Tc-99m-pyrophosphate myocardial scintigraphy for the detection of acute myocardial infarction. Clin Nucl Med 5:9, 1980.
14. Olson, HG, Lyons, KP, Butman, S, et al: Validation of technetium-99m stannous pyrophosphate myocardial scintigraphy for diagnosing acute myocardial infarction more than 48 hours old when serum creatine kinase-MB has returned to normal. Am J Cardiol 52:245, 1983.
15. Corbett, JR, Lewis, M, Willerson, JT, et al: 99m Tc-pyrophosphate imaging in patients with acute myocardial infarction: Comparison of planar imaging with single-photon scintigraphy with and without blood pool overlay. Circulation 69:1120, 1984.
16. Powers, TA, Tyler, JL, and Kulkarni, MV: Efficacy of technetium Tc 99m pyrophosphate imaging in patients with equivocal myocardial infarction. South Med J 76:338, 1983.
17. Corbett, JR, Lewis, SE, Wolfe, CL, et al: Measurement of myocardial infarct size by technetium pyrophosphate single-photon tomography. Am J Cardiol 54:1232, 1984.
18. Jansen, DE, Corbett, JR, Wolfe, CL, et al: Quantification of myocardial infarction: A comparison of single photon-emission computed tomography with pyrophosphate to serial plasma MB-creatine kinase measurements. Circulation 72:327, 1985.
19. Khaw, BA, Beller, GA, Haber, E, et al: Localization of cardiac myosin-specific antibody in myocardial infarction. J Clin Invest 58:439, 1976.

20. Khaw, BA, Gold, HK, Leinbach, RC, et al: Early imaging of experimental myocardial infarction by intracoronary administration of ^{131}I-labelled anticardiac myosin $(Fab)_2$ fragments. Circulation 58:1137, 1978.
21. Khaw, BA, Fallon, JT, Beller, GA, et al: Specificity of localization of myosin-specific antibody fragments in experimental myocardial infarction. Circulation 60:1527, 1979.
22. Khaw, BA, Strauss, HW, Carvalho, A, et al: Technetium-99m labeling of antibodies to cardiac myosin Fab and to human fibrinogen. J Nucl Med 23:1011, 1982.
23. Khaw, BA, Mattis, JA, Melincoff, G, et al: Monoclonal antibody to cardiac myosin: Imaging of experimental myocardial infarction. Hybridoma 3:11, 1984.
24. Khaw, BA, Gold, HK, Yasuda, T, et al: Scintigraphic quantification of myocardial necrosis in patients after intravenous injection of myosin-specific antibody. Circulation 74:501, 1986.
25. Braat, SH, de Zwaan, C, Teule, J, et al: Value of indium-111 monoclonal antimyosin antibody for imaging in acute myocardial infarction. Am J Cardiol 60:725, 1987.
26. Klausner, SC, Botvinick, EH, Shames, D, et al: The application of radionuclide infarct scintigraphy to diagnose perioperative myocardial infarction following revascularization. Circulation 56:173, 1977.
27. Lowenthal, IS, Parisi, AF, Tow, DE, et al: Diagnosis of acute myocardial infarction in patients undergoing open heart surgery: A comparison of serial myocardial imaging with cardiac enzymes, electrocardiography, and vectorcardiography. J Nucl Med 18:770, 1977.
28. Burdine, JA, DePuey, EG, Orzan, F, et al: Scintigraphic, electrocardiographic, and enzymatic diagnosis of perioperative myocardial infarction in patients undergoing myocardial revascularization. J Nucl Med 20:711, 1979.
29. Force, T, Kemper, AJ, Bloomfield, P, et al: Non-Q-wave perioperative myocardial infarction: Assessment of the incidence and severity of regional dysfunction with quantitative two-dimensional echocardiography. Circulation 72:781, 1985.
30. Schofer, J, Stritzke, P, Montz, R, et al: Assessment of myocardial necrosis immediately after intracoronary thrombolysis by intracoronary injection of technetium-99m pyrophosphate. Eur Heart J 5:617, 1984.
31. Wheelan, K, Wolfe, C, Corbett, J, et al: Early positive technetium-99m stannous pyrophosphate images as a marker of reperfusion after thrombolytic therapy for acute myocardial infarction. Am J Cardiol 56:252, 1985.
32. Hashimoto, T, Kambara, H, Fudo, T, et al: Early estimation of acute myocardial infarction size soon after coronary reperfusion using emission computed tomography with technetium-99m pyrophosphate. Am J Cardiol 60:952, 1987.
33. Geltman, EM, Abendschein, DR, and Devries, SR: Assessment of coronary thrombolysis. Cardiol Clin 5:55, 1987.
34. Manyari, DE, Thompson, CR, Duff, HJ, et al: Usefulness of early positive technetium-99m stannous pyrophosphate scan in predicting reperfusion after thrombolytic therapy for acute myocardial infarction. Am J Cardiol 61:16, 1988.
35. Gibson, RS and Watson, DD: Clinical applications of myocardial perfusion imaging with thallium-201. In Yu, P and Goodwin, JF (eds): Progress in Cardiology. Lea & Febiger, Philadelphia, 1984, vol 12, pp 67–106.
36. Gibson, RS, Taylor, GJ, Watson, DD, et al: Prognostic significance of resting anterior thallium-201 defects in patients with inferior myocardial infarction. J Nucl Med 21:1015, 1980.
37. Henning, H, Schelbert, HR, Righetti, A, et al: Dual myocardial imaging with technetium-99m pyrophosphate and thallium-201 for detecting, localizing and sizing acute myocardial infarction. Am J Cardiol 40:147, 1977.
38. Wackers, FJT, Sokole, EB, Samson, G, et al: Value and limitations of thallium-201 scintigraphy in the acute phase of myocardial infarction. N Engl J Med 295:1, 1976.
39. Parkey, RW, Bonte, FJ, Stokely, EM, et al: Acute myocardial infarction imaged with ^{99m}technetium-stannous pyrophosphate and 201 thallium: A clinical evaluation. J Nucl Med 17:771, 1976.
40. Smitherman, TC, Osborn, RC, and Narahara, KA: Serial myocardial scintigraphy after a single dose of thallium-201 in men after acute myocardial infarction. Am J Cardiol 42:177, 1978.
41. Wackers, FJT, Lie, KI, Liem, KL, et al: Potential value of thallium-201 scintigraphy as a means of selecting patients for the coronary care unit. Br Heart J 41:111, 1979.
42. Dunn, RF, Kelly, DT, Freedman, SB, et al: Serial thallium-201 myocardial perfusion scanning in acute myocardial infarction. Aust NZ J Med 10:629, 1980.
43. Becker, LC: Enhanced reduction of thallium-201 defects in acute myocardial infarction by nitroglycerin treatment: Initial results of a prospective randomized trial. Clin Res 26:219A, 1978.

44. Schwartz, JS, Ponto, RA, Forstrom, LA, et al: Decrease in thallium-201 image defect size after permanent coronary occlusion. Am Heart J 106:1082, 1983.
45. Zaret, BL and Wackers, FJ: Radionuclide methods for evaluating the results of thrombolytic therapy. Circulation 76(Suppl 2):8, 1986.
46. Schwarz, F, Schuler, G, Katus, H, et al: Intracoronary thrombolysis in acute myocardial infarction: Correlations among serum enzyme, scintigraphic and hemodynamic findings. Am J Cardiol 50:32, 1982.
47. Schuler, G, Schwarz, F, Hofmann, M, et al: Thrombolysis in acute myocardial infarction using intracoronary streptokinase: Assessment by thallium-201 scintigraphy. Circulation 66:658, 1982.
48. DeCoster, PM, Melin, JA, Detry, JMR, et al: Coronary artery reperfusion in acute myocardial infarction: Assessment by pre- and postintervention thallium-201 myocardial perfusion imaging. Am J Cardiol 55:889, 1985.
49. Melin, JA, DeCoster, PM, Renkin, J, et al: Effect of intracoronary thrombolytic therapy on exercise-induced ischemia after acute myocardial infarction. Am J Cardiol 56:705, 1985.
50. Fung, AY, Lai, P, Juni, JE, et al: Prevention of subsequent exercise-induced ischemia by emergency coronary angioplasty in acute myocardial infarction: Comparison with intracoronary streptokinase. J Am Coll Cardiol 8:496, 1986.
51. Topol, EJ, Juni, JE, O'Neill, WW, et al: Exercise testing three days after onset of acute myocardial infarction. Am J Cardiol 60:958, 1987.
52. Gibson, RS: Detection and quantification of residual ischemia after acute uncomplicated myocardial ischemia by thallium-201 scintigraphy. In Califf, R, Mark, D, and Wagner G (eds): Acute Coronary Care in the Thrombolytic Era. Martinus-Nijhoff Publishers, The Hague/Boston/London, 1988 (in press).
53. Gibson, RS and Beller, GA: Should exercise electrocardiographic testing be replaced by radionuclide methods? In Rahimtoola, SH, Brest, AN (eds): Controversies in Coronary Artery Disease. FA Davis, Philadelphia, 1983, pp 1–32.
54. Gibson, RS, Watson, DD, Craddock, GB, et al: Predicting cardiac events after uncomplicated acute myocardial infarction: A prospective study comparing predischarge exercise thallium-201 scintigraphy and coronary angiography. Circulation 68:321, 1983.
55. Gibson, RS: The prognostic value of predischarge exercise thallium-201 scintigraphy after acute myocardial infarction. J Cardiovasc Rehabil 5:28, 1985.
56. Gibson, RS, Beller, GA, and Kaiser, DL: Prevalence and clinical significance of painless ST segment depression during early postinfarction exercise testing. Circulation 75(Suppl 5):36, 1987.
57. Leppo, JA, O'Brien, J, Rothender, JA, et al: Dipyridamole thallium-201 scintigraphy in the prediction of future cardiac events after acute myocardial infarction. N Engl J Med 310:1014, 1984.
58. Gibson, RS: Diagnostic and prognostic value of exercise ECG and radionuclide markers of ischemia in asymptomatic and symptomatic populations. In Morganroth, J and Moore, EN (eds): Silent Myocardial Ischemia. Martinus-Nijhoff Publishers, The Hague/Boston/London, 1988, p 25.
59. Varma, SK and Gibson, RS: Predischarge exercise ECG versus thallium-201 in predicting prognosis after non-Q-wave myocardial infarction. Circulation 76(Suppl 4):321, 1987.
60. Schelbert, HR: Current status and prospects of new radionuclides and radiopharmaceuticals for cardiovascular nuclear medicine. Sem Nucl Med 17:145, 1987.
61. Sia, STB and Holman, BL: Dynamic myocardial imaging in ischemic heart disease: Use of technetium-99m isonitriles. Am J Card Image 1:125, 1987.
62. Okada, RD, Glover, D, Gaffney, T, et al: Myocardial kinetics of technetium-99m-hexakis-2-methoxy-2-methylpropyl-isonitrile. Circulation 77:491, 1988.
63. Corbett, JR, Dehmer, GJ, Lewis, SE, et al: The prognostic value of submaximal exercise testing with radionuclide ventriculography before hospital discharge in patients with recent myocardial infarction. Circulation 64:535, 1981.
64. Nicod, P, Corbett, JR, Firth, BG, et al: Prognostic value of resting and submaximal exercise radionuclide ventriculography after acute myocardial infarction in high-risk patients with single and multivessel disease. Am J Cardiol 52:30, 1983.
65. Morris, KG, Palmeri, ST, Califf, RM, et al: Value of radionuclide angiography for predicting specific cardiac events after acute myocardial infarction. Am J Cardiol 55:318, 1985.
66. Borer, JS, Miller, D, Schreiber, T, et al: Radionuclide cineangiography in acute myocardial infarction: Role in prognostication. Semin Nucl Med XVII:89, 1987.
67. Merhige, ME and Rowe, RW: Positron emission tomography. Pract Cardiol 14(2):51, 1988.
68. Marshall, RC, Tillisch, JH, Phelps, ME, et al: Identification and differentiation of resting myo-

cardial ischemia in man with positron computed tomography: ^{18}F-labelled fluordeoxyglucose and N-13 ammonia. Circulation 67:766, 1983.
69. Ter-Pogossian, MM, Klein, MS, Markham, J, et al: Regional assessment of myocardial metabolic activity in vivo by positron emission tomography with ^{11}C-labeled palmitate. Circulation 61:242, 1980.
70. Geltman, EM, Biello, D, Welch, MJ, et al: Characterization of nontransmural myocardial infarction by positron emission tomography. Circulation 65:747, 1982.
71. Schwaiger, M, Brunken, R, Grover-McKay, M, et al: Regional myocardial metabolism in patients with acute myocardial infarction assessed by positron emission tomography. J Am Coll Cardiol 8:800, 1986.
72. Schwaiger, M, Schelbert, HR, Ellison, D, et al: Sustained regional abnormalities in cardiac metabolism after transient ischemia in the chronic dog model. J Am Coll Cardiol 6:336, 1985.
73. Brunken, R, Tissisch, J, Schwaiger, M, et al: Regional perfusion, glucose metabolism and wall motion in patients with chronic electrocardiographic Q-wave infarctions: Evidence for persistence of viable tissue in some infarct regions by positron emission tomography. Circulation 73:951, 1986.
74. Brunken, R, Schwaiger, M, Grover-McKay, M, et al: Positron emission tomography detects tissue metabolic activity in myocardial segments with persistent thallium perfusion defects. J Am Coll Cardiol 10:557, 1987.
75. Tillisch, J, Brunken, R, Marshall, R, et al: Prediction of the reversibility of cardiac wall motion abnormalities using positron tomography-^{18}flurodeoxyglucose and ^{13}N-ammonia. N Engl J Med 314:884, 1986.

CHAPTER 8

Unrecognized Myocardial Infarction

Barry D. Bertolet, M.D.
James A. Hill, M.D.

Although myocardial infarction (MI) is often associated with a constellation of symptoms easily recognized by physicians and lay persons, a substantial number of infarctions go unrecognized by both the patient and physician. Although not a new entity, being first described in 1912 by Herrick,[1] clinically unrecognized MI has been the subject of much research and controversy. As will be discussed, unrecognized MI seems to comprise a large percentage of the total number of infarctions and carry approximately the same prognosis as recognized MI. Thus, a better understanding and recognition of this problem are important.

DEFINITION

Unrecognized MI is an infarction in which symptoms that occur are so atypical that even the medically sophisticated patient and physician do not realize that they are related to acute myocardial damage. Silent MI, by the strictest definition, is an infarction in which there is clinical evidence of myocardial damage yet the patient is devoid of symptoms and is unaware of the event, even in retrospect.[2] Regardless of whether MI is associated with atypical symptoms or devoid of symptoms, it goes undetected and treatment is either delayed or directed to some other condition. Therefore, in a practical sense, it is useful to consider unrecognized and silent MI as a single entity.

WHY ARE MYOCARDIAL INFARCTIONS SILENT?

Why MI is clinically silent in some people and not others and why the same individual can have both silent and symptomatic infarction is not known. In 1934, Libman[3] postulated that the fact that some patients have higher pain thresholds accounted for the difference. In 1968, Keele[4] quantitated Libman's studies through the use of an algometer measuring the amount of pressure applied in kilograms. He measured the pain thresholds of patients who had had an MI and correlated this to the intensity and duration of cardiac pain, and the amount of morphine required to control it. He found a close correlation between these parameters, and he noted that a patient's pain threshold was quite constant. Droste and Roskamm[5] examined several variables in patients with asymptomatic ST segment depression and silent myocardial ischemia, and compared them with patients who had typical angina with ST segment depression. Despite similarities of the groups in functional ability, angiographic data, and risk factors, marked variability was found in various experimental pain measures. Patients with silent ischemia had significantly higher pain tolerance to electrical shock, cold, and ischemia compared with the symptomatic ischemia group. Results from neuropsychiatric testing were very similar except for a lower score in the asymptomatic group for nervousness and excitability and a higher score in masculinity. These differences may account for social or cultural differences concerning the acceptability and, thus, the perception of pain in this group. However, this supports the theory that these people have an altered sensitivity to pain in general.

The central transmission of painful stimuli may vary in an individual as well. In 1965, Melzack and Wall[6] proposed a "gate control theory of pain" in which painful stimuli are modulated at a central location. This theory provides the basis of many recent observations and studies. Endogenous opiodes, endorphins, may vary in different patients and may contribute to differences in pain perception. Preliminary data from Van Rijn and Rabkin[7] have shown that after injections of naloxone, a specific opioide antagonist, provocable angina occurred with less exertion. They performed a double-blind randomized clinical trial on men aged 50 to 56 years with effort-induced angina using exercise treadmill tests. Using placebo control, the patients were found to have angina significantly earlier on testing after naloxone compared with placebo. Results of this study were reinforced by Sheps and coworkers[8] who studied 25 patients with coronary artery disease and exercise-induced myocardial ischemia. Pre-exercise endorphin levels were drawn, the patient was exercised to the point of ischemia or fatigue, and postexercise endorphin levels were drawn. A significant positive correlation was noted between postexercise endorphin levels and time-to-onset of angina, with strong negative correlations between postexercise endorphin levels and duration of exercise as well as presence of angina. Postexercise endorphin levels were significantly lower in patients with angina during exercise than in those with ischemia without angina. These data suggest that endorphins may play a role in individual variations in pain perception.

Another potential mechanism for the lack of pain during myocardial ischemia or infarction is the destruction of nociceptive pathways from the heart by MI or polyneuropathies, or by surgical interruption after coronary artery bypass or transplantation. However, data from the Mayo Clinic[9] suggest that a previous MI does not influence the ability to diagnose a subsequent one. Patients with diabetes mellitus, a major cause of polyneuropathy, do not seem to have more silent MI than others with coronary heart disease. The majority of patients who have undergone cardiac surgery also seem to be able to perceive ischemic pain and MI. Cardiac transplant patients have not been studied specifically regarding perception of ischemia and incidence of MI, but they represent a small subset of patients with ischemic heart disease. These variables may help explain painless infarction in some groups, but they do not explain painless and painful infarction in the same patient and do not account for the majority.

The effects of anesthesia or postoperative pain medications may obscure ischemic pain in patients in the perioperative setting. In a prospective study of 496 randomly selected patients undergoing noncardiac surgery, Driscoll and associates[10] obtained ECGs prior to, and 12 and 72 hours after surgery. A total of 12 MIs were identified (2.4 percent). Only two patients complained of pain typical of myocardial ischemia. Four others could have been suspected based on prolonged hypotension (three) or respiratory distress (one). Therefore, 50 percent had a clinically unsuspected MI. In a retrospective study, Becker and Underwood[11] reviewed 30,000 surgical cases over a 5-year period and identified 28 cases of perioperative MI. Eleven (39 percent) had symptoms typical of myocardial ischemia. Patients receiving sedatives, pain medications, or neuroleptics for various medical ailments may have altered perceptions of ischemic pain, which may explain some silent MIs. It seems also that this subgroup explains only a small percentage of the total number of MIs.

How exactly silent myocardial ischemia relates to silent MI is unknown, but there seems to be a correlation. In the study of Droste and Roskamm,[5] of the 20 patients in the asymptomatic ischemia group, 16 had previous infarctions (4 without symptoms, 6 with atypical symptoms, 6 with typical symptoms at the time of MI). In the 22 patients with typical angina there were 17 MIs, of which only 2 (11.7 percent) were silent. In the Mayo autopsy study, of the 37 patients with a symptomatic MI, 34 (92 percent) had a history of angina pectoris. Of the 26 patients with silent MI, only 7 (27 percent) had a history of symptomatic myocardial ischemia. These data were also confirmed by the Framingham study[14] in which 13 of 72 men (18 percent) and 9 of 42 women (21 percent) with unrecognized MI had a history of prior angina pectoris.

CLINICAL PRESENTATION

Symptoms of patients with unrecognized MI are variable. Symptoms reported or noted in retrospect include dyspnea, nausea, syncope, cough, paroxysmal nocturnal dyspnea, bronchospasm, orthopnea, insomnia, ankle edema, tender hepatomegaly, atrial fibrillation, fatigue, chest pain related to meals and relieved by belching, heartburn, and palpitations. In the Framingham study,[12–14] it was found that one-half of patients with clinically unrecognized MI had atypical symptoms and one-half were totally asymptomatic. In a Boston City Hospital study[15] in which 102 consecutive patients with MI were studied, 25 percent presented without chest pain. Of these, 15 had dyspnea (acute in 14), 6 had abdominal complaints, 4 had extreme fatigue, 1 had intractable nausea and vomiting, and 1 had syncope. In unrecognized perioperative MI, unstable blood pressure and tachycardia were the two signs most often noted.[10,11]

Diagnosis of silent MI can be made by noting regional wall motion abnormalities on echocardiogram, radionuclide angiogram, or contrast ventriculogram, or nonreversible defects by thallium perfusion imaging in the absence of clinical events. Usually, however, typical changes noted on a routine ECG is the most common method employed for diagnosing silent MI. Retrospective diagnosis of MI by ECG may not be that sensitive, however. Cox and Lond[16] found that in a series of men who survived their first MI without reinfarction during the 4-year study period, the ECG reverted to normal in 10.9 percent at 1 year and 13.3 percent at 2 years. Abnormal Q waves had disappeared in 10.6 percent of ECGs at 2 years. Similar changes were noted in the Aspirin Myocardial Infarction Study[17] in which 4230 patients with Q wave MI were identified and followed with serial ECGs. The Q waves disappeared from 12.5 percent of the ECGs at 1 year and 13.3 percent at 2 years. We have identified 24 patients with regional wall motion abnormalities by radionuclide ventriculography and nonreversible defects on thallium perfusion scanning. In only one patient was a pathologic Q wave found, and in two other patients suggestive changes (poor R wave progression or T wave inversion) were noted. It appears, therefore, that the ECG is an insensitive tool for MI detection when used in retrospect, and it is likely that the studies using this tool for retrospective diagnosis underestimate the true incidence of MI.

INCIDENCE

The incidence of silent MI has been estimated in several retrospective and prospective studies. The Western Collaborative Group study[18,19] evaluated 3524 men aged 39 to 59 years. On screening exam, 113 had coronary heart disease, of which 42 (37 percent) had previously unrecognized MI by ECG criteria. Annual followup studies on 3182 of the initially well subjects over 4.5 years revealed new coronary heart disease in 133—104 suffered an MI and 29 developed angina. Thirty-one of these 104 (29.8 percent) were clinically unrecognized.

The Framingham cohort of 5127 subjects, aged 30 to 62 years and initially free of coronary heart disease, were followed biennially. During the 30-year followup period, 708 MIs occurred—469 in men and 239 in women. Of these, 130 (28 percent) in men and 83 (35 percent) in women were clinically unrecognized at the time, an overall incidence of 30 percent. Of note is that one-half of these people could not recall any symptoms, atypical or otherwise, suggestive of MI.

The Israeli Heart Attack Study[20] followed 9764 subjects aged 40 and older and free of coronary heart disease for 5 years. They noted 427 MIs, of which 170 (40 percent) were unrecognized. As in the Framingham study, 50 percent of persons with unrecognized MI were totally asymptomatic. Combining these three prospective cohort studies, 414 of the 1239 (33 percent) MIs were not recognized by patient or physician.

A retrospective study from the Mayo Clinic[9] reviewed 1267 necropsies over a 2-year period. Acute or healed MI was found in 143. In 80 of 143 (56 percent), healed infarcts alone were found; in 30 of 143 (21 percent), acute infarcts alone were found; and in 33 of 143 (23 percent) both healed and acute infarcts were noted. Of the 113 healed infarcts, 56 (50 percent) had not been diagnosed or suspected prior to death. Of the 63 acute infarcts, 25 (40 percent) were not diagnosed or suspected. In the 113 subjects with healed MI, clinical histories were reviewed and subdivided into fair, good, and excellent. Histories were excellent in 33 percent, that is, the patient was seen frequently (at least yearly) and had undergone extensive investigations including repeated ECGs. In these 37 patients with excellent histories and followup, 17 (46 percent) had no diagnosis of prior MI. In this particular study combining both healed and acute MI, 81 of 176 infarctions (46 percent) were neither diagnosed nor suspected prior to death (Table 8–1).

The 46 percent incidence of silent MI noted by autopsy study is substantially higher than the cohort studies using living subjects, in which the average was 33 percent. These differences may be accounted for by an underestimation of the true incidence of silent MI by prospective studies. These studies excluded MIs without persistent ECG changes, episodes of silent MI that resulted in out-of-hospital

Table 8–1.

Reference	Cases	Total MIs	MI Incidence (%)	Unrecognized MI				Duration of Study Period
				Men	Women	Total	% of All MIs	
PROSPECTIVE STUDIES								
Rosenman[18,19]	3182	104	3.3	31	—	31	29.8	4.5 y.
Kannel and Margolis[12–14]	5127	708 (469M, 239F)	13.8	130	83	213	30	30 yr
Medalie[20]	9764	427	4.4	170	—	170	39.8	5 yr
TOTAL		1239				445	33	
RETROSPECTIVE STUDIES								
Johnson[9]	1267	176				81	46	2 yr
		63 Acute				25	39.7	
		113 Healed				56	49.5	

Table 8–2.

Study	Cases	Def. of Sudden Death	% Symptoms at Death	Incidence Acute MI (%)
Reichenbach[21]	87	w/i 12 hr	36% w/i week prior	5
Baba and Bashe[22,23]	121	w/i 24 hr	—	12
Friedman[24]	27	w/i 30 sec	—	0
Friedman[24]	37	w/i 24 hr	92	21
Perper[25]	169	w/i 24 hr	—	11
Lie and Titus[26]	120	w/i 6 hr	100	33
Schwartz[27]	19	Not defined	—	32
Phillips[28]	19	w/i 1 hr	—	0
Titus[29]	86	Not defined	—	40
Liberthson[30]	80	SCD in hospital, monitored and defibrillated	18	39
Liberthson[30]	70	SCD in hospital, monitored and autopsied	20	27
Liberthson[30]	150	SCD outside hospital, witnessed and autopsied	25	27
TOTAL	1105			(Mean) 20

death, and patients who only had enzyme evidence of MI or did not meet rigid criteria ECG criteria. For example, of the first 214 acute MIs noted in the Framingham study, 26 (12 percent) were documented by enzyme changes alone or autopsy and were not included in further analysis.[14] The incidence of MI causing sudden death varies from 0 percent to 40 percent[21–30] (Table 8–2). The number of those patients who had a truly unrecognized MI is unknown, but autopsy and history data suggest that at least some had silent MI. Approximately one-third of all acute MIs never manifest a diagnostic Q wave.[31,32] Therefore, it seems reasonable to assume that 40 percent to 45 percent of all MIs are unrecognized.

WHO IS AT RISK?

Patients who are likely to have an MI that is unrecognized seem to be no different from those with symptomatic MI. In the Boston City Hospital study, those patients diagnosed with MI but who had atypical presentations without chest pain tended to be older (mean 69.1 versus 58.7 years) and to have no prior history of angina (96 percent versus 63 percent) when compared with patients with typical presentations of MI. However, no difference in the incidence of diabetes, cigarette smoking, hypertension, patient reliability, sex, race, or activity level at the onset of symptoms was noted. The Western Collaborative Group Study found that a parental history of MI was significantly associated with the emergence of silent MI when compared with symptomatic MI. The Framingham study showed the proportion of unrecognized MI was higher in women except in the elderly group (age 75 or older), and in men the incidence was higher in the age 75-or-older group. The incidence of silent MI was also higher in those people without a previous history of angina. In the Israeli study, risk factors associated with the emergence of silent MI were age greater than 60, left axis deviation and/or left ventricular hypertrophy on ECG, cigarette smoking, and both systolic and diastolic hypertension. Diabetes mellitus and hypercholesterolemia did not predispose subjects studied to silent MI.

In the autopsy series of the Mayo Clinic, approximately 48 percent of the patients who died and had unrecognized MI had no history of angina. Again, older patients tended to have a greater incidence of silent MI, but equal ratios were noted between men and women in recognized and unrecognized infarctions. A history of a previous infarct did not interfere with the diagnosis of an acute infarct. A previous history of congestive heart failure, hypertension, or diabetes did not alter the incidence of unrecognized as compared with recognized infarction. It is apparent from both the prospective and retrospective studies that no clear differentiation can be made as to the risk factors that predispose to unrecognized MI. Patients' risk factors tend to be similar to those with typical MI, that is, hypertension, family history, diabetes, age, and cigarette smoking, with the possible exception of hypercholesterolemia and male sex. It is noteworthy that diabetes and history of previous infarction did not predispose to silent MI as commonly thought.

PROGNOSIS

The prognosis of patients with unrecognized MI varies somewhat depending on the population studied. The Framingham Study, after 30 years of followup, found that men with unrecognized MI were more likely to have a recurrence than those with recognized MI, 23 percent versus 13 percent. This association was not found in women; in fact, the reverse was true. In other morbidity except for angina, men were just as likely to develop cardiac failure and stroke regardless of whether their MI was recognized or not. Women with previous unrecognized MI tended to have less morbid events than men, but this was not statistically significant. In those patients who survived the initial MI, the average mortality for both symptomatic and unrecognized MI was 4 percent to 5 percent per year. After 10 years, 45 percent of patients with unrecognized MI were dead as compared with 39 percent of those with recognized MI. Women had a higher mortality rate with recognized MI than with unrecognized MI. In the Mayo autopsy study, MI recurrence was more likely noted in those patients with prior unrecognized MI compared with those with symptomatic MI (69 percent versus 41 percent). Also, a higher incidence of cardiac failure was noted in the unrecognized MI group. In the Boston City Hospital study, the mortality rate in the patients with atypical presentation of MI was 50 percent as opposed to 18 percent in the typical group. The cause of death in this atypical group was cardiogenic shock, myocardial rupture, and arrhythmias, which were more frequent compared with those with a typical presentation. The Israeli study does not agree with these figures. They found a mortality rate of 17.3/1000 in silent MI patients and 36.3/1000 in recognized MI patients over an 8.5-year followup. Although the mortality figures differ among studies, it is clear that morbidity and mortality from unrecognized MI is significant and in no way does the lack of recognition of the problem imply a benign prognosis.

EVALUATION AND FOLLOWUP

Regardless of how they come to medical attention, patients in whom previously unrecognized MI is identified should be evaluated in a similar manner as those with symptomatic MI. As with any ischemic heart disease patient, they should undergo evaluation for any cardiac risk factors that can be modified and, once identified, aggressively treated. Data from several prospective risk factor intervention studies support this. The Lipid Research Clinics Trial[33] found that cardiovascular mortality was substantially increased by hypercholesterolemia, smoking, hypertension, and hyperglycemia, especially in those patients with an abnormal exercise test that suggested myocardial ischemia. Subsequent reduction in at least some of these risk factors reduced cardiovascular mortality. The Multiple Risk Factor Intervention Trial (MRFIT)[34] revealed that intensive modification of cardiac risk factors in men with abnormal exercise tests suggesting myocardial ischemia decreased subsequent coronary heart disease deaths.

Active myocardial ischemia seems to predispose the patient to reinfarction,[12,35] malignant arrhythmias,[36] and sudden death.[37,38] Standard exercise testing can be used to identify residual ischemia after MI, which can be predictive of subsequent mortality. This relationship can be shown early as well as late after MI. The MILIS Study Group[39] investigators performed maximal exercise treadmill tests on 473 patients 6 months after MI and followed them for the next 12 months. Their results indicated that mortality was increased significantly in any patient who could not perform the test owing to cardiac limitations, had ST segment elevation of 1 mm or more, demonstrated inadequate blood pressure response during exercise, developed premature ventricular contractions (PVCs) during or after exercise, or could not exercise beyond stage 1 of the modified Bruce protocol. Residual ischemia should be treated.

Even in the absence of residual ischemia, patients with silent MI should be considered for beta blocker and aspirin therapies, which have been shown in various studies using various protocols to be effective prophylaxis against subsequent MI and death. Although only studied in symptomatic MI patients, these therapies also may provide effective prophylaxis for the unrecognized MI patient. As has been pointed out, patients with unrecognized MI have the same risk factors and morbidity, and the same, perhaps higher, mortality. Thus, it seems logical that they may benefit from the same prophylactic therapy. Clinical judgment must guide any such therapy, however, pending confirmation by appropriate investigation.

SUMMARY

MI is frequently unrecognized for reasons that are unknown, comprising approximately 40 percent of all MIs that occur. Although many unrecognized MIs are accompanied by symptoms of some sort, probably half are totally asymptomatic. Patients with unrecognized MI seem to be similar to those with typical presentations, with similar risk factors and other characteristics. It appears that MI carries the same prognosis whether clinically apparent or not and, therefore, warrants management in both cases. Therapy for silent MI should be aimed at (1) identification and modification of risk factors, (2) identification and treatment of residual ischemia, and (3) attempts at reducing the risk of reinfarction with subsequent morbidity and mortality. As we develop a better understanding of silent ischemic heart disease, hopefully the optimal management strategy for these patients will emerge.

REFERENCES

1. Herrick, JB: Clinical features of sudden obstruction of the coronary arteries. JAMA 59:2015, 1912.
2. Bayliss, RIS: Clinical recognition and significance of silent myocardial infarction. Practical Cardiology 12:41, 1986.
3. Libman, E: Observations on individual sensitiveness to pain. JAMA 102:335, 1934.
4. Keele, KD: Pain complaint threshold in relation to pain of cardiac infarction. Br Med J 1:670, 1968.
5. Droste, C and Roskamm, H: Experimental pain measurement in patients with asymptomatic myocardial ischemia. J Am Coll Cardiol 1(3):940, 1983.
6. Melzack, R and Wall, PD: Pain mechanisms: A new theory. Science 150:971, 1965.
7. Van Rijn, T and Rabkin, SW: Effect of naloxone, a specific opioid antagonist on exercise induced angina pectoris. Circulation 64(Suppl 4):IV-149, 1981.
8. Sheps, DS, et al: Endorphins are related to pain perception in coronary artery disease. Am J Cardiol 59:523, 1987.
9. Johnson, WJ, et al: Unrecognized myocardial infarction. Arch Intern Med 103:253, 1959.
10. Driscoll, AC, et al.: Clinically unrecognized myocardial infarction following surgery. N Engl J Med 264:633, 1961.
11. Becker, RC and Underwood, DA: Myocardial infarction in patients undergoing noncardiac surgery. Cleve Clin J Med 54:25, 1987.
12. Kannel, WB and Abbott, RD: Incidence and prognosis of unrecognized myocardial infarction. N Engl J Med 311:1144, 1984.
13. Margolis, JR, et al.: Clinical features of unrecognized myocardial infarctions—silent and symptomatic. Am J Cardiol 32:1, 1973.
14. Kannel, WB, et al: The unrecognized myocardial infarction. Geriatrics 25:75, 1970.
15. Uretsky, BF, et al: Symptomatic myocardial infarction without chest pain: Prevalence and clinical course. Am J Cardiol 40:498, 1977.
16. Cox, CJ and Lond, MB: Return to normal of the electrocardiogram after myocardial infarction. Lancet 1:1194, 1967.
17. Wasserman, AG, et al: Prognostic implications of diagnostic Q waves after myocardial infarction. Circulation 65:1451, 1982.
18. Rosenman, RH, et al: Clinically unrecognized myocardial infarction in the Western Collaborative Group Study. Am J Cardiol 19:776, 1967.
19. Rosenman, RH, et al: Coronary heart disease in the Western Collaborative Group Study. J Chronic Dis 23:173, 1970.
20. Medalie, JH and Goldbourt, U: Unrecognized myocardial infarction: Five year incidence, mortality, and risk factors. Ann Intern Med 84:526, 1976.
21. Reichenbach, DD, et al: Pathology of the heart in sudden cardiac death. Am J Cardiol 39:865, 1977.
22. Baba, Nobuhisa, et al: Pathology of atherosclerotic heart disease in sudden death. II. Organizing thrombosis and acute coronary vessel lesions. Circulation 51,52(Suppl III):III-53, 1975.
23. Bashe, Jr, Winslow, J, et al: Pathology of atherosclerotic heart disease in sudden death. II. The significance of myocardial infarction. Circulation 51,52(Suppl III):III-63, 1975.
24. Friedman, M, et al: Instantaneous and sudden deaths. JAMA 225:1319, 1973.
25. Perper, JA, et al: Arteriosclerosis of coronary arteries in sudden unexpected deaths. Circulation 51,52(Suppl III):III-27, 1975.
26. Lie, JT, et al: Pathology of myocardium and the conduction system in sudden coronary death. Circulation 51,52(Suppl III):III-41, 1975.
27. Schwartz, CJ and Gerrity, RG: Anatomical pathology of sudden unexpected cardiac death. Circulation 51,52(Suppl III):III-18, 1975.
28. Phillips, M, et al: Sudden cardiac death in Air Force recruits. JAMA 256:2696, 1986.
29. Titus, JL, et al: Sudden unexpected death as the initial manifestation of ischemic heart disease. Clinical and pathologic observations. Am J Cardiol 26:662, 1970.

30. Liberthson, RR, et al: Pathophysiologic observations in prehospital ventricular fibrillation and sudden cardiac death. Circulation 49:790, 1974.
31. Horan, LG, et al: Significance of the diagnostic Q wave of myocardial infarction. Circulation 43:428, 1971.
32. Madias, JE, et al: A comparison of transmural and nontransmural acute myocardial infarction. Circulation 49:498, 1974.
33. Gordon, DJ, et al: Predictive value of the exercise tolerance test for mortality in North American men: The Lipid Research Clinics Mortality Follow-up Study. Circulation 74:252, 1986.
34. Multiple Risk Factor Intervention Trial Research Group: Exercise electrocardiogram and coronary heart disease mortality in the Multiple Risk Factor Intervention Trial. Am J Cardiol 55:16, 1985.
35. Gibson, RS, et al: Prevalence and clinical significance of painless ST segment depression during early postinfarction exercise testing. Circulation 75(Suppl II):II-36, 1987.
36. Hong, RA, et al: Life-threatening ventricular tachycardia and fibrillation by painless myocardial ischemia during exercise testing. JAMA 257:1937, 1987.
37. Warnes, CA and Roberts, WC: Sudden coronary death: Relation of amount and distribution of coronary narrowing at necropsy to previous symptoms of myocardial ischemia, left ventricular scarring and heart weight. Am J Cardiol 54:65, 1984.
38. Sharma, Bimlendra, et al: Demonstration of exercise induced ischemia without angina in patients who recover from out-of-hospital ventricular fibrillation. Am J Cardiol 47:445, 1981.
39. Stone, PH, et al: Prognostic significance of the treadmill exercise test performance 6 months after myocardial infarction. J Am Coll Cardiol 8:1007, 1986.

CHAPTER 9

Q-Wave Versus Non-Q-Wave Myocardial Infarction*

James T. Willerson, M.D.
L. Maximilian Buja, M.D.

Myocardial infarction occurring without the development of new Q waves has been called "subendocardial," "nontransmural," and "non-Q-wave" infarction. Myocardial infarcts occurring with "Q waves" have been called "transmural," or "Q-wave," infarcts. Howevever, the correlation between the electrocardiographic findings of transmural and subendocardial myocardial infarcts and the postmortem anatomic changes is not perfect.[1–3] Some patients with postmortem-determined transmural infarctions have no Q waves or loss of R waves, and some patients with nontransmural or subendocardial myocardial infarcts have Q waves or R wave loss on their electrocardiograms. Therefore, although most transmural infarcts are "Q-wave" infarcts and most nontransmural infarcts are "non-Q-wave" infarcts, it is common today to refer to acute myocardial infarcts based on what is actually observed on the electrocardiogram (i.e., as being "Q-wave" and "non-Q-wave" myocardial infarcts). The pathophysiology, clinical consequences, and treatment of these types of infarction are different and these differences will be reviewed in this chapter.

PATHOPHYSIOLOGY

Most Q-wave myocardial infarcts are caused by an occlusive coronary thrombus at the site of a relatively proximal and severe coronary artery stenosis, and the thrombus develops as a consequence of endothelial injury—often as a result of plaque fissuring and ulceration.[4–9] In contrast, most non-Q-wave myocardial infarcts are associated with multivessel coronary artery stenoses and transient reductions in coronary blood flow without a permanent and completely obstructing coronary thrombus.[6,10] On the basis of extensive clinical and experi-

*This work was supported in part by NHLBI Ischemic SCOR HL 17669 and the Moss Heart Fund of Dallas, Texas.

mental animal studies, we and our colleagues have suggested that endothelial injury at sites of coronary artery stenosis is associated with platelet aggregation and the release of the platelet-derived mediators, thromboxane A_2 and serotonin, which cause further platelet aggregation and dynamic increases in coronary vascular resistance and decreases in coronary blood flow[11–28] (Fig. 9–1). We have speculated that endothelial injury, usually at sites of narrowed coronary arteries, is the location for platelet aggregation and subsequently white blood cell attachment and release of thromboxane and serotonin (and possibly other mediators, including platelet-derived growth factor, platelet activating factor, prostaglandin D_2, endothelin, and/or selected leukotrienes resulting from white blood cell and mast cell infiltration into the injured endothelial region); this sequence causes dynamic vasoconstriction and further platelet aggregation and thrombus development leading to mechanical obstruction and dynamic stenoses that are important factors in the conversion from chronic stable to unstable angina (see Fig. 9–1).[11,12] When these pathophysiological alterations reduce coronary blood flow for periods of 20 minutes to approximately 2 hours, non-Q-wave infarcts may develop (see Fig. 9–1).[11,12] When a critical reduction in coronary blood flow is maintained for periods longer than 2 hours, a Q-wave myocardial infarction may occur.[11,12] Others have also shown an important role for platelet aggregation at sites of endothelial injury and coronary artery narrowing, leading to abrupt reductions in coronary blood flow, as well as protection against myocardial infarction and death in patients with unstable angina who are treated with the cyclo-oxy-

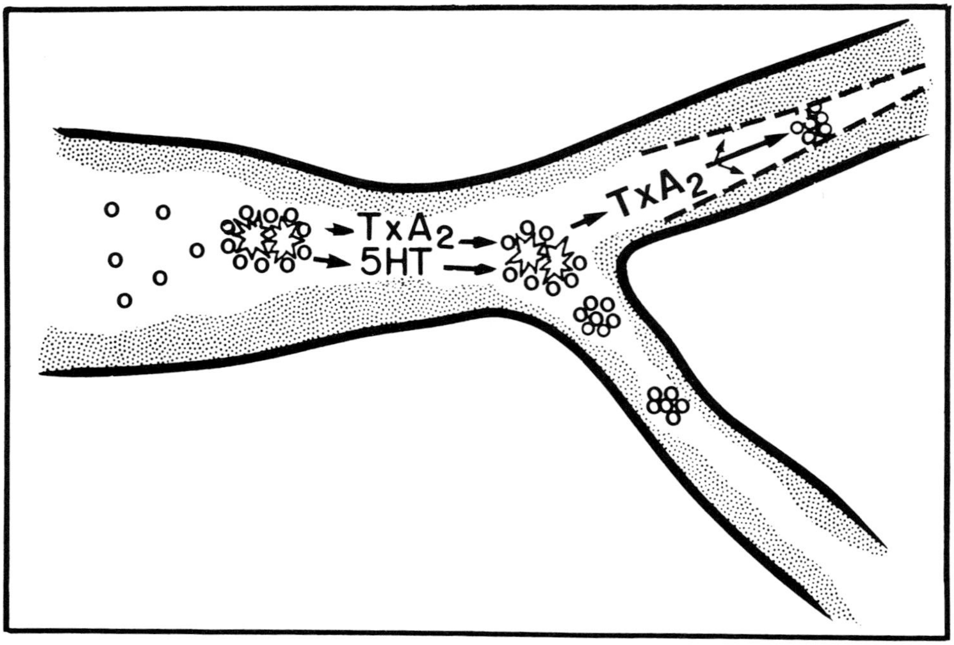

Figure 9–1. A schematic diagram indicating the possible mechanisms by which thromboxane A_2 (TxA_2) and serotonin ($5HT_2$) promote platelet aggregation and decreases in coronary blood flow in the patient with angina. Aggregating platelets *(stars)* release thromboxane A_2 and serotonin, which cause further platelet aggregation downstream and dynamic reductions in coronary luminal diameter. (Reproduced by permission from the Journal of the American College of Cardiology 8:248, 1986.)

genase inhibitor, aspirin.[29–37] The importance of the accumulation of platelet-derived mediators in causing enhanced coronary vasoconstriction and possibly contributing to the conversion from chronic to acute coronary heart disease is almost certainly increased in circumstances in which the injured endothelium possesses less ability to vasodilate as a consequence of having reduced concentrations of endothelial-derived relaxing factor, tissue plasminogen-activating factor, and/or prostacyclin.[11,12] Non-Q-wave infarcts also may be caused by a severe increase in myocardial oxygen demand or severe, generalized impairment in coronary perfusion.[6] The precipitating events in such cases are usually apparent clinically.

GENERAL RECOGNITION OF Q-WAVE AND NON-Q-WAVE MYOCARDIAL INFARCTS

Most patients with acute myocardial infarction have severe left precordial chest pain. Nausea and vomiting occur in many patients. Some patients describe a sensation of weakness, and most patients appear anxious and in distress. Population studies have suggested that between 20 percent and 60 percent of nonfatal myocardial infarcts may be unrecognized or misinterpreted by the patient and are discovered only on subsequent routine electrocardiographic or postmortem evaluations.[38–40]

Patients with anterior Q-wave myocardial infarcts are generally the ones with clinical evidence of severe heart failure and/or hypotension, inasmuch as these infarcts tend to be the largest and result in the most severe left ventricular dysfunction.[41–44] Patients with inferior Q-wave myocardial infarcts and those with non-Q-wave infarcts generally have smaller amounts of myocardium damaged by the infarction and less commonly develop hypotension or clinical evidence of serious heart failure with their first infarcts. However, in the patient with an inferior Q-wave myocardial infarction and extensive infarction of the right ventricle, hypotension and/or clinical signs and symptoms that simulate pericardial tamponade may develop as a consequence of severe right ventricular dysfunction.[45–47] In patients with previous myocardial infarcts, a new infarction in any location may cause hypotension and/or severe heart failure because even a small new infarct superimposed on extensive previous infarction may damage enough of the ventricle to result in pump failure.

ECG Recognition

In general, patients with Q-wave infarcts present with prominent T waves and/or hyperacute ST segment elevation that evolves in the subsequent few minutes, hours, or sometimes days to a pattern of significant Q waves (the electrocardiographic correlate of myocardial necrosis) and T wave inversion in the leads reflecting the site of myocardial infarction. Typically, patients with acute non-Q-wave myocardial infarcts present with T wave inversion and/or ST segment depression of varying magnitude that subsequently reverts to a normal pattern in the hours to days thereafter. Whereas the electrocardiogram may be used to recognize acute Q-wave myocardial infarcts with relative certainty in most patients, the ECG changes in patients with non-Q-wave infarcts are not specific for this entity; subendocardial ischemia, rapid heart rates, electrolyte abnormalities, intraventricular conduction defects, and the use of certain medications (notably digitalis preparations) may cause the same ECG changes. Moreover, as mentioned earlier, some patients with transmural myocardial infarcts do not develop Q waves or R wave loss on their electrocardiograms, and some patients with nontransmural myocardial infarcts demonstrate ST segment elevation initially (usually no more than 1 to 2 mm) and/or subsequently develop R wave loss and/or Q waves. Thus, the electrocardiogram does not separate transmural and nontransmural infarcts with certainty, but, in general, Q-wave infarcts (and/or infarcts associated with more than 50 percent R wave loss in the ECG leads reflecting the infarction) are transmural infarcts, and those without subsequent Q waves or R wave loss presenting with ST segment depression and T wave inversion initially are usually nontransmural myocardial infarcts.

Enzymatic Recognition

The diagnosis of acute myocardial infarction is supported by demonstrating increases in serum creatine kinase (CK) and the relatively specific myocardial isoenzyme of creatine kinase, the MB isoenzyme. This finding is particularly important in patients with non-Q-wave myocardial infarcts, inasmuch as the electrocardiogram does not provide a specific means to detect this type of infarction. One should obtain blood samples at 4- to 6-hour intervals for a period of 18 to 24 hours to identify increases in CK and CK-MB isoenzyme, which evolve in a typical pattern suggestive of infarction, to help document its occurrence, especially in patients with non-Q-wave myocardial infarcts.

CLINICAL CONSEQUENCES

Acute mortality in patients with non-Q-wave infarcts is approximately one-half that of patients with Q-wave infarcts.[42,43] If in-hospital infarct extension or reinfarction occurs, mortality becomes similar for patients with Q-wave and non-Q-wave myocardial infarcts.[48,49] Infarct extension occurs in approximately 10 percent of patients with acute myocardial infarcts during the first 10 days.[48–52] Infarct extension is usually associated with severe and prolonged chest pain occurring after the original infarct, often associated with new ECG changes—ST elevation for Q-wave infarct extension and ST segment depression for non-Q-wave infarct extension. Infarct extension is generally documented by a re-elevation of CK-MB in the serum after the initial peak.[49,50] Mortality is increased in patients in whom infarct extension occurs.[50,51] Infarct extension may occur more frequently in obese females, in patients with non-Q-wave infarcts, in patients with diabetes mellitus, in those with a previous myocardial infarction, and in patients with an early peaking CK-MB value (i.e., less than 15 hours).[49,51,52] An increased mortality associated with infarct extension is most likely related to the larger mass of myocardium that is injured and a consequent further deterioration of ventricular function. Patients with non-Q-wave infarcts generally have smaller infarcts initially than patients with anterior Q-wave infarcts.[42,44,53–55] Consequently, the frequency of heart failure early after non-Q-wave infarction is less than with anterior Q-wave infarcts, but postinfarction angina is more frequent in patients with non-Q-wave infarcts, presumably related to the presence of viable myocardium with marginal blood supply.[43,53,54] Thus, uncomplicated non-Q-wave myocardial infarcts are not benign conditions in many patients.[53–58] Approximately 60 percent of patients with non-Q-wave infarcts have significant obstructions in two or three of the major coronary arteries, and approximately 20 percent of patients with non-Q-wave infarcts have a new Q-wave infarction within 3 months of the non-Q-wave event.[54] In one series, approximately one-half of the patients with non-Q-wave infarcts developed unstable angina during a followup period averaging 11 months.[60] Hutter and associates have reported high early and late reinfarction rates in patients with "subendocardial infarctions" and comparable late mortalities in patients with subendocardial and transmural infarctions.[42] In-hospital extension of a non-Q-wave infarction appears to increase long-term risk, with an almost doubling of 1-year mortality in one study.[61]

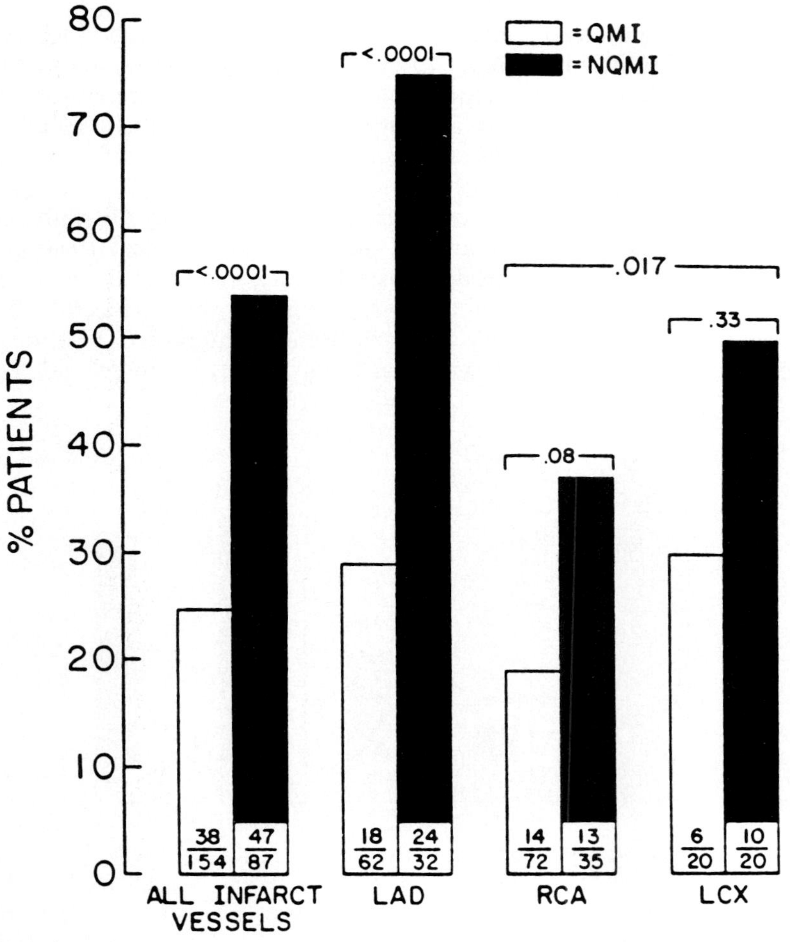

Figure 9–2. Prevalence of open infarct-related vessels 11 ± 3 days after onset of clinical infarction. Patency rates are higher for left anterior descending (LAD) and non-LAD right coronary artery (RCA) and left circumflex (LCx) combined in patients with non-Q-wave myocardial infarctions. (Reproduced by permission from the American Heart Association [Circulation 73:1190, 1986].)

Prediction of Future Prognosis

The development of postinfarct angina at rest or low levels of activity in the hours to several days after the initial event identifies the patients at risk for future coronary events. These patients are treated vigorously with antianginal medications, especially ones that increase coronary blood flow (nitrates and selected calcium antagonists). Diltiazem administration has been shown to decrease the frequency of reinfarction in patients with non-Q-wave myocardial infarcts in one recent study.[62] In the patients with postmyocardial infarction angina at rest or low levels of activity, we believe that coronary arteriography is generally indicated, and subsequent coronary revascularization, either percutaneous transluminal coronary angioplasty (PTCA) or coronary artery revascularization, is indicated when the patient's coronary anatomy is suitable. However, a substantial number of patients at risk for future coronary events do not have rest angina or angina at low levels of activity, and additional means of identifying them need to be employed. Gibson and coworkers studied 241 patients 65 years of age or younger with an acute uncomplicated myocardial infarction and obtained followup coronary angiography, radionuclide ventriculography, 24-hour Holter monitoring, and quantitative thallium-201 scintigraphy during treadmill exercise 10 ± 3 days after infarction.[53] One hundred and fifty-four of these patients had Q-wave infarcts and 87 non-Q-wave infarcts. The prevalence of open infarct-related vessels 11 ± 3 days after the Q-wave and non-Q-wave infarcts in these patients is shown in Figure 9–2. Figure 9–3 demonstrates the frequency of death, recurrent myocardial infarction, unstable angina, and need for revascularization among these 241 patients. These studies demonstrated an increased risk for future myocardial infarction, the development of unstable angina, and the need for coronary revascularization, either coronary artery revascularization or PTCA, for patients with acute non-Q-wave infarcts (see Figs. 9–2 and 9–3).[53] Gibson and colleagues

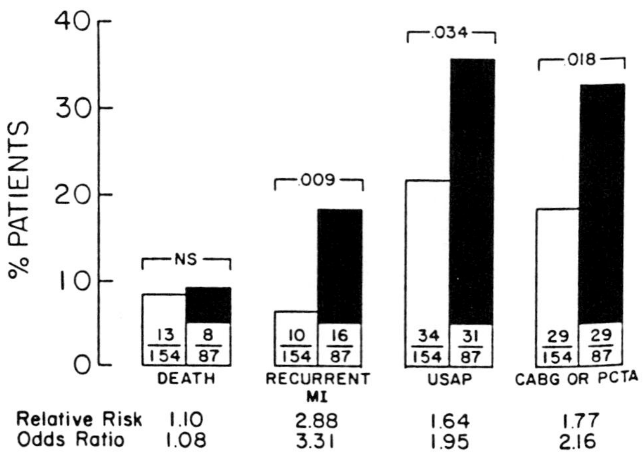

Figure 9–3. Incidence of death, recurrent myocardial infarction, unstable angina, and the subsequent need for bypass surgery or percutaneous transluminal coronary angioplasty (PTCA) in 241 patients with uncomplicated acute infarctions. Relative risk values and odds ratios are presented as guides to the magnitude of the associations (e.g., the risk of experiencing an event for patients with non-Q-wave myocardial infarcts relative to patients with Q-wave myocardial infarcts). (Reproduced by permission from the American Heart Association [Circulation 73:1192, 1986].)

demonstrated that many of the patients at risk for future events had specific thallium-201 scintigraphic abnormalities at low-level exercise prior to hospital discharge (Fig. 9–4). Thus, low-level exercise testing with thallium-201 scintigraphy, especially with single photon emission computed tomography (SPECT), provides a means to identify many of the patients with non-Q-wave infarcts at risk for future coronary events (see Figs. 9–2 through 9–4).[53]

An alternative noninvasive means for identifying patients at risk for future coronary events, including sudden death, new myocardial infarction, and/or the development of unstable angina or severe heart failure is the use of submaximal exercise with radionuclide ventriculography. Corbett and coworkers[63,64] have

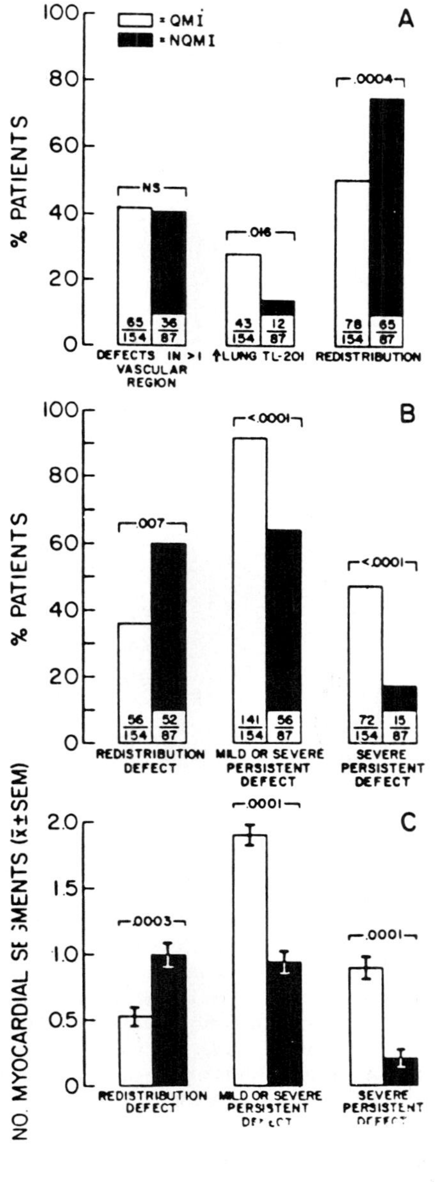

Figure 9–4. (*A*) Prevalence of high-risk thallium-201 scintigraphic patterns among patients with Q-wave myocardial infarcts and non-Q-wave myocardial infarcts. (*B*) Prevalence of thallium-201 redistribution and persistent defects in infarct-related segments. (*C*) Number of scan segments in infarct zones with thallium-201 redistribution and persistent defects. (Reproduced by permission from the American Heart Association [Circulation 73:1192, 1986].)

demonstrated that one may identify patients at risk for future coronary events after acute myocardial infarction by detecting patients whose left ventricular ejection fractions decrease and/or left ventricular end-systolic volumes increase at low-level exercise approximately 2 weeks after myocardial infarction (Figs. 9–5 and 9–6). Thus, one may also use submaximal exercise testing and radionuclide ventriculography to predict future prognosis after myocardial infarction in patients, irrespective of the location of the myocardial infarction, and including patients with non-Q-wave myocardial infarcts.

Therefore, one has several alternatives as regards attempting to predict future prognosis in patients with non-Q-wave infarcts after their initial recovery. In patients who continue to have angina at rest or low levels of activity, coronary arteriography and some form of revascularization is generally indicated. In patients who appear stable on an individually appropriate medical regimen, low-level exercise testing with either perfusion imaging (thallium-201 or, in the future, possibly with technetium-labeled isonitrile analogues) or radionuclide ventricu-

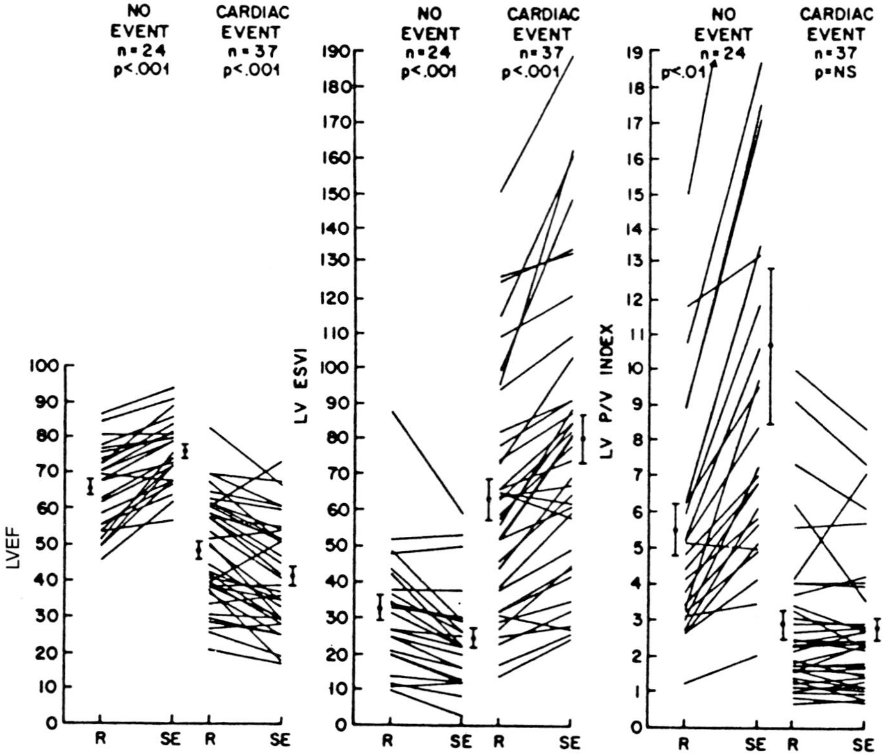

Figure 9–5. Left ventricular ejection fractions (LVEF), left ventricular end-systolic volume indexes (LVESVI), and left ventricular pressure-volume (P/V) indexes at rest (R) and during submaximal exercise (SE). The mean ± SEM are shown to the sides of each graph; p values are for the comparisons of mean values at rest and during submaximal exercise within each group. Patients are classified according to 6-month followup. The patients without future cardiac events had significant increases in their LVEFs and P/V indexes and decreases in their LVESVIs; whereas those with subsequent cardiac events had decreases in their LVEFs, increases in their LVESVIs, and no change in their P/V indexes. (Reproduced by permission from the American Heart Association [Circulation 64:540, 1981].)

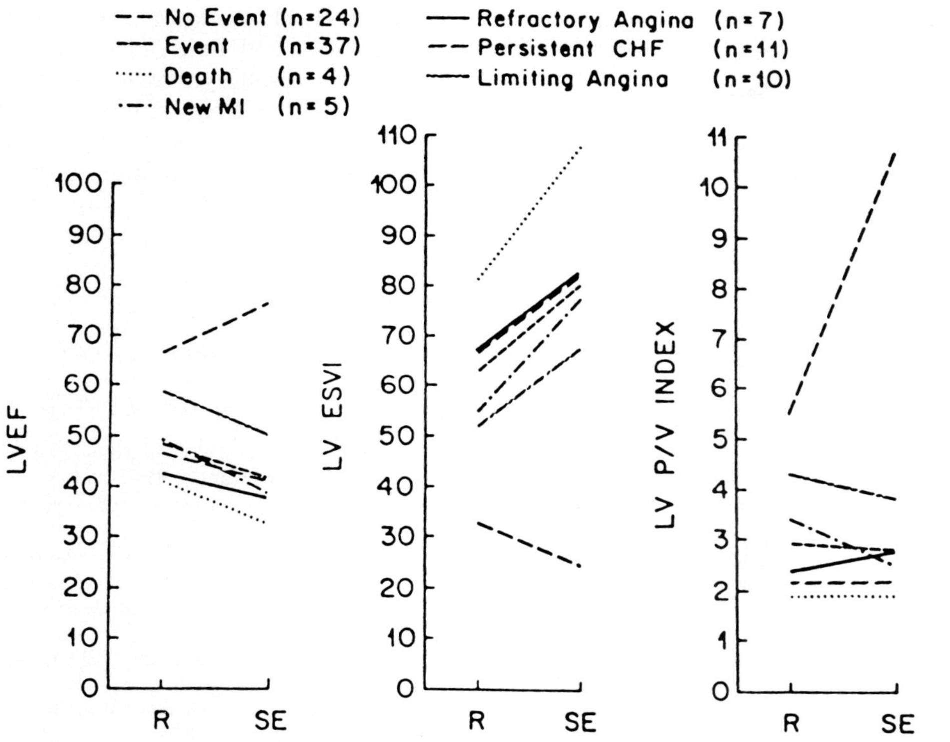

Figure 9–6. Submaximal exercise-induced alterations in mean left ventricular ejection fractions (LVEFs), left ventricular end-systolic volume indexes (LVESVIs), and pressure-volume (P/V) indexes. MI = myocardial infarction; CHF = congestive heart failure. (Reproduced by permission from the American Heart Association [Circulation 64:540, 1981].)

lography helps to identify patients at risk for future coronary events. In these individuals, if maximal medical therapy does not change this risk, coronary arteriography and, subsequently, coronary artery revascularization are usually indicated.

Differences in Therapy

Thrombolytic therapy is probably the treatment of choice for patients with acute Q-wave myocardial infarcts seen within the first 6 hours of the onset of symptoms.[65–79] Effective thrombolytic therapy given within the first 3 hours of the onset of symptoms suggestive of myocardial infarction generally preserves segmental ventricular function. Successful thrombolysis in patients with anterior Q-wave myocardial infarcts within the first 6 hours of the onset of symptoms reduces mortality.[65] However, patients with acute non-Q-wave myocardial infarcts are not generally treated with thrombolytic interventions presently, inasmuch as only a subset have persistent and completely occlusive coronary thrombi.[6,10] Instead, they are usually treated with platelet-active agents and interventions that improve coronary blood flow, including nitrates and calcium antagonists. In addition, some patients with non-Q-wave infarcts are treated with heparin with the hope that this may maintain patency of narrowed coronary arteries where recent platelet aggregation and platelet-derived mediator release have occurred. However, one needs to identify those patients with non-Q-wave infarcts (and those with Q-wave infarcts) at risk for future coronary events, including reinfarction, using the approaches identified earlier in this chapter. In patients at risk for future coronary events, more aggressive therapeutic approaches are warranted, including intensive medical therapy and, when appropriate, coronary arteriography and subsequent coronary artery revascularization.

REFERENCES

1. Phibbs, B: "Transmural" versus "subendocardial" myocardial infarction: An electrocardiographic myth. J Am Coll Cardiol 1:561, 1983.
2. Levine, HD: Subendocardial infarction in retrospect: Pathologic, cardiographic, and ancillary features. Circulation 72:790, 1985.
3. Spodick, DH: Q-wave infarction versus S-T infarction: Nonspecificity of electrocardiographic criteria for differentiating transmural and nontransmural lesions. Am J Cardiol 51:913, 1983.
4. Herrick, MB: Clinical features of sudden obstruction of the coronary arteries. JAMA 59:2015, 1912.
5. Blumgart, HL, Schlesinger, MJ, and Davis, D: Studies on the relation of the clinical manifestations of angina pectoris, coronary thrombosis, and myocardial infarction to the pathologic findings with particular reference to the significance of the collateral circulation. Am Heart J 19:1, 1940.
6. Buja, LM and Willerson, JT: Clinicopathologic correlates of acute ischemic heart disease syndromes. Am J Cardiol 47:343, 1981.
7. DeWood, MA, Spores, J, Notske, R, et al: Prevalence of total coronary occlusion during the early hours of transmural myocardial infarction. N Engl J Med 303:897, 1980.
8. Silver, MD, Baroldi, G, and Mariani, F: The relationship between acute occlusive coronary thrombi and myocardial infarction studied in 100 consecutive patients. Circulation 61:219, 1980.
9. Davies, MD and Thomas, AC: Plaque-fissuring—the cause of acute myocardial infarction, sudden ischaemic death, and crescendo angina. Br Heart J 53:363, 1985.
10. DeWood, MD, Stifter, WF, Simpson, CS, et al: Coronary arteriographic findings soon after non-Q wave myocardial infarction. N Engl J Med 315:417, 1986.
11. Willerson, JT, Campbell, WB, Winniford, MD, et al: Conversion from chronic to acute ischemic heart disease: Speculation regarding mechanisms (editorial). Am J Cardiol 5:1349, 1984.
12. Willerson, JT, Hillis LD, Winniford, JD, and Buja, LM: Speculation regarding mechanisms responsible for acute ischemic heart disease syndromes. J Am Coll Cardiol 8:245, 1986.
13. Bush, LR, Campbell, WB, Tilton, GD, et al: Effects of the selective thromboxane synthetase inhibitor dazoxiben on variations in cyclic blood flow in stenosed canine coronary arteries. Circulation 69:1161, 1984.
14. Bush, LR, Campbell, WB, Kern, K, et al: The effects of $alpha_2$ adrenergic and serotonergic receptor blockade on platelet aggregation in stenosed canine coronary arteries. Circ Res 55:642, 1984.
15. Apprill, P, Schmitz, JM, Campbell, WB, et al: Cyclic blood flow variations induced by platelet activating factor in stenosed canine coronary arteries despite inhibition of thromboxane synthetase, serotonin receptors, and alpha-adrenergic receptors. Circulation 72:397, 1985.
16. Schmitz, JM, Apprill, PG, Buja, LM, et al: Vascular prostaglandin and thromboxane production in a canine model of myocardial ischemia. Circ Res 57:223, 1985.
17. Ashton, JH, Benedict, CR, Fitzgerald, C, et al: Serotonin is a mediator of cyclic flow variations in stenosed canine coronary arteries. Circulation 73:572, 1986.
18. Buja, LM and Willerson, JT: The role of coronary artery lesions in ischemic heart disease: Insights from recent clinicopathologic coronary arteriographic and experimental studies. Hum Pathol 18:451, 1987.
19. Ashton, JH, Schmitz JM, Campbell, WB, et al: Inhibition of cyclic flow variations in stenosed canine coronary arteries by thromboxane A_2/prostaglandin H_2 receptor antagonists. Circ Res 59:568, 1986.
20. Apprill, PG, Ashton, J, Guerrero, J, et al: Ancrod decreases the frequency of cyclic flow variations and causes thrombolysis following acute coronary thrombosis. Am Heart J 113:898, 1987.

21. Ashton, JH, Ogletree, ML, Michel, IM, et al: Serotonin and thromboxane A_2/prostaglandin H_2 receptor activation cooperatively mediate cyclic flow variations in dogs with severe coronary artery stenoses. Circulation 76:952, 1987.
22. Golino, PG, Ashton, JH, Glas-Greenwalt, P, et al: Thromboxane A_2 and serotonin mediate reocclusion after thrombolysis with tissue-type plasminogen activator in a canine model of coronary thrombosis. Circulation, in press, 1988.
23. Golino, PG, Ashton, JH, Buja, LM, et al: Local platelet activation causes vasoconstriction of large epicardial canine coronary arteries in vivo. Thromboxane A_2 and serotonin are possible mediators. Circulation (in press), 1989.
24. Golino, PG, Buja, LM, Ashton, JH, et al: Effect of thromboxane and serotonin receptor antagonists on intracoronary platelet deposition in dogs with experimentally stenosed coronary arteries. Circulation 78:701, 1988.
25. Ashton, JH, Golino, P, McNatt, JM, et al: Serotonin S_2 receptor blockade (LY53857) combined with thromboxane A_2/prostaglandin H_2 receptor blockade (SQ29,548) provide protection against epinephrine-induced intermittent thrombosis in severely narrowed canine coronary arteries. Submitted for publication.
26. van den Berg, EK, Schmitz, JM, Benedict, CR, et al: Transcardiac serotonin concentration is increased in selected patients with limiting angina and complex coronary lesion morphology. Circulation (in press),1989.
27. Hirsh, PD, Hillis, LD, Campbell, WB, et al: Release of prostaglandins and thromboxane into the coronary circulation in patients with ischemic heart disease. N Engl J Med 304:685, 1981.
28. Hirsh, PD, Campbell, WB, Willerson, JT, and Hillis, LD: Prostaglandins and ischemic heart disease. Am J Med 71:1009, 1981.
29. Gorlin, R, Fuster, V, and Ambrose, JA: Anatomic-physiologic links between acute coronary syndromes (editorial). Circulation 74:6, 1986.
30. Folts, JD, Crowell, EB, and Rowe, GG: Platelet aggregation in partially obstructed vessels and its elimination with aspirin. Circulation 54:365, 1976.
31. Folts, JD, Gallagher, K, and Rowe, GG: Blood flow reductions in stenosed canine coronary arteries: Vasospasm or platelet aggregation. Circulation 65:248, 1982.
32. Aiken, JW, Gorman, RR, and Shebuski, RJ: Prevention of blockage of partially obstructed coronary arteries with prostacyclin correlates with inhibition of platelet aggregation. Prostaglandins 17:483, 1979.
33. Bolli, R, Ware, JA, Brandon, TA, et al: Platelet-mediated thrombosis in stenosed canine coronary arteries: Inhibition by nicergoline, a platelet-active alpha-adrenergic antagonist. J Am Coll Cardiol 3:1417, 1984.
34. Fitzgerald, DJ, Roy, L, Catella, F, and Fitzgerald, GA: Platelet activation in unstable coronary disease. N Engl J Med 315:983, 1986.
35. Chesebro, JH and Fuster, V: The therapeutic challenge of plaque rupture: Value of biochemical markers. J Am Coll Cardiol 10:1005, 1987.
36. Lewis, HD, Davis, JW, Archibald, DG, et al: Protective effects of aspirin against acute myocardial infarction and death in men with unstable angina. N Engl J Med 309:396, 1983.
37. Cairns, JA, Gent, M, Singer, J, et al: Aspirin, sulfinpyrazone, or both in unstable angina. Results of a Canadian multicenter trial. N Engl J Med 313:369, 1985.
38. Roseman, MD: Painless myocardial infarction: A review of the literature and analysis of 220 cases. Ann Intern Med 41:1, 1954.
39. Margolis, JR, Kannel, WB, Feinleib, M, et al: Clinical features of unrecognized myocardial infarction—silent and symptomatic. Eighteen-year follow-up: The Framingham Study. Am J Cardiol 32:1, 1973.
40. Sullivan, W, Vlodaver, Z, Tuna, N, et al: Correlation of electrocardiographic and pathologic findings in healed myocardial infarction. Am J Cardiol 42:724, 1978.
41. Stone, PH, Raabe, DS, Jaffe, AS, et al, and the MILIS Study Group: Prognostic significance of location and type of myocardial infarction: Independent adverse outcome associated with anterior location. J Am Coll Cardiol. In press, 1988.
42. Hutter, AM, Jr, DeSanctis, RW, Flynn, T, and Yeatman, LA: Nontransmural myocardial infarction: A comparison of hospital and late clinical course of patients with that of matched patients with transmural anterior and transmural inferior myocardial infarction. Am J Cardiol 48:595, 1981.
43. Nicholson, MR, Roubin, GS, Bernstein, L, et al: Prognosis after an initial non-Q-wave myocardial infarction related to coronary arterial anatomy. Am J Cardiol 52:462, 1983.

44. Nicod, P, Corbett, J, Sanford, CF, et al: Comparison of the influence of acute transmural and nontransmural myocardial infarction on ventricular function. Am Heart J 107:28, 1984.
45. Isner, JM and Roberts, WC: Right ventricular infarction complicating left ventricular infarction secondary to coronary heart disease: Frequency, location, associated findings, and significance from analysis of 236 necropsy patients with acute or healed myocardial infarction. Am J Cardiol 42:885, 1978.
46. Cohn, JN, Guiha, NH, Broder, MI, and Limas, CJ: Right ventricular infarction. Clinical and hemodynamic features. Am J Cardiol 33:209, 1974.
47. Lorell, B, Leinbach, RC, Pohost, GM, et al: Right ventricular infarction: Clinical diagnosis and differentiation from cardiac tamponade and pericardial constriction. Am J Cardiol 43:465, 1979.
48. Buda, AJ, Macdonald, IL, Dubbin, JD, et al: Myocardial infarct extension: Prevalence, clinical significance, and problems in diagnosis. Am Heart J 105:744, 1983.
49. Muller, JE, Rude, RE, Braunwald, E, et al, and the MILIS Study Group: Myocardial infarct extension: Occurrence, outcome, and risk factors in the Multicenter Investigation of Limitation of Infarct Size. Ann Intern Med 108:1, 1988.
50. Rothkopf, M, Boerner, J, Stone, MJ, et al: Detection of myocardial infarction extension in patients by CK-B radioimmunoassay. Circulation 59:268, 1979.
51. Baker, JT, Bramlet, DA, Lester, RM, et al: Myocardial infarct extension: Incidence and relationship to survival. Circulation 65:918, 1982.
52. Marmor, A, Sobel, BE, and Roberts, E: Factors presaging early recurrent myocardial infarction ("extension"). Am J Cardiol 48:603, 1981.
53. Gibson, RS, Beller, GA, Gheorghiade, M, et al: The prevalence and clinical significance of residual myocardial ischemia 2 weeks after uncomplicated non-Q wave infarction: A prospective natural history study. Circulation 73:1186, 1986.
54. Connolly, DC and Elveback, LR: Coronary heart disease in residents of Rochester, Minnesota. VI. Hospital and posthospital course of patients with transmural and subendocardial myocardial infarction. Mayo Clin Proc 60:375, 1985.
55. Rigo, R, Murray, M, Taylor, DR, et al: Hemodynamic and prognostic findings in patients with transmural and nontransmural infarction. Circulation 51:1064, 1975.
56. Madias, JE and Gorlin, R: The myth of "mild" myocardial infarction. Ann Intern Med 86:347, 1977.
57. Zema, MJ: Q-wave, S-T segment, and T-wave myocardial infarction. Am J Med 78:391, 1985.
58. Goldberg, RJ, Gore, JM, Alpert, JS, et al: Non-Q wave myocardial infarction: Recent changes in occurrence and prognosis—a community-wide perspective. Am Heart J 113:273, 1987.
59. Madias, JE, Chahine, RA, Gorlin, R, et al: A comparison of transmural and nontransmural acute myocardial infarction. Circulation 49:498, 1974.
60. Madigan, NP, Rutherford, BD, and Frye, RL: The clinical course, early prognosis and coronary anatomy of subendocardial infarction. Am J Med 60:634, 1976.
61. Maisen, AS, Ahnve, S, Gilpin, E, et al: Prognosis after extension of myocardial infarct: The role of Q-wave or non-Q-wave infarction. Circulation 71:211, 1985.
62. Gibson, RS, Boden, WE, Theroux, P, et al, and the Diltiazem Reinfarction Study Group: Diltiazem and reinfarction in patients with non-Q wave myocardial infarction. Results of a double-blind randomized, multicenter trial. N Engl J Med 315:423, 1986.
63. Corbett, JR, Dehmer, GJ, Lewis, SE, et al: The prognostic value of submaximal exercise testing with radionuclide ventriculography prior to hospital discharge in patients with recent myocardial infarction. Circulation 64:535, 1981.
64. Corbett, JR, Nicod, P, Lewis, SE, et al: Prognostic value of submaximal exercise radionuclide ventriculography following acute transmural and nontransmural myocardial infarction. Am J Cardiol 52:82A, 1983.
65. Gruppo Italiano Per Lo Studio Della Streptochinasi Nell'Infarcto Miocardico (GISSI): Effectiveness of intravenous thrombolytic treatment in acute myocardial infarction. Lancet 1:397, 1986.
66. Yusuf, S, Collins, R, Peto, R, et al: Intravenous and intracoronary fibrinolytic therapy in acute myocardial infarction: Overview of results on mortality, reinfarction, and side effects from 33 randomized control trials. Eur Heart J 6:556, 1985.
67. Laffel, GL and Braunwald, E: Thrombolytic therapy. A new strategy for treatment of acute myocardial infarction. N Engl J Med 311:710, 770, 1984.
68. Bergmann, SR, Lerch, RA, Fox, KAA, et al: The temporal dependence of beneficial effects of coronary thrombolysis characterized by positron tomography. Am J Med 73:573, 1982.

69. Reimer, KA and Jennings, RB: The wavefront phenomenon of myocardial ischemic cell death. II. Transmural progression of necrosis within the framework of ischemic bed size (myocardium at risk) and collateral flow. Lab Invest 40:633, 1979.
70. Braunwald, E and Kloner, RA: Myocardial reperfusion: A double-edged sword? J Clin Invest 76:1713, 1985.
71. Smalling, RW, Fuentes, F, Matthews, MW, et al: Factors affecting outcome of coronary reperfusion with intracoronary streptokinase in acute myocardial infarction. Am J Cardiol 59:505, 1987.
72. Mathey, DG, Sheehan, FH, Schofer, J, and Dodge, HT: Time from onset of symptoms to thrombolytic therapy: A major determinant of myocardial salvage in patients with acute transmural infarction. J Am Coll Cardiol 6:581, 1985.
73. The TIMI Study Group: The thrombolysis in myocardial infarction (TIMI) trial. Phase I findings. N Engl J Med 312:932, 1985.
74. Verstraete, M, Bory, M, Collen, D, et al: Randomized trial of intravenous recombinant tissue-type plasminogen activator versus intravenous streptokinase in acute myocardial infarction. Lancet 1:842, 1985.
75. Badger, RS, Brown, BG, Kennedy, JW, et al: Usefulness of recanalization to luminal diameter of 0.6 millimeter or more with intracoronary streptokinase during acute myocardial infarction in predicting "normal" perfusion status, continued arterial patency and survival at one year. Am J Cardiol 59:519, 1987.
76. Simoons, ML, Brands, M, De Zwaan, C, et al: Improved survival after early thrombolysis in acute myocardial infarction. Lancet 2:578, 1985.
77. Gold, HK, Leinbach, RC, Garabedian, HD, et al: Acute coronary reocclusion after thrombosis with recombinant human tissue-type plasminogen activator: Prevention by a maintenance infusion. Circulation 73:347, 1986.
78. Bush, LR, Samowitz, W, Buja, LM, et al: Recovery of left ventricular segmental function after long-term reperfusion following temporary coronary occlusion in conscious dogs: Comparison of 2- and 4-hour occlusions. Circ Res 53:248, 1983.
79. Bush, LR, Buja, LM, Tilton, G, et al: Effects of propranolol and diltiazem alone and in combination on the recovery of left ventricular segmental function after long-term reperfusion following temporary coronary occlusion in conscious dogs. Circulation 72:413, 1985.

CHAPTER 10

Myocardial Infarction in the Young and in Women

Deborah A. Jalowiec, M.D.
James A. Hill, M.D.

Ischemic heart disease in the young population occurs with relatively low frequency in comparison with older individuals. However, it attracts attention, owing to the potential for premature death and long-term disability with resulting consequences for society. The available reports discussing premature coronary artery disease and myocardial infarction use different definitions of young age, ranging from 30 to 56 years, and thus present a mixed picture. The purpose of this chapter is to examine the problem of coronary artery disease (CAD) and myocardial infarction (MI) in men younger than 40 and in women younger than 46.

INCIDENCE AND ETIOLOGY

Data have shown that about 2 percent to 6 percent of MIs occur in patients less than 40 years of age.[1–3] In men under 40 years of age, an incidence of 0.1 to 0.9 MIs/1000 individuals/year has been shown.[1] The large majority of these patients with MI have severe coronary atherosclerosis, accounting for 80 percent to 85 percent of patients.[4] However, in addition to single and multivessel CAD, occasional patients are found with normal coronary arteries and left ventricular wall motion abnormalities. Moreover, several types of coronary artery anomalies occur and have particular significance in adults. Anomalous origin of the coronary arteries from the pulmonary artery occurs in approximately 0.4 percent of all patients with congenital cardiac anomalies.[5] Approximately 15 percent of such patients survive into adulthood, owing to adequate intracoronary collaterals, and may present with myocardial ischemia or injury.[6] Origin of both coronary arteries from the left or right sinus of Valsalva occurred in slightly greater than 1 percent of a large group of patients undergoing coronary angiography.[7] When both the right and left coronary arteries arise from the right sinus of Valsalva, it is thought that flow to the left coronary artery may be diminished and may lead to myocardial ischemia. The suggested mechanism involves narrowing and/or compression of the proximal left coronary artery.[8] Congenital coronary arteriovenous fistulas often present in the fifth or sixth decades with myocardial ischemia and symptoms of left ventricular failure.[9] Fistulas of the right coronary artery occur more frequently than the left coronary artery and involve the right atrium, coronary sinus, or right ventricle.[9] Although these coronary anomalies are of interest, they account for a very small number of patients with MI.

Interest in CAD in the young was stimulated by findings of Yater, Enos, and their colleagues[10–12] from the late 1940s to the mid 1950s. Autopsy studies evaluated 300 American soldiers killed in battle with an average age of 22 years and found significant CAD in 77 percent.[13] An early report of angiographic findings in young men evaluated for chest pain was published in 1970.[14] Forty-nine percent of these 357 men were found to have 50 percent or greater narrowing of one or more coronary arteries. Subsequent studies included clinical and historical information in addition to anatomic data.[15] These investigations have led to an increased interest in the identification of risk factors and clinical variables in order to provide guidelines for the diagnosis and management of CAD and MI in this younger subset.

RISK FACTORS

Much attention has been focused on the evaluation of conventional risk factors in young patients with MI. Although the etiology of CAD appears to be multifactorial in all age groups, an increased number of risk factors has been observed in this younger population. Uhl and Farrell[16] compared male MI patients under age 40 with MI patients over age 40. They showed significantly more risk factors in the younger group compared with the older group.

A correlation between the mean number of risk factors per patient and the extent of vessel involvement has been demonstrated repeatedly in this young population.[16–18] Values range from 1.3 risk factors per patient[17] for single vessel disease to 3.5 risk factors per patient[18] in those with triple-vessel disease. Moret and coworkers[17] observed that young patients with more than three risk factors have a high probability for severe CAD and a poorer long-term prognosis with respect to postinfarction angina and recurrence of infarction. However, Gohlke and associates[18] have suggested that unique mechanisms may account for premature coronary disease in the young, which is not explained exclusively by the presence of a large number of risk factors. They evaluated 844 patients under the age of 40 with documented transmural MI. When this group was divided into patients under 30 years, 30 to 34 years, and 35 to 39 years, the lowest prevalence of risk factors was noted in the youngest age group (Fig. 10–1).

Cigarette smoking is uniformly the most common risk factor in young MI patients, with an incidence ranging from 61 percent to 93 percent in various studies.[16–21] Weinberger's[19] study of 30 patients under 30 years of age with acute MI demonstrated smoking to be the only risk factor of importance, with a low prevalence of the other conventional risk factors. In fact, 23 percent of his patients had none of the other conventional risk factors.

Following tobacco use, there is less consistency in the prevalence of other risk factors. Hyperlipidemia, including hypercholesterolemia and/or hypertriglyceridemia, is defined as cholesterol levels >250 mg% and triglyceride levels >150

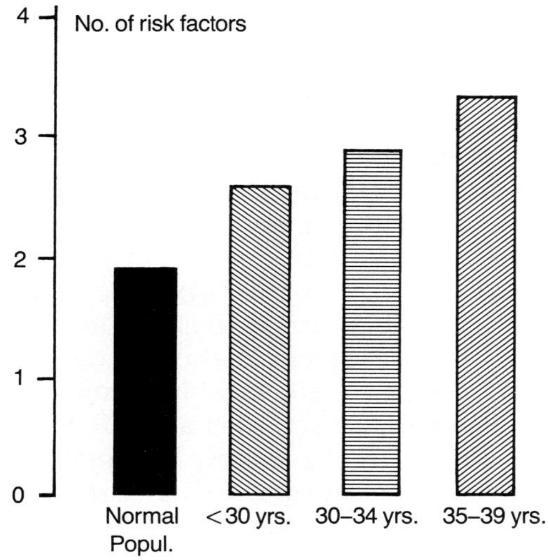

Figure 10–1. Mean number of risk factors in patients with transmural MI in the three different age groups, compared with normal controls. (From Gohlke, H, Sturzenhofecker, P, Thilo, A, et al: Coronary angiographic findings and risk factors in postinfarction patients under the age of 40. In Roskamm, H (ed): Myocardial Infarction at Young Age. Springer-Verlag, Heidelberg, 1981, p 69, with permission.)

mg%. The prevalence of hyperlipidemia in young MI patients ranged from 41 percent to 80 percent in numerous studies[16–21] and has generally been shown to be one of the three most important risk factors in the young population. Data from Uhl and Farrell[16] and Gofman and colleagues[22] suggest that hyperlipidemia is a more reliable predictor of recurrent MI in patients aged 30 to 39 than in older age groups.

A positive family history, defined as premature incidence of overt CAD in a first-degree relative, has a wide range of prevalence in this young population, varying from 14 percent to 69 percent.[16–21] Most often, it is one of the three major risk factors. Rissanen and Nikkila[23] determined that the younger the patient is when the first MI occurs, the more common was CAD in relatives. In addition, they demonstrated up to a tenfold excess risk of developing CAD in siblings of patients who suffered an MI before the age of 46 years. Twin studies also suggest a strong inherited component in early onset compared with a late onset of MI.[24]

Whereas obesity is variably regarded as a risk factor for CAD, it appears to be related to the occurrence of CAD and MI in the young. Defined as body weight exceeding ideal body weight by 20 percent or more, obesity was found in 30 percent to 58 percent of young patients with ischemic heart disease.[16–18,20] Its prevalence was significantly greater compared with an older age group with CAD[16] and a similar age control group.[17,18,20] It should be pointed out that obesity is frequently present with hyperlipidemia, hypertension, or diabetes mellitus.

Hypertension and diabetes mellitus, established risk factors for CAD,[25] appear to have less importance in younger than in older patients. Although the presence of hypertension is greater in a population of young patients with MI than in those without MI, it is lower compared with older patients with MI. The prevalence of hypertension in young patients with MI ranges from 14 percent to 30 percent.[16–18,20,21] It is possible that duration of hypertension may be more important than the presence of hypertension as a risk factor for MI. The prevalence of diabetes mellitus in young patients with CAD, although greater than in the normal controls, is low, being less than 10 percent in several studies.[16,17,19,21]

There is increasing evidence that cocaine use is associated with occurrence of MI in young patients and is not limited to intravenous use.[26,27] The evidence is based on a temporal association between the use of cocaine and subsequent MI in patients with and without preexisting fixed coronary disease.[26,28] There are several speculations as to the involved mechanism. Myocardial ischemia secondary to increased sympathetic activity in patients with fixed atherosclerotic lesions and coronary constriction have been suggested. Other possibilities include endothelial thrombotic effects due to the drug itself or its contaminants, or direct cardiovascular effects of contaminants, including quinidine, procainamide, amphetamines, and talc.[28] Prognosis for a patient who survives an MI related to cocaine appears to be excellent if cocaine use is discontinued.

Although not truly a risk factor, physical activity preceding MI is an important consideration in young patients. Several studies have determined that extreme physical exertion at the time of MI is more common in the younger age group and may have a role in etiology. Uhl and Farrell[16] noted that in 32 percent of the young patients, MI was associated with physical stress, compared with 20 percent of the older patients. Gohlke[29] and Roskamm[30] and their colleagues showed a greater incidence of physical exertion in patients without severe CAD but with documented MI compared with patients with multivessel CAD (27 percent versus 12 percent and 25 percent versus 10 percent, respectively). One possible explanation for this difference may be that younger people are more likely to be engaged in heavy physical exertion than older people. It is not clear whether degree of physical activity is a risk factor for CAD per se.

In summary, young MI patients generally have more of the conventional risk factors than older patients. A direct correlation between the number of risk factors and severity of atherosclerosis has been demonstrated repeatedly. Cigarette smoking is overwhelmingly the most prevalent risk factor in this subset of patients.

CORONARY ANGIOGRAPHIC FINDINGS

Single vessel CAD is the most common angiographic finding in young patients with MI.[3,16,18,19,21,30–33,39] The left anterior descending artery is most commonly involved, followed by the right, circumflex, and left main coronary arteries.[4,41] Despite the involvement of only one vessel, the extent of left ventricular dysfunction appears as great as in older patients with more extensive CAD. This suggests that MI in the young occurs secondary to rapid occlusion of the coronary artery, without time for establishment of collateral pathways.[4] Multivessel CAD occurs in 30 percent to 40 percent of young patients with MI,[3,16,18,19,21,31–33,39] but this does not seem to correlate with numerous clinical and ECG parameters. Vanhaecke and coworkers[36] found that results of exercise treadmill stress testing, serum cholesterol, smoking habits, and the presence of angina before or after infarction all proved to be poor predictors of multivessel disease in young men who have survived an MI. Sheldon and coworkers[39] suggested that a higher prevalence of multivessel disease is found in survivors.

Starzenhofecker and colleagues,[35] in their followup angiograms of young MI patients, demonstrated little progression of atherosclerosis in patients with one vessel disease over an average of 3.5 years of followup (24 percent versus 37.7 percent). This finding was in contrast to the high frequency of progression in patients with multivessel disease diagnosed at the time of MI. Regression was found in 16 percent of the patients with one-vessel disease as compared with 7 percent of those with multivessel disease. Regression of CAD occurred predominantly in the proximal left anterior descending artery. Whether this represents true regression or only recanalization is uncertain. Two different patterns of CAD progression in patients with multivessel disease have been proposed by Kapoor.[34] In one, the progression of disease is slower, which allows for development of intracoronary collaterals. This pattern is more consistent with that encountered in an older population. In the second type, there is diffuse and extensive atherosclerosis, and disease is relentlessly progressive. These patients often have a familial history of atherosclerosis and hyperlipidemia.

NORMAL CORONARY ARTERIES WITH LEFT VENTRICULAR WALL MOTION ABNORMALITIES

An interesting subset of patients with MI are those without severe CAD noted by subsequent angiogram. The incidence of normal coronary arteries in all patients with MI ranges from 1 percent to 15 percent.[38,43] In young patients, the incidence has been reported to be as high as 32 percent, but in most studies ranges between 8 percent and 17 percent (Table 10–1).[3,16,18,19,21,30–33,39] These patients often have few or no risk factors and no angina prior to MI.[3,16,18,19,38] Infarction location is variable, and different studies show either an inferior wall predilection[16] or an almost equal division between anterior, inferior, and lateral walls.[19] In an autopsy series of these patients, the size of the infarcted area ranged from 5 percent to 33 percent of the myocardium. The prognosis for survival after the acute event in such patients is usually excellent; however, fatalities have been reported.[34] The majority of such patients subsequently have normal exercise stress tests, and only a small number develop angina or recurrent infarction.[38,39]

Several mechanisms have been proposed for the occurrence of myocardial infarction with normal coronary arteries. Coronary vasospasm, spontaneous lysis

Table 10–1. Extent of CAD in Young Patients

Study	Total Number of Patients	3VD (%)	2VD (%)	1VD (%)	No CAD (%)
Uhl[16]	81	31	35	23	11
Sheldon[39]	236	8	28	63	3
Weinberger[19]	25	24	8	36	32
Kennelly[21]	50	20	22	52	4
Bergstrand[3]	18	11	11	56	17
Koskennou[33]†	19		< 89 >		11
Vojacek[32]‡	96	< 32 >		43	26*
Roskamm[30]‡	679	< 34 >		57	8.4
Robert[31]†	22		< 92 >		8
	619	15	19	58	8
Gohlke[18]					

*Includes insignificant CAD.

†Further breakdown of individual vessels involved not given.

‡No further division made for multivessel disease.

of a coronary thrombus on a small nonobstructing plaque, coronary embolism from the endocardium or heart valve, and angiographically indiscernible coronary lesions have all been implicated.

SEVERITY OF CLINICAL COURSE

The presence of preinfarction angina is variable in young patients, ranging from 16 percent to 53 percent.[16,19,33,37] In a large comparison study with older MI patients, the incidence was statistically less common in the younger patients.[37] However, Uhl and Farrell[16] found no difference between the two groups. A significantly larger number of inferior MIs occur in younger patients compared with older patients, but there is no difference in the frequency of anterior MI. Transmural MI with associated left ventricular wall motion abnormality is more common than subendocardial infarction. In addition, young patients have been shown to have more extensive MIs, based on peak enzyme levels.[37]

Complications during MI occur with equal or less frequency in the younger population.[16,37] Common complications include arrhythmias, with ventricular arrhythmias being more common in the young group than in the older group,[37] and congestive heart failure in 17 percent to 20 percent of the young patients.[16,19]In-hospital mortality has been found to be significantly lower for the younger age group (2.5 percent to 3 percent).[16,37]

PROGNOSIS

Long-term survival of young patients who survive an infarction as determined by one study showed that 77.3 percent of patients were alive at the end of the 16-year study.[44] This corresponds to a mortality rate of 5 percent a year as determined from the Framingham study in patients uncontrolled for age.[45] Extended long-term followup studies, for up to 16 years, determined that 34 percent to 45 percent of a group of young MI patients develop a recurrence.[42,44] The second MI was fatal in over half of these patients (56 percent).[44] Postinfarction angina occurs in approximately 50 percent of surviving individuals.[19,34,42] As expected, the presence of postinfarction angina has been associated with multivessel CAD.[36] Progression of atherosclerosis over a 7-year time span has been found to be significantly more frequent in patients with multivessel disease at initial diagnosis as compared with those having single-vessel involvement (34.3 percent versus 3.6 percent).[35] In young MI patients, 96 percent were able to return to work after the initial recovery period, with 78 percent resuming their former positions, compared with an 85 percent employment rate in the Framingham study.[44,45] It is unknown how modern aggressive management and risk factor reduction will change the prognosis.

MYOCARDIAL INFARCTION IN WOMEN

The low incidence of MI in women, particularly those of young age, has limited the ability to investigate this entity adequately. The majority of studies have addressed CAD and angina in combination with MI. Coronary artery disease, as used in this section, will refer to the spectrum of disease, including MI.

Coronary artery disease accounts for approximately one-third of all deaths in women, ranking second only to neoplasms in most Western nations for the age group 25 to 64 years.[46] The annual mortality rate secondary to CAD increases with aging up to 70 years, whereas it levels off at age 50 years in men.[40] Coronary artery disease in women is more apt to present as angina than MI or sudden death.[46] Conventional risk factors associated with MI in men have similar implications in women, with oral contraceptives being an additional consideration. At comparable levels of risk factors, however, the risk of MI in women is only one-half that in men of similar age.[46] In an angiographic study of young women with chest pain, significant CAD was found in 55 percent of the women with more than two risk factors but only in 7 percent of those with less than two risk factors ($p \leq 0.001$).[47]

As with men, cigarette smoking correlates significantly with the extent of CAD. The risk of MI appears to increase with the number of cigarettes smoked, even in the absence of other predisposing factors. Slone and colleagues[48] have demonstrated a sevenfold increase in MI risk for young women smoking less than 24 cigarettes per day. For those smoking more than 35 cigarettes per day, the risk escalates twentyfold over women who never smoked.

Familial aggregation of CAD occurs more commonly in families of female index patients. Slack and Evans[50] found a sevenfold increase in CAD among female relatives of female patients with premature CAD, while Thordarsson and Fridriksson[52] found the greatest risk among first-degree male relatives of female index patients.[51]

Oral contraceptives influence carbohydrate and lipid metabolism. An increase in serum triglycerides, and to a lesser extent serum cholesterol, occurs with high estrogen dosage but appears not to occur with low estrogen preparations.[49,52] In addition, oral contraceptives have been found to increase blood pressure and predispose to thrombotic events. Duration of use has also been shown to increase risk of cardiac and vascular disease.[53] The presence of other risk factors and increasing age have additive effects in increasing an individual's cardiac risk. Women who have at least one coronary risk factor and are birth control pill users may have up to a fourfold increase in the likelihood of sustaining an MI.[46] However, noncontraceptive estrogen use does not augment the risk of atherosclerosis and may even have a protective effect in young women who have undergone oophorectomy.[54,55]

Serum cholesterol is generally lower in women than in men until the sixth decade, but then the reverse is true. High-density lipoprotein levels are also higher among women, which impart an additional favorable effect in women without other risk factors.

After the age of 45, both hypertension and diabetes mellitus tend to be more prevalent in women than in men.[46] A cross-sectional study has shown a twofold increase in prevalence of CAD in women with blood pressure and blood sugar levels in the highest quartile.[56] Hypertension and diabetes mellitus were found by Waters and associates[47] to be at least twice as frequent in women with significant CAD than in those with normal coronary arteries. In the Framingham study, a twofold risk for CAD persisted even after adjustment for additional risk factors.[57]

Women who sustain an MI have a poorer prognosis than men. There is a 75 percent greater mortality in the first month after infarction in women compared with men.[46] The 1-year mortality and risk of reinfarction are more than double in women compared with men.[46] The long-term prognosis is also less favorable.

During 12 years of followup of women up to age 60 with MI, a mortality rate of about 50 percent was shown.[58]

In the absence of risk factors, CAD is uncommon in young women. When the disease occurs, angina pectoris is more likely to be the initial presentation rather than MI or sudden death. After MI, however, both the acute and long-term prognosis are unfavorable.

SUMMARY

Although only 2 percent to 6 percent of MIs occur in young patients, this disorder represents a major cause of long-term disability in this group. In these patients, an increased number of conventional risk factors has been observed, with cigarette smoking being the most prevalent. Angiography in young patients with MI most often demonstrates single-vessel CAD and slow progression of atherosclerosis. When multivessel CAD is found, the long-term prognosis is less favorable.

In women, CAD is more likely to present as angina than MI or sudden death. Cigarette smoking and oral contraceptive use are important risk factors. Although MIs in women occur less often than in men, women experience a less favorable acute and long-term prognosis.

REFERENCES

1. Lamm, G: The epidemiology of acute myocardial infarction in young age groups. In Roskamm, H (ed): Myocardial Infarction at Young Age. Springer-Verlag, Heidelberg, 1981.
2. Simonson, E and Berman, R: Myocardial infarction in young people—experience in the USSR. Am Heart J 84(6):814, 1972.
3. Bergstrand, R, Vedin, A, Wilkelmsson, C, et al: Myocardial infarction among men below age 40. Br Heart J 40:783–788, 1978.
4. Kapoor, AS: Assessment, risk stratification and prognosis of young patients after myocardial infarction. Cardiovasc Rev Reports 7:1, 14–28, 1986.
5. Wesselhoeft, H, Fawcett, JS, and Johnson, AL: Anomalous angina of the left coronary artery from the pulmonary trunk: Its clinical spectrum, pathology and pathophysiology based on a review of 140 cases with 7 further cases. Circulation 38:403, 1968.
6. Chaitman, BR, Lesperance, J, Sahiel, J, and Bourassa, MG: Clinical, angiographic and hemodynamic findings in patients with anomalous origin of coronary arteries. Circulation 53:122, 1976.
7. Kimbiris, D, Iskandrian, AS, Segal, BL, and Bemis, E: Anomalous aortic origin of the coronary arteries. Circulation 58:606, 1978.
8. Chertlin, MD, DeCostro, CM, and McAllister, HA: Sudden death as a complication of anomalous left coronary origin from the anterior sinus of Valsalva. A not-so-minor congenital anonaly. Circulation 50:780, 1974.
9. Liberthson, RR, Sagar, K, Berkobev, JP, et al: Congenital coronary arteriovenous fistula: Report of 13 patients, reviews of the literature and delineation of management. Circulation 59:849, 1979.
10. Yater, W, Traum, A, Brown, W, et al: Coronary artery disease in men 18–39 years of age. Am Heart J 36:334, 1948.
11. Yater, W, Welsh, P, Stapelton, J, et al: Comparison of clinical and pathologic aspects of coronary artery disease in men of various age groups. Ann Intern Med 34:352, 1951.
12. Enos, W, Beyer, J, and Holmes, R: Pathogenesis of coronary disease of American soldiers killed in Korea. JAMA 158:912, 1955.
13. Blackburn, H: Progress in epidemology and prevention of coronary heart disease in YU PN. In Goodwin, JF (ed): Progress in Cardiology. Lea & Febiger, Philadelphia, 1974.
14. Welch, C, Proudfit, W, Sones, F, et al: Cinecoronary arteriography in young men. Circulation 42:647–652, 1970.

15. Davia, J, Hallal, F, Cheitlin, M, et al: Coronary artery disease in young patients: Anteriographic and clinical review of 40 cases aged 35 and under. Am Heart J 87:689–696, 1974.
16. Uhl, G and Farrell, P: Myocardial infarction in young adults: Risk factors and natural history. Am Heart J 105:548, 1983.
17. Moret, P, Gutziviller, F, and Junod B: Coronary artery disease in young adults under 35 years old: Risk factors (Swiss Surgery). In Roskamm, H (ed): Myocardial Infarction at Young Age. Springer-Verlag, Heidelberg, 1981.
18. Gohlke, H, Sturzenhofecker, P, Thilo, A, et al: Coronary angiographic findings and risk factors in postinfarction patients under the age of 40. In Roskamm, H (ed): Myocardial Infarction at Young Age. Springer-Verlag, Heidelberg, 1981.
19. Weinberger, F, Rotenberg, Z, Fiechs, J, et al: Myocardial infarction in young adults under 30 years: Risk factors and clinical course. Clin Cardiol 10:9–15, 1987.
20. Nitter-Hauge, S, Erikssen, J, Thaulow, E, et al: Angiographic and risk factor characteristics of subjects with early onset ischemic heart disease. Br Heart J 46:325–330, 1981.
21. Kennelly, BM, Gersh, BJ, Lane, GK, et al: The relationship between angiographic findings and risk factors in young men with myocardial infarction. S Afr Med J 61:508, 1982.
22. Gofman, JW, Young, W, and Tandy, R. Ischemic heart disease, atherosclerosis and longevity. Circulation 34:679, 1966.
23. Rissanen, AM and Nikkila, EE: Role of family history in coronary heart disease at young age. In Roskamm, H (ed): Myocardial Infarction at Young Age. Springer-Verlag, Heidelberg, 1981.
24. deFaire, U, Friberg, L, and Lundman, T: Concordance for mortality with special reference to ischemic heart disease and cerebrovascular disease. A study on the Swedish twin registry. Prev Med 4:509–517, 1975.
25. Kannel, WB, Sorlie, P, and McNamara, PM: Prognosis after initial myocardial infarction: The Framingham Study. Am J Cardiol 44:53, 1979.
26. Isner, JM, Estes, NAM, Thompson, PB, et al: Acute cardiac events temporally related to cocaine abuse. N Engl J Med 315(23):1438, 1986.
27. Pasternack, PF, Colvin, SB, and Baumann, FG: Cocaine-induced angina pectoris and acute myocardial infarction in patients younger than 40 years. 55:847, 1985.
28. Mathias, DW: Cocaine-associated myocardial ischemia. Am J Med 81:675, 1986.
29. Gohlke, H, Gohlke-Barwolf, C, Sturzenhofecker, P, et al: Myocardial infarction at young age—correlation of angiographic findings with risk factors and history in 619 patients. Circulation 62(Suppl III):39, 1980.
30. Roskamm, H, Gohlke, H, Sturzenhofecker, P, et al: Myocardial infarction at a young age (under 40 years). Int J Sports Med 5:1, 1984.
31. Robert, JPJ, Massabuav, P, Cassagneau, B, et al: Infarctus du myocarde avant l'age de 35 ans. Aspects cliniques et coronarographiques. La Presse Medicale 12:1911, 1983.
32. Vojacek, J, Fabian, J, and Belan, A: Myocardial infarction in men under 40. Risk factors, coronary angiography and long-term prognosis (abstr). Eur Heart J 5(Suppl 1):230, 1984.
33. Koskenvuo, K, Karvonen, MJ, and Rissanen, V: Death from ischemic heart disease in young Finns aged 15–24 years. Am J Cardiol 42:114, 1978.
34. Eliot, RS, Baroldi, G, and Leone, A: Necropsy studies in myocardial infarction with minimal or no coronary luminal reduction due to atherosclerosis. Circulation 49:1127, 1974.
35. Starzenhofecker, P, Samek, L, Droste, C, et al: Prognosis of coronary heart disease and progression of coronary atherosclerosis in post infarction patients under the age of 40. In Roskamm, H (ed): Myocardial Infarction at Young Age. Springer-Verlag, Heidelberg, 1981.
36. Vanhaecke, J, Piessens, J, Williams, J, et al: Coronary arterial lesions in young men who survived a first myocardial infarction: Clinical and electrocardiographic predictors of multivessel disease. Am J Cardiol 47:810, 1981.
37. Hoit, BD, Gilpin, EA, Henning, H, et al: Myocardial infarction in young patients: An analysis by age subsets. Circulation 74(4):712–721, 1986.
38. Arnett, EN and Roberts, WC: Acute myocardial infarction and angiographically normal coronary arteries. An unproven combination. Circulation 53:395, 1976.
39. Sheldon, WC, Razavi, M, and Lim, VJ: Coronary arteriographic findings in younger survivors of acute myocardial infarction including those with normal coronary arteries. In Roskamm, H (ed): Myocardial Infarction at Young Age. Springer-Verlag, Heidelberg, 1981.
40. Johansson, S, Vedin, A, and Wilhelmsson, C: Myocardial infarction in women. Epidemiol Rev 5:67, 1983.

41. Virami, R and McAllister, HA: Coronary heart disease at young age: A report of 187 autopsy patients who died of severe coronary atherosclerosis. Cardiovasc Rev Reports 5(8):799, 1984.
42. Gertler, MM, White, PD, Simon, R, and Gottsch, L: Long-term follow up study of young coronary patients. Am J Med Sci 247:145, 1964.
43. Thomspon, SI, Vieweg, WVR, Alpert, JS, et al: Incidence and age distribution of patients with myocardial infarction and normal coronary arteriograms. Cathet Cardiovasc Diagn 3:1–9, 1977.
44. Roth, O, Berki, A, and Wolff, GD: Long range observation in fifty-three young patients with myocardial infarction. Am J Cardiol 19:331, 1967.
45. Kannel, W, Sorlie, P, and McNamara, P: Prognosis after initial myocardial infarction: The Framingham Study. Am J Cardiol 44:53, 1979.
46. Wenger, NK: Coronary disease in women. Annu Rev Med 36:285, 1985.
47. Waters, DD, Halphen, C, Theroux, P, et al: Coronary artery disease in young women: Clinical and angiographic features and correlation with risk factors. Am J Cardiol 42:41, 1978.
48. Slone, D, Shapiro, S, Rosenberg, L, et al: Relation of cigarette smoking to myocardial infarction in young women. N Engl J Med 298:1273, 1978.
49. Stokes, T and Wynn, V: Serum lipids in women on oral contraceptives. Lancet 2:677, 1971.
50. Slack, J and Evans, KA: The increased risk of death from ischemic heart disease in first degree relatives of 121 men and 91 women with ischemic heart disease. J Med Genet 3:239, 1966.
51. Thordarsson, O and Fridriksson, S: Aggregation of death from ischemic heart disease among first and second degree relatives of 108 males and 42 females with MI. Acta Med Scand 205:493, 1979.
52. Wynn, V, Adams, PW, Godsland, T, et al: Comparison of effects of different combined oral contraceptive formulations on carbohydrate and lipid metabolism. Lancet 1:1045, 1979.
53. Royal College of General Practioners' Oral Contraceptive Study: Mortality among oral contraceptive users. Lancet 2:729, 1977.
54. Bain, C, Wilett, W, Hennekens, CH, et al: Use of postmenopausal hormones and risk of myocardial infarction. Circulation 64:42, 1981.
55. Rosenberg, L, Slone, D, Shapiro, S, et al: Noncontraceptive estrogens and myocardial infarction in young women. JAMA 244(4):339, 1980.
56. Epstein, PH, Ostrander, LD, Johnson, BC, et al: Epidemiolgic studies of cardiovascular disease in a total community—Tecumseh, Michigan. Ann Intern Med 62:1170, 1965.
57. Kannel, WB and McGee, DL: Diabetes and cardiovascular disease: The Framingham Study. JAMA 241:2035, 1979.
58. Lapidus, L: Ischemic heart disease, stroke and total mortality in women. Acta Med Scand [suppl] 705:1, 1985.

PART 4

Management

CHAPTER 11

Thrombolytic Therapy for Acute Myocardial Infarction

Allan M. Ross, M.D.

Angiographic evidence for the causative role of intracoronary thrombosis in myocardial infarction restimulated the current enthusiam for thrombolytic therapy in this prevalent syndrome. The major recent clinical trials, which have in general advanced our knowledge and provided some definitive answers to central questions (but as always generated new and important additional questions), fall into three categories (Table 11–1). In the early years of this decade, studies evaluated the lytic potential of intracoronary installation of routinely available lytic agents (streptokinase and urokinase). The next cluster of trials evaluated the clinical benefit and reperfusion rates of these agents delivered intravenously and examined also the potential of "second generation" thrombolytic substances (notably tissue plasminogen activator and acylated streptokinase). The third cluster of clinical trials, many ongoing at this time, are intended to refine combination strategies that begin with lytic therapy, but then include other pharmacologic adjuncts as well as mechanical interventions (most notably coronary angioplasty).

INTRACORONARY THROMBOLYSIS

It was perhaps predictable inasmuch as the angiographic laboratory provided the definitive proof that intracoronary thrombus was present in up to 85 percent of acute infarction victims studied within the first few hours of the symptom onset,[1] that the angiographers themselves modified the diagnostic procedure intent on providing definitive therapy at the time of catheterization. Initial reports, first from Western Europe,[2,3] and soon thereafter from the United States, demonstrated that clot lysis could be achieved utilizing relatively low-dose selective intracoronary instillation of (usually) streptokinase and (occasionally) urokinase. Up to 75 percent of totally occluded coronary arteries were reopened employing this approach, often within an hour of starting the selective lytic infusion, which typically consisted of 250,000 units (SK) administered over 10 to 90 minutes. Occasionally, pharmacological thrombolysis was augmented by guide

Table 11–1. Clinical Trials of Thrombolytic Therapy for Acute Myocardial Infarction

Intracoronary thrombolysis	(1980–1983)
Intravenous thrombolysis	(1983–1987)
Combination strategies	(1987–)

wire perforation of the clot, and some investigators utilized a small infusion catheter within the angiographic catheter to enter affected branches and accomplish subselective (or supraselective) infusion.

The efficacy of these interventions was analyzed predominantly by quantifying an improving left ventricular ejection fraction from the day of infarct to followup at hospital discharge or somewhat later.

Initial publications reported consecutive patients managed in this fashion and demonstrated improved outcome ejection fraction in many, thus confirming the mechanism of reperfusion leading to the salvage of jeopardized but not yet fully necrotic myocardium. These studies further demonstrated an important relationship between duration of complete occlusion and magnitude of ultimate benefit. Just as investigators in animal research laboratories had observed, very early reperfusion was associated with dramatic infarct size reduction, whereas later reperfusion was associated with relatively unimpressive gains. Exceptions, however, were observed—particularly the expanded "therapeutic window" available when well-established collaterals were present (unfortunately not common in acute infarction patients)[2] and when the infarct took a "stuttering" course possibly indicative of short recurrent periods of total thrombotic occlusion interspersed with spontaneous partial reperfusion.

Endpoints other than global left ventricular (LV) ejection fraction were considered, including infarct sizing by enzyme analysis and by ECG criteria, but these indices generally were not highly satisfactory. In patients without global LV improvement, regional analysis of the infarct zone was utilized to document smaller benefits and to compensate for the confounding effects of observed hyperkinesis in the unaffected zones of the infarcting ventricle.

Controlled clinical trials of selective intracoronary thrombolysis were then instituted with rigid entry criteria and true randomized controls. Multiple reports[4–6] soon became available, but disappointingly they documented only minimal or even absent group benefit from this costly and resource-consuming therapeutic approach.

Table 11–2 displays the change in global LV ejection fraction for treated patients and controls in some of the randomized trials of intracoronary thrombolysis. In the absence of substantial left ventricular functional benefit attendant to this therapy, it perhaps came as no surprise that the desired benefit in acute infarction mortality associated with these efforts was meager also. In his compilation of published randomized trials of intracoronary streptokinase, Furberg[7] found no difference in early and intermediate-term mortality rates comparing treated groups with controls.

Closer analysis established the obvious difficultly in generally accomplishing coronary reperfusion (by a method requiring triage, transportation to a catheter-

Table 11–2. Clinical Trials of Intracoronary Thrombolysis for Acute Myocardial Infarction: Improvement in Global LV Ejection Fraction from Admission to Followup

Author	Treated (%)	Controls (%)
Anderson	+4	−3
Leiboff	−1	−3
Kennedy	+1	+1
Khaja	0	+1
Rentrop	+2	−1

ization laboratory, and selective angiography before the therapeutic intervention could begin), within the time frame required to salvage large quantities of jeopardized myocytes. In most reporting centers, time from symptom onset to diagnostic angiography was in the 4- to 5-hour range. Even in centers particularly cognizant of the time factor and geared to rapid mobilization, time to actual reperfusion was usually late.

These important but disappointing studies led directly to the second phase of thrombolysis investigations, namely, the application of lytic drugs administered much earlier in the infarct course by utilizing the simpler intravenous route.

INTRAVENOUS THROMBOLYSIS

Several decades before coronary angiography became routinely available, acute coronary thrombosis was considered to be the proximate cause of myocardial infarction. Subsequently, pathologists were misled (and, therefore, in turn misled clinicians) by finding a much lower-than-expected incidence of thrombotic coronary occlusion in hospitalized patients who later died of infarct sequelae. These observations, however, antedated the current understanding that in up to half the patients with infarction, intrinsic thrombolytic mechanisms result in clot dissolution in the hours, days, and weeks after infarct onset. Not until 1979 was the etiological role of the clot fully re-established. Shortly before the coronary thrombosis theory fell out of favor, a number of intravenous thrombolytic and anticoagulant trials were undertaken.[8] These studies, performed two decades (or more) ago, suffered from lack of information regarding the time factor in limiting myocardial necrosis, and further from the lack of endpoint techniques available to current investigators. While on the right track, the potential benefits of such efforts were, therefore, not established to the satisfaction of the clinical-care community.

Toward the middle of this present decade, two realities rekindled interest in the application of intravenous thrombolytic therapy for acute myocardial infarction (MI), and for the launching of a second generation of clinical trials of these efforts—first, the aforementioned need for faster reperfusion than could be accomplished with the time-consuming catheterization-laboratory-based intracoronary treatment, and, second, the recognition that a majority of infarct patients enter the health care system remote from tertiary care centers where the interventional angiographic approach is unavailable. Thus, even if safely transportable, most infarct patients would still be outside the range from which triage, transfer, and treatment could all be accomplished within a time frame likely to justify the undertaking.

Two kinds of clinical trials of intravenous (IV) thrombolysis ensued. Large studies were begun administering intravenous lytic therapy and comparing outcome LV function and mortality to randomized controls. Smaller studies initiated at about the same time were aimed at angiographically defining the frequency of successful reperfusion when streptokinase (and subsequently other agents) were delivered intravenously, and carefully examining sophisticated endpoints. These investigations, by necessity, also often were catheterization-laboratory-based, and, therefore, treatment commonly was still delayed to allow for pretreatment angiography to establish agent-specific lysis rates.

The first very large clinical trial, performed in Italy,[9] nearly eclipsed the others by virtue of sheer size. In this 12,000-patient trial of 1.5 million units of intravenous streptokinase versus randomized controls, a nearly 50 percent 21-day mortality benefit was afforded to infarct patients treated within the first hour of symptoms (Table 11–3), a 25 percent mortality benefit overall for treatment within 3 hours of symptom onset, and a 17 percent benefit if treatment was begun between the third and sixth hour of infarction. No statistically significant benefit was obtained from treatment starting beyond six hours. Other large and more-or-less similar trials include the ISAM study,[10] and the ISIS II trial.[11] After 4000 patients were randomized to IVSK or control in fewer than 4 hours, the ISIS study group announced an interim end-point analysis in which control group mortality was 12 percent and treatment group mortality was 8 percent, representing a 33 percent reduction in MI-related early death.

The ISAM study was not as large and not as dramatic in outcome. Only 477 patients were randomized within 4 hours of symptom onset. The control-group 30-day mortality was uncharacteristically low at 6.5 percent, and the treatment-group mortality was 5.2 percent. It must be appreciated in considering the ISAM outcome data, as well as subsequent smaller and intermediate size trials, that if selection criteria result in a study population in which the control or placebo-treated group has a remarkably low mortality rate, then the benefits of thrombolysis (or any other therapy) will be difficult to recognize (statistically). In such studies endpoint data, such as regional or global ventricular function, are generally sought, as opposed to raw mortality rates. One such study recently reported by White and coworkers[12] from Auckland, New Zealand, relies upon clinically important improvement in ejection fraction to argue for the efficacy of early lytic

Table 11–3. GISSI: Randomized Controlled Trial of Intravenous Thrombolysis in Myocardial Infarction

Time from Symptom Onset to Treatment (hr)	21-Day Mortality			
	IVSK	Control	N	P
<1	8.2	15.4	1277	<0.0001
≤3	9.2	12.0	6094	<0.0005
3–6	11.7	14.1	3649	<0.03

therapy. Although in this study, a mortality benefit also was observed, the authors highlight the broad confidence limits of prime death rates when the sample size is limited.

The AIMS trial[13] is thus far the only mortality study that compares a modified streptokinase preparation, APSAC, with placebo. APSAC was developed with the goal of modifying streptokinase by acetylation so that it would have fewer systemic effects and thus be more "clot specific." Experience to date, however, suggests that to accomplish competitive reperfusion rates, the quantity required (about 30 units) is, in fact, a systemic fibrinolytic and fibrinogenolytic dose. Nonetheless, the agent is attractive in part because it can be given rapidly as an IV bolus as opposed to most other agents used as prolonged infusions. In the AIMS study, an important 30-day mortality benefit was observed with treatment instituted less than 6 hours from the onset of infarction symptoms; the mortality rate for treated patients was 6.4 percent—a 48 percent reduction compared with the 12.2 percent mortality observed in the control group.

Despite the aforementioned substantial clinical efficacy (on mortality rate) of intravenous streptokinase, catheterization-laboratory-based investigators had observed only a modest frequency of prompt drug-induced clot lysis with intravenous SK. Noninvasive "markers" of successful thrombolysis (such as ECG changes, relief of pain, and sudden arrhythmias) satisfied some researchers that the lysis rate was sufficiently high, but among patients who had pre- and post-therapy coronary angiograms the results were only fair and were clustered around the 50 percent efficacy level.[14] These findings, in part, may be related to dosage and may be somewhat ascribable also to the recognition that as the duration of clot presence increases, the chances of achieving lysis with SK diminish.

Simultaneously, other investigative efforts were undertaken to produce better lytic agents for intravenous use. Goals included higher lysis rates, absence of antigenicity (an occasionally important problem with SK), and a favorable safety profile. The "second generation" lytic agent that captured the greatest enthusiasm, and thus far the most extensively validated data, is the molecularly engineered (recombinant) tissue plasminogen activator (rt-PA). This naturally occurring mammalian serine protease is unique in its high affinity for fibrin and, thus, was expected to show biologic activity selectively concentrated at the site of the pathogenic coronary thrombus. Preliminary data established markedly reduced systemic activity (circulating fibrinogenolysis) and the predicted affinity for clot fibrin. Subsequently, the National Heart Lung and Blood Institute (NHLBI) cooperative trial "Thrombolysis in Myocardial Infarction" (TIMI) investigative group elected to perform a direct comparison of the new agent with IV streptokinase.[15] A similar collaborative group undertook such an evaluation in Western Europe. In the TIMI trial, infarct patients with symptoms up to 7 hours in duration, who after immediate angiography demonstrated lack of antegrade coronary flow, were randomly treated with 80 mg of double chain rt-PA and an SK placebo or SK 1.5 million units and an rt-PA placebo. Study angiographers documented the presence of successful reperfusion (while blinded to drug allocation). At the dose of SK given, generally thought to be the highest reasonable dose, only 36 percent of occluded arteries opened within 90 minutes. With what may be considered a moderate dosing schedule of rt-PA, twice as many (66 percent) occluded coronaries reperfused. Further analysis by the TIMI group has established that SK appears to be relatively more effective if given in the first 3 to 4 hours of infarct (near 50 percent clot lysis) than if given later (5 to 7 hours, about 25 percent), and that TPA, now expressed as a single chain molecule, when given at 100 mg results in a 2-hour post-treatment patency rate of about 80 percent. The European Study Group SK-TPA comparison closely parallels the TIMI experience.[16]

Other clinical trials currently are evaluating the lysis ability of urokinase and of other second- (or third-) generation fibrinolytics including APSAC and pro-urokinase. It remains speculative as to whether any developmental lytic agent will equal or exceed the success experienced with rt-PA, particularly without sacrifice of relative clot specificity. Common to any thrombolytic therapy is the risk of also lysing unrecognized thrombi that may serve a patient benefit. Most notable among such possibly "good clots" are those that form when the integrity of the cerebral vasculature is breached. Hemorrhagic cerebrovascular accidents especially and gastrointestinal hemorrhage secondly are the most hazardous of the nonpuncture site related bleeding complications incident to the use of lytic drugs and anticoagulants. A hemorrhagic CVA incidence of 1.6 percent observed by the TIMI investigators in over 1000 patients using 150 mg of single-chain rt-PA prompted a reduction in dosage to 100 mg. With subsequent experience in a similarly large number of patients, the rate of this complication has fallen to the range of 0.5 percent. It remains possible and even probable that when utilizing any antithrombotic strategy, clinicians will face a trade-off of efficacy versus hemorrhagic complications.

Other current or ongoing clinical trials of rt-Pa include smaller studies of its benefits measured in terms of left ventricular function and larger trials aimed at defining the mortality benefit of rt-PA versus placebo and versus streptokinase.

Major LV functional benefits associated with t-PA use have been reported in the Australian "TICO" trial[17] and the study from Johns Hopkins.[18] The major mortality studies utilizing rt-PA are still in the patient recruitment phase.

CLINICAL TRIAL OF COMBINATION STRATEGIES IN ACUTE MYOCARDIAL INFARCTION

Despite the breakthrough nature of effective lytic therapy in reducing the morbidity and mortality of acute myocardial infarction, a number of questions remain and a number of residual shortcomings are recognized. These issues form the most current and the future round of clinical trials in this fast-moving field. The largest trials of lytic efficacy in MI show benefits for "all comers" meeting entry criteria (usually prolonged pain and ST elevation) when treated early (under 4 hours). When stratified by infarct site, anterior versus inferior, in most trials it is the anterior infarct patients who benefit the most. It may be a reasonable hypothesis that the control group mortality rate phenomenon (discussed earlier in relation to the ISAM trial) is at work. The low intrinsic fatality incidence after inferior MI will presumably augment the difficulty in demonstrating a favorable treatment trend. It is ironic perhaps that in the longer term followup in ISAM, inferior infarct patients did benefit, as they did in the New Zealand trial of outcome LV function. Even more problematic is the value of treatment in non-Q wave MI patients (virtually unstudied to date except for ISIS II), and in the elderly in whom complication rates are expected to be higher. Future clinical trials may provide better treatment guidelines for these and other MI subgroups.

The largest number of current and ongoing clinical trials in thrombolysis arise from the cognizance that there are quantifiable shortcomings to therapy of

Table 11–4. Shortcomings of Lytic Therapy

Failure to reperfuse
Limited myocardial salvage
Recurrent occlusion and reinfarction
Recurrent ischemia

MI with thrombolytic drugs and anticoagulation (Table 11–4). These shortcomings relate to the status of the infarct artery after the lytic drug is given, and to its status over the subsequent days and weeks.

Even utilizing the most effective of agents (i.e., rt-PA), at least 15 percent to 20 percent of patients will be left with a persistently occluded infarct artery. Strategies to reopen this residual subgroup using mechanical means (usually angioplasty but conceivably other, more specific, thrombectomy devices) are underway. The strategies are persistently hampered, however, by the absence of highly reliable nonangiographic markers of reperfusion.

Even after successful thrombolysis, many patients are left with a high-grade atherosclerotic obstruction at the site of recent occlusion. This residual stenosis results, predictably, in an important subsequent incidence of reocclusion, reinfarction, and postinfarction angina. Almost paradoxical is the fulfilled prediction that the more effective the initial lytic strategy, the more common the late recurrences of reinfarction and ischemia, because more arteries are opened and more myocardium supplied by stenotic vessels is salvaged. The frequency of reinfarction and recurrent ischemia after rt-PA treatment may be estimated at 15 percent and 35 percent, respectively, and somewhat lower after SK treatment. Additionally, there is experimental and clinical evidence to support the notion that greater reperfusion coronary flow (i.e., less severe residual stenosis) may lead to greater myocardial salvage.[19,20] These observations provide the rationale for application of angioplasty as part of a combination strategy in treating myocardial infarction. If a residual tight stenosis limits salvage and leads to reocclusion and/or recurrent ischemia, then PTCA should provide a larger infarct artery lumen and overcome these lytic therapy shortcomings.

Some experience has accrued using percutaneous transluminal coronary angioplasty (PTCA) as the reperfusion method without pharmacologically induced lysis.[21] Whereas this approach might serve the occasional patient in the exceptionally well-equipped and well-staffed treatment setting, the concept in general suffers from the same limitations previously discussed regarding intracoronary thrombolytic infusion. For most infarct patients, such facilities are simply not available, and for most of the remainder the time delay in accomplishing such therapy will likely limit the ultimate benefit.

Nonetheless, angioplasty after initial reperfusion with IV lytic therapy has become a highly attractive combination strategy which, in fact, has worked its way (prematurely?) into widespread clinical practice. Recently reported or still ongoing clinical trials have tested the outcome of PTCA immediately after, or days to a week after lytic therapy. In the TAMI trial,[22] patients randomized to immediate post-rt-PA PTCA showed (surprisingly?) no evident reduction in final reocclusion rate nor benefit in ventricular function augmentation compared with patients whose post-lytic PTCA was delayed a week (or not performed at all).

Recently published data from the European cooperative study[23] indicate that patients treated with rt-PA alone may have a better short- and intermediate-term outcome than those whose rt-PA therapy is followed by PTCA. This observation in part is due to a higher complication rate, particularly hemorrhage, and need for transfusions, in those randomized to early angioplasty. Importantly, in both the TAMI and the European trials, immediate post-lytic dilatation did not result in better outcome LV function, in less reocclusion, or in a lower mortality rate. Investigators from both groups conclude that after t-PA-induced reperfusion, cardiac catheterization and angioplasty should be deferred. It was particularly apparent in both trials that the goal of improving the prognosis of those in whom drug therapy failed to produce reperfusion was not achieved for the group in toto. Nonetheless, exceptions to such general recommendations clearly exist. Investigators in the field are nearly unanimous in advocating early intervention in patients who clinically are not faring well, particularly those with unstable hemodynamics or recurrent ischemic signs. What the trials have shown is that the most aggressive early strategies do not produce group benefits for "all comers." They have also shown, unfortunately, that we have no reliable selection criteria to allow stratification of the large infarct population into those whose early post-lytic drug course should be conservative, and those in whom early angiography, angioplasty, or bypass surgery would be a preferred strategy. The largest trial of its kind, TIMI II, is still in the recruitment phase and may be expected to contribute significantly to this unsettled issue. Preliminary information from this trial, however, supports the conclusions of TAMI and the European Cooperative Study (i.e., angiography and PTCA, if undertaken, should be delayed at least a day or two after lytic therapy.)[24] A unique aspect of the TIMI II trial is a comparison, in more than 3,000 patients, of delayed cardiac catheterization and PTCA versus a conservative, symptom-directed, post-lytic management scheme. The results of this trial are expected by the end of 1988.

A glimpse toward the future reveals numerous other strategies to be interrogated by clinical trial techniques, including earlier lytic therapy in the prehospital phase of care (ambulance treatment ?), combinations of lytic and anticoagulant drugs with different properties, and studies of other methods to protect jeopardized cardiac myocytes including agents that inhibit oxygen free-radical-mediated injury as well as the more standard agents that reduce oxygen demand (e.g., beta blockers).

The most recent data in the field of thrombolytic therapy involve two major trials, the ECSG t-PA versus placebo, and the ISIS II study, which were completed in the spring of 1988, and provide important new information relevant to the issues herein discussed.

The ECSG randomized 700 patients to receive either 100 mg of t-PA, or placebo, within 4 hours of infarct symptom onset. Although designed primarily to interrogate the endpoints of infarct size by enzyme analysis and outcome LV functions, the investigators reported an approximately 50 percent reduction in mortality rate at hospital discharge associated with the use of IV t-PA. This benefit becomes ever more striking when one considers that it was achieved despite the notably low mortality rate (6 percent) of the control group.

The ISIS II study is more difficult to characterize in a short space and without full details in published form available thus far for scrutiny. This study was of overwhelming size (more than 17,000 patients treated in more than 400 hospitals). It is different from all previous thrombolytic trials in that suspicion of infarction was the entry criterion resulting in major cohorts of study patients in whom the usual ECG criteria for infarct were absent. It seems likely that ISIS II was a trial in patients with unstable angina as well as infarct patients. Treatment consisted of IV streptokinase, aspirin at 160 mg per day, both drugs, or neither drug. Additionally, against the recent trial trends, patients were accepted for entry as late as 24 hours after their symptom onset. The major findings of ISIS II included confirmation of the mortality benefit of SK given early, demonstration of an independent mortality and reinfarction benefit for aspirin, and a synergistic effect of the two agents given together. Highly fascinating also is the information that although of lower magnitude, a mortality benefit attended active therapy in every subgroup defined by time from pain onset to treatment assignment (as late as 24 hours). This information has rekindled interest in the occasionally stated notion that infarct-related arterial patency may be of value for long-term prognosis even when accomplished too late to effect recognizable early ventricular function benefit.

SUMMARY

This decade has witnessed the establishment of thrombolysis, the most widely available therapeutic intervention that specifically treats the direct cause of myocardial infarction and leads to biologically and clinically compelling patient outcome benefits. The next series of investigational tasks will refine issues such as patient and drug selection and optimal postlysis strategies.

REFERENCES

1. DeWood, MA, Spores, J, Notske, RN, et al: Prevalence of total coronary occlusion during the early hours of transmural myocardial infarction. N Engl J Med 303:897, 1980.
2. Rentrop, KT, Blanke, H, Karsch, KR, and Kreuzer, H: Initial experience with transluminal recanalization of the recently occluded infarct-related coronary artery in acute myocardial infarction. Comparison with conventionally treated patients. Clin Cardiol 2:92, 1979.
3. Mathey, DG, Kuck, KH, Tilsner, V, et al: Nonsurgical coronary artery recanalization in acute transmural myocardial infarction. Circulation 63:489, 1981.
4. Khaja, F, Walton, JA Jr, Brymer, JF, et al: Intracoronary fibrinolytic therapy in acute myocardial infarction. Report on a prospective randomized trial. N Engl J Med 308:1305, 1983.
5. Anderson, JL, Marshall, HW, Bray, BE, et al: A randomized trial of intracoronary streptokinase in the treatment of acute myocardial infarction. N Engl J Med 308:13, 1983.
6. Leiboff, RH, Katz, RS, Wasserman, AG, et al: A randomized angiographically controlled trial of intracoronary streptokinase in acute myocardial infarction. Am J Cardiol 53:404, 1984.
7. Furberg, CD: Clinical value of intracoronary streptokinase (editorial). Am J Cardiol 53:626, 1984.
8. Yusuf, S, Collins, R, Peto, R, et al: Intravenous and intracoronary fibrinolytic therapy in acute myocardial infarction: Overview of results on mortality, reinfarction and side-effects from 33 randomized controlled trials. Eur Heart J 6:556, 1985.
9. The Italian Group for the Study of Streptokinase in Myocardial Infarction (GISSI): Effectiveness of intravenous thrombolytic treatment in acute myocardial infarction. Lancet 1:397, 1986.
10. The ISAM Study Group: A prospective trial of intravenous streptokinase in acute myocardial infarction (ISAM). Mortality, morbidity, and infarct size at 21 days. N Engl J Med 314:1465, 1986.
11. Randomized trial of intravenous streptokinase, oral aspirin, both or neither (ISIS-2). Lancet 2:349, 1988.
12. White, HD, Norris, RM, Brown, MA, et al: Effect of intravenous streptokinase on left ventricular function and early survival after acute myocardial infarction. N Engl J Med 317:850,1987.
13. AIMS Trial Study Group: Effect of intravenous APSAC on mortality after acute myocardial infarction: Preliminary report of a placebo-controlled clinical trial. Lancet 1:545,1988.

14. Anderson, JL: Streptokinase and acylated streptokinase: Biochemical properties and clinical effects. In Topol, E (ed): Acute Coronary Intervention, pp 3–23, Alan R Liss, NY, 1988.
15. Chesebro, JH, Knatterud, G, Roberts, R, et al: Thrombolysis in myocardial infarction (TIMI) trial, phase I: A comparison between intravenous tissue plasminogen activator and intravenous streptokinase. Circulation 76:142, 1987.
16. Verstraete, M, Bernard, R, Bory, M, et al: Randomized trial of intravenous recombinant tissue-type plasminogen activator versus intravenous streptokinase in acute myocardial infarction. Lancet 1:842, 1985.
17. O'Rourke, M and Norris, R, for Sydney/Auckland Thrombolysis in Coronary Occlusion (TICO) Group: Improved LV ejection fraction at 21 days following coronary occlusion treated by early intravenous rt-PA infusion. J Am Coll Cardiol 11:105A, 1988.
18. Guerci, AD, Gerstenblith, G, Brinker, JA, et al: A randomized trial of intravenous tissue plasminogen activator for acute myocardial infarction with subsequent randomization to elective coronary angioplasty. N Engl J Med 317:1613, 1987.
19. Schmidt, SB, Varghese, PJ, Bloom, S, et al: The influence of residual coronary stenosis on size of infarction after reperfusion in a canine preparation. Circulation 73:1354, 1986.
20. O'Neill, W, Timmis, GC, Bourdillon, PD, et al: A prospective randomized clinical trial of intracoronary streptokinase versus coronary angioplasty for acute myocardial infarction. N Engl J Med 324:812, 1986.
21. Rothbaum, DA, Linnemeier, TJ, Landin, RJ, et al: Emergency percutaneous transluminal coronary angioplasty in acute myocardial infarction: A 3 year experience. J Am Coll Cardiol 10:264, 1987.
22. Topol, EJ, Califf, RM, George, BS, et al, and the Thrombolysis and Angioplasty in Myocardial Infarction Study Group: A randomized trial of immediate versus delayed elective angioplasty after intravenous tissue plasminogen activator in acute myocardial infarction. N Engl J Med 317:581, 1987.
23. Simoons, ML, Betriu, A, Col, J, et al: Thrombolysis with tissue plasminogen activator in acute myocardial infarction: No additional benefit from immediate coronary angioplasty. Lancet 1:197,1988.
24. Presented at the American Heart Association Annual Scientific Sessions, Dallas, Texas, November, 1987.

CHAPTER 12

Interventional Therapy in Acute Myocardial Infarction

Andrew Zalewski, M.D.
Sheldon Goldberg, M.D.

The idea that coronary artery thrombi are involved in the pathogenesis of acute myocardial infarction was first proposed by Herrick in 1912.[1] In subsequent years, the cause of acute myocardial infarction was widely debated until 1980, when DeWood and coworkers described the results of coronary arteriography in patients with evolving myocardial infarction.[2] These investigators demonstrated that acute myocardial infarction was associated with total occlusion of the infarct-related artery in 87 percent of patients who underwent cardiac catheterization within 4 hours after symptom onset (Figs. 12–1*A*, 12–2*A*, 12–3*A*, 12–4*A*, 12–5*A*, 12–6*A*). In addition, coronary thrombi were retrived in 52 of 59 patients undergoing emergency coronary artery bypass graft surgery. In contrast, in patients undergoing cardiac catheterization more than 12 hours after symptom onset, the incidence of complete coronary artery occlusion decreased to 65 percent, as a result of spontaneous recanalization by the body's intrinsic fibrinolytic system.

In 1979, Rentrop and associates reported that the intracoronary administration of streptokinase during evolving transmural infarction resulted in reperfusion of the infarct-related artery in four of five patients.[3] Subsequent investigators confirmed the efficacy of intracoronary thrombolysis, with successful reperfusion reported to be between 60 percent and 85 percent.[4–12] The rate of coronary recanalization was found to be higher in patients with persistent ischemic discomfort[12] and in those who were treated relatively early after symptom onset.[12,13] Reperfusion was generally established within 30 minutes of intracoronary drug infusion, with greater efficacy reported by investigators using subselective techniques.[5]

Because the goal of reperfusion during acute myocardial infarction is myocardial salvage, the end points for measuring the results of coronary thrombolysis should include indices of left ventricular function as well as mortality statistics. However, reports of changes in left ventricular function after intracoronary thrombolysis showed that there was either a modest improvement[6] or no sub-

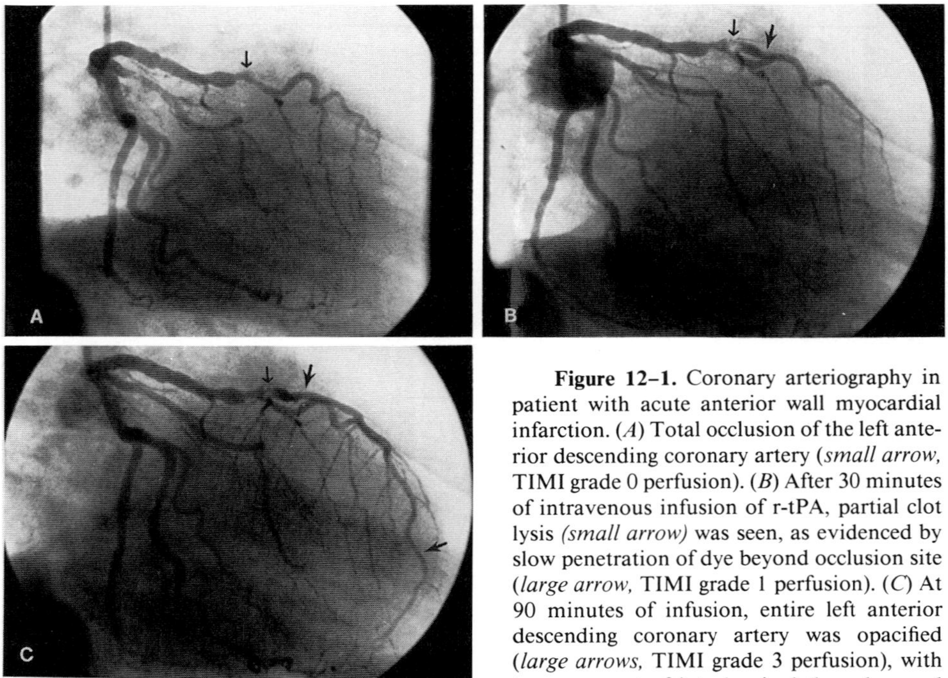

Figure 12–1. Coronary arteriography in patient with acute anterior wall myocardial infarction. (*A*) Total occlusion of the left anterior descending coronary artery (*small arrow,* TIMI grade 0 perfusion). (*B*) After 30 minutes of intravenous infusion of r-tPA, partial clot lysis *(small arrow)* was seen, as evidenced by slow penetration of dye beyond occlusion site (*large arrow,* TIMI grade 1 perfusion). (*C*) At 90 minutes of infusion, entire left anterior descending coronary artery was opacified (*large arrows,* TIMI grade 3 perfusion), with large amount of intraluminal thrombus and residual stenosis at the site of previous occlusion *(small arrow).*

stantial alteration.[7–9] These findings were in part due to the relatively late administration of the drug, which was inherent with the intracoronary route. Several predictors of recovery of left ventricular function have been identified (Table 12–1) such as early spontaneous[14] or treatment-related reperfusion within the first 2 to 4 hours after symptom onset,[15,16] the presence of residual flow to the infarcting zone,[17] and the extent of initially compromised left ventricular function.[11] It is also conceivable that the severity of the residual stenosis after successful thrombolysis can influence recovery of wall motion.[16]

The effects of intracoronary streptokinase on mortality were reported in the Western Washington Randomized Trial,[7,18] which showed a significant reduction in the 30-day mortality from 11.2 percent in patients treated with placebo versus 3.7 percent in patients treated with intracoronary streptokinase.[7] Although this difference in mortality was no longer statistically significant at 1 year, the treated patients had a 44 percent lower mortality when compared with the placebo group.[18]

Because of the time delays inherent with the *intracoronary* route of administration of thrombolytic agents, investigators sought to study the effects of *intravenous* agents in patients with acute myocardial infarction. Intravenous thrombolytic therapy seemed especially attractive, inasmuch as therapy could be started earlier in the course of a myocardial infarction and could be applied to a larger patient population. If intravenous treatment proved effective in achieving coronary reperfusion, the effects on myocardial salvage and mortality might be expected to be superior to intracoronary drug delivery. However, the results of

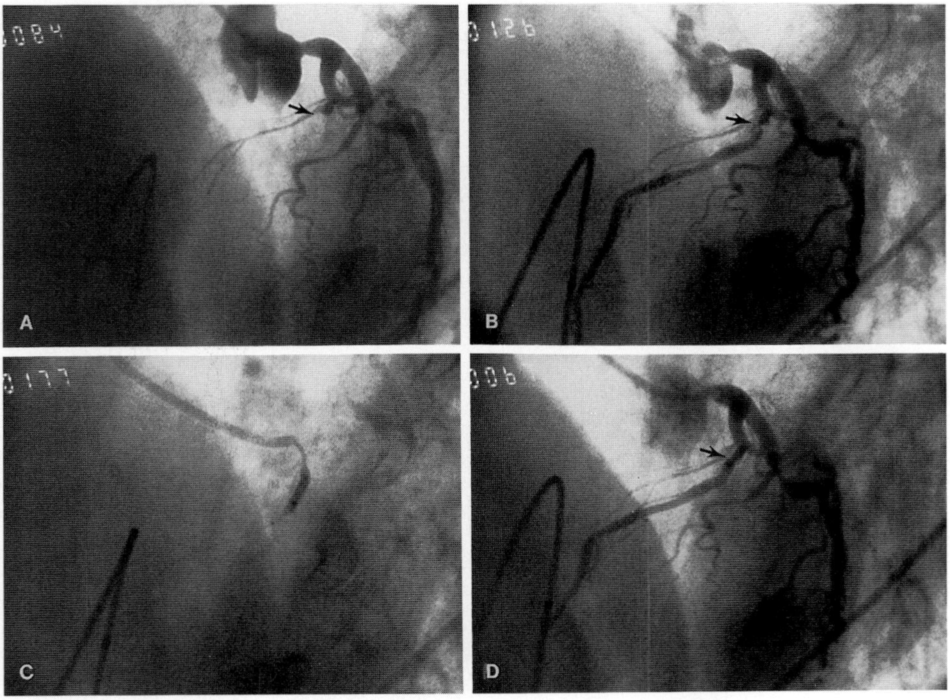

Figure 12–2. Coronary arteriography in patient with acute anterior wall myocardial infarction. (*A*) Total occlusion of the left anterior descending coronary artery (*arrow,* TIMI grade 0 perfusion). (*B*) At 90 minutes of intravenous r-tPA infusion, angiography showed successful reperfusion of the infarct-related artery (TIMI grade 2 perfusion), with a 95 percent residual stenosis *(arrow)* and intraluminal thrombus at the site of occlusion. (*C*) Immediate PTCA was performed—angioplasty balloon inflated at the site of stenosis. (*D*) Final angiogram showed reduction of lesion to luminal irregularities *(arrow)* and excellent flow in the distal portion of the left anterior descending artery (TIMI grade 3 perfusion).

various randomized trials using intravenous streptokinase showed reperfusion rates that were significantly lower than those achieved with intracoronary streptokinase: recanalization was reported to vary between 31 percent and 55 percent.[19,20] The majority of trials that reported higher reperfusion rates lacked pretreatment angiography and, therefore, included patients with subtotal occlusions of the infarct-related artery. However, some studies have shown improvement in left ventricular function,[21] despite the lower rate of coronary reperfusion with the

Table 12–1. Determinants of Recovery of Left Ventricular Function

1. Spontaneous early reperfusion or treatment-related reperfusion less than 4 hours from symptom onset
2. Presence of residual flow to infarcting zone (i.e., collaterals, subtotal occlusion)
3. Extent of initially compromised left ventricular function
4. Severity of residual stenosis after thrombolysis

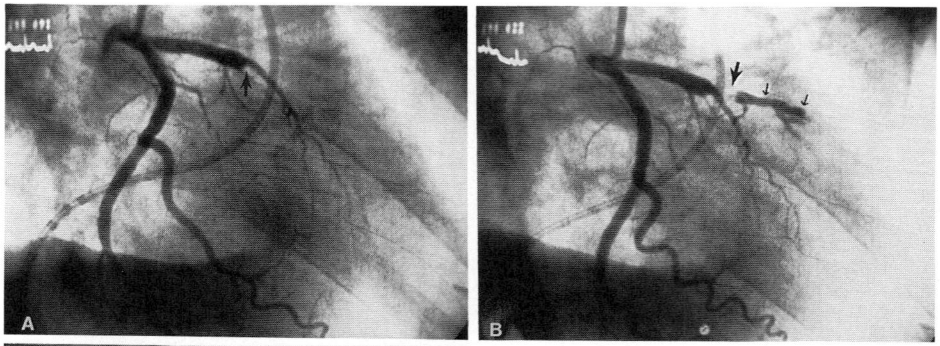

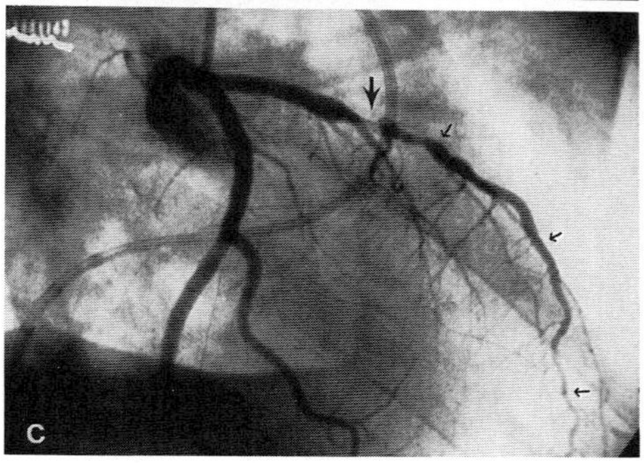

Figure 12–3. Coronary arteriography in patient with acute anterior wall myocardial infarction. (*A*) Initial angiogram showed complete occlusion (*arrow*, TIMI grade 0 perfusion) of the left anterior descending coronary artery. (*B*) At 30 minutes of intravenous r-tPA infusion, subtotal occlusion *(large arrow)* of the infarct-related artery was present with only minimal penetration of dye beyond occlusion (*small arrows*, TIMI grade 1 perfusion). (*C*) At 90 minutes of infusion, coronary flow to mid and distal portion of the infarct-related artery was restored (*small arrows*, TIMI grade 3 perfusion). "Hazy" appearance at site of previous occlusion *(large arrow)* and residual stenosis are typical findings after thrombolysis.

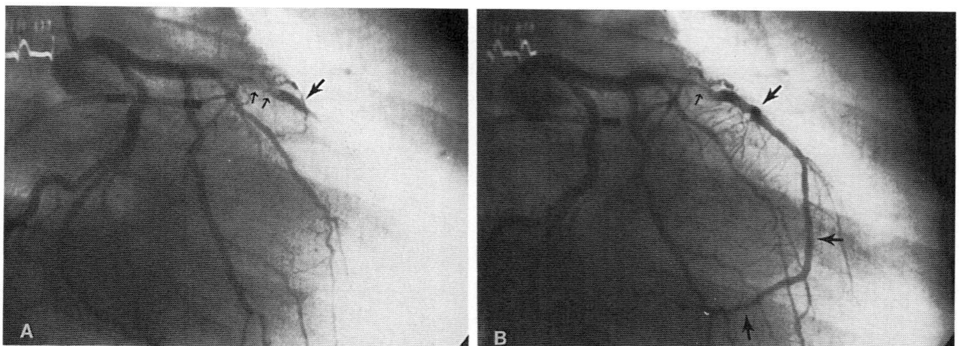

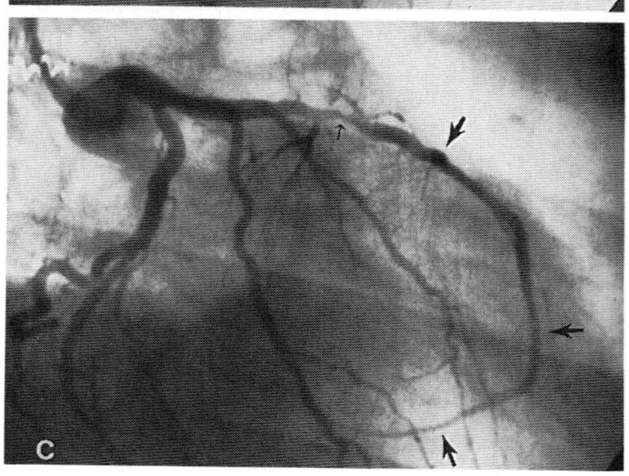

Figure 12–4. Coronary arteriography in patient with acute anterior wall myocardial infarction. (*A*) Initial angiogram showed occlusive thrombus *(small arrows)* in the proximal portion of the left anterior descending coronary artery with only minimal penetration of dye (*large arrow*, TIMI grade 1 perfusion) beyond occlusion. (*B*) At 90 minutes of intravenous r-tPA infusion, the artery is reperfused *(large arrows)* with moderately severe residual stenosis (*small arrow*, TIMI grade 3 perfusion). (*C*) Two days later, further improvement in coronary arterial patency *(small arrow)* was noted, which alleviated the need for PTCA.

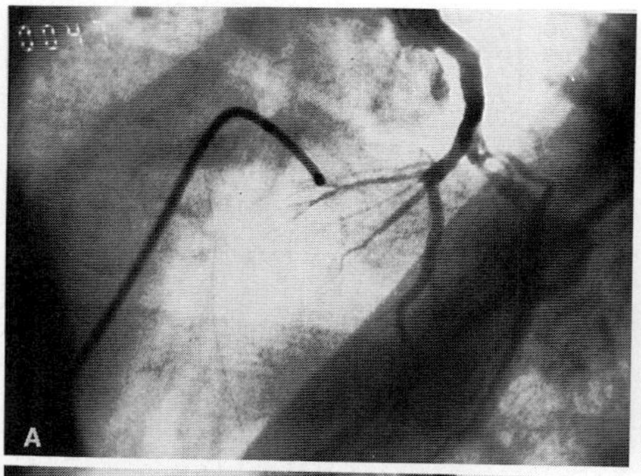
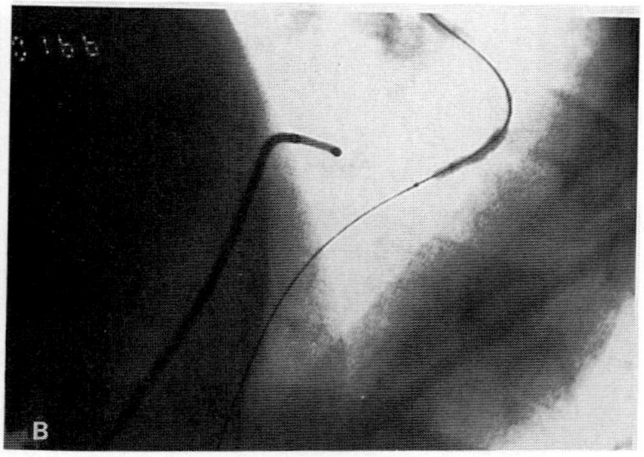
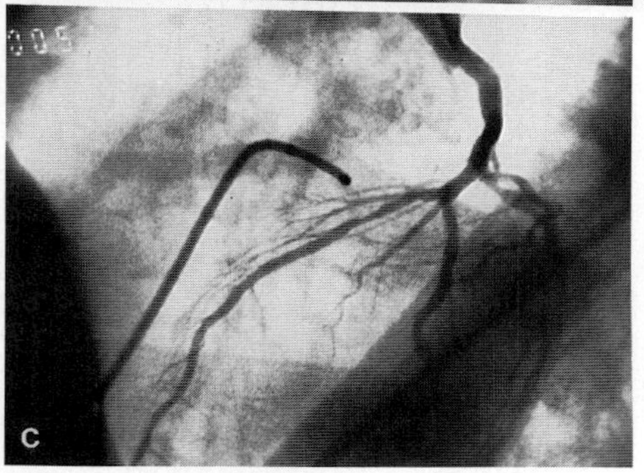

Figure 12–5. Coronary arteriography in patient with acute anterior wall myocardial infarction. (*A*) Coronary angiogram obtained at 90 minutes of intravenous r-tPA infusion showing persistent occlusion of the left anterior descending coronary artery, that is, failure of thrombolytic therapy (TIMI grade 0 perfusion). (*B*) Emergency PTCA was performed. (*C*) Final angiogram showed restored patency of the left anterior descending coronary artery and excellent flow in the distal portion of the vessel (TIMI grade 3 perfusion).

use of intravenous streptokinase. The results of intravenous thrombolysis trials using mortality as an end point are conflicting. The Intravenous Streptokinase in Acute Myocardial Infarction trial (ISAM) and the Western Washington Intravenous Streptokinase trial failed to demonstrate improved survival in treated patients.[22,23] This failure was most likely related to the lower reperfusion rates achieved with intravenous streptokinase and the inclusion of low-risk patients (mortality less than 10 percent in the control group).[22,23] In contrast, the GISSI study,[24] in which 11,712 patients were randomized to placebo or intravenous streptokinase, demonstrated an 18 percent reduction in inhospital mortality in the treated group ($p = 0.0002$). The beneficial effect of intravenous streptokinase on mortality was more pronounced in patients treated very early after symptom onset.[24]

More recently, the Second International Study of Infarct Survival (ISIS-2) demonstated significant reduction in 5-week vascular mortality after intravenous streptokinase in patients with suspected myocardial infarction. Interestingly, combined treatment with intravenous streptokinase and oral aspirin produced an additive effect. Mortality in the control group was 13.2 percent, whereas mortality in the aspirin plus streptokinase group was significantly reduced to 8 percent.[(42)]

As a means of increasing the probability of successful coronary recanalization, investigators began experimenting with a new generation of thrombolytic agents, the most notable being recombinant tissue-type plasminogen activators (r-tPA).[25] Administration of these relatively fibrin-specific, short half-life agents resulted in significantly higher coronary reperfusion rates than did treatment with intravenous streptokinase. Using the 90-minute coronary arteriogram as the end point, successful reperfusion was achieved in 62 percent to 75 percent of patients treated with intravenous r-tPA.[19,20,26,27]

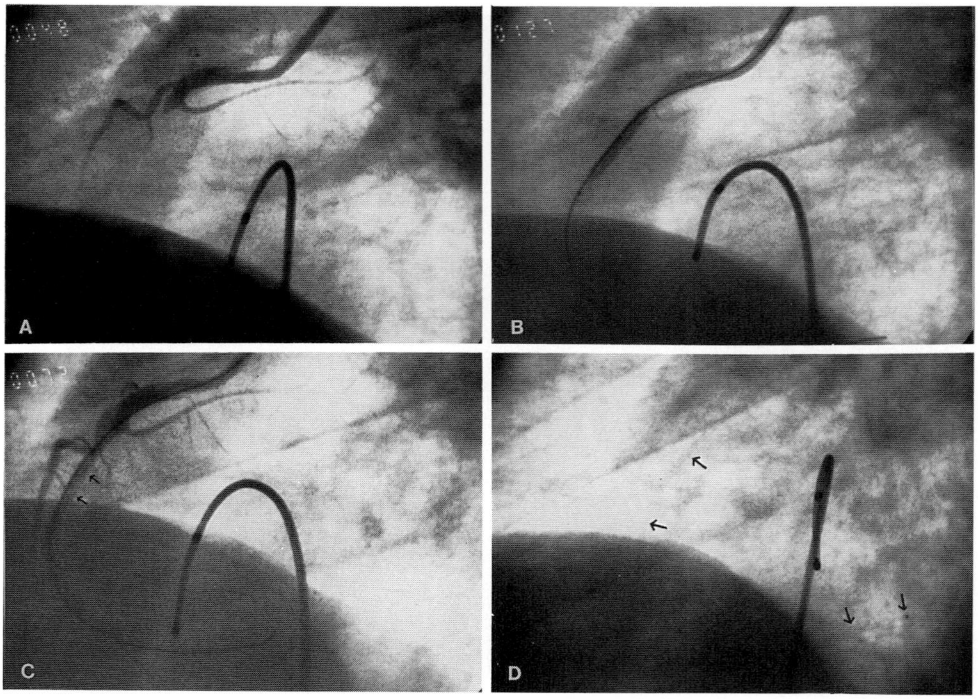

Figure 12–6. Coronary arteriography in patient with acute inferior wall myocardial infarction. (*A*) Coronary angiogram at 90 minutes of intravenous r-tPA infusion showed complete occlusion of the right coronary artery (TIMI grade 0 perfusion). (*B*) Emergency PTCA was performed after failed thrombolytic therapy. (*C*) Coronary angiogram after several balloon inflations showed large residual intraluminal thrombus *(arrows)* with poor penetration of dye beyond occlusion (TIMI grade 1 perfusion), representing failure of PTCA. (*D*) Perfusion catheter *(arrows)* with multiple sideholes was advanced into the right coronary artery, which allowed for temporary perfusion with arterial blood from the aorta of the ischemic region. The patient underwent emergency bypass surgery.

Following successful coronary thrombolysis, high-grade residual coronary stenosis of the infarct-related artery is frequently the problem that results in reocclusion in 13 percent to 45 percent of patients (Figs. 12–1*B*, *C*; 12–2*B*; 12–3*B*, *C*; and 12–4*B*, *C*).[26,28–30] In order to assess the optimal therapeutic strategy in acute myocardial infarction, studies on the efficacy of PTCA were undertaken. PTCA can be used either as the primary treatment[31–33] or in conjunction with thrombolytic agents.[26,27,29,31,34,35] If used in the latter situation, PTCA can be performed during or immediately after thrombolysis, or the procedure can be performed in a delayed, elective manner.[26,27]

When PTCA was used as a primary treatment, marked improvement in coronary arterial lumen diameter was accompanied by significant improvement in left ventricular ejection fraction.[32] In one report,[32] when PTCA was compared directly with intracoronary streptokinase infusion, the rates of coronary recanalization were similar in both treatment groups, as were the times required to achieve reperfusion. However, in patients treated with primary PTCA, the residual coronary stenosis was significantly less severe than in the group treated with intracoronary streptokinase. In addition, left ventricular function was superior in the PTCA-treated patients: when serial contrast left ventriculograms were compared, both the changes in absolute ejection fraction and regional wall motion at 7 to 10 days showed greater improvement in the group treated with PTCA.

The timing of PTCA, when used in conjunction with thrombolysis has remained an important concern. This subject was addressed in the Thrombolysis and Angioplasty in Myocardial Infarction trial.[26] The trial compared the efficacy of immediate versus delayed PTCA at 7 to 10 days after coronary thrombolysis with intravenous r-tPA. The moderate improvement in regional wall motion was similar for both treatment groups. However, the rate of emergency coronary angioplasty because of recurrent ischemia or reinfarction was significantly higher for patients assigned to the delayed PTCA strategy. This finding would suggest that earlier PTCA (i.e., 2 to 3 days after reperfusion) may be a safer therapeutic option.[27]

The Thrombolysis in Myocardial Infarction (TIMI IIA) Study group sought to compare the effects of immediate PTCA, that is, performed within 2 hours after the start of rt-PA, with delayed PTCA, that is, 18 to 48 hours after rt-PA treatment. Preliminary data indicate that immediate PTCA was associated with higher in-hospital morbidity and did not result in significantly better recovery of left ventricular function.[(43)]

MODES OF CLINICAL PRESENTATION

The cardiologist may be called upon to decide on therapeutic strategies when patients present in one of several clinical settings (Table 12–2):

1. Patients with acute evolving transmural myocardial infarction
2. Patients with recent transmural myocardial infarction in a stable state during the first 2 weeks after thrombolytic therapy
3. Patients with postinfarction angina or reinfarction after thrombolytic treatment has already been administered

PATIENTS PRESENTING WITH ACUTE TRANSMURAL MYOCARDIAL INFARCTION

The decision whether or not to attempt thrombolysis with urgent or delayed cardiac catheterization is made on the basis of a combination of clinical factors including: (1) the duration of symptoms, (2) the hemodynamic status of the patient (e.g., the majority of patients with cardiogenic shock should undergo urgent catheterization), (3) the findings of persistent chest discomfort accompa-

Table 12–2. Interventional Therapy in Myocardial Infarction: Clinical Indications

1. Acute myocardial infarction (<6 hours' duration) with clinical (i.e., chest pain) and electrocardiographic (i.e., ST segment elevation) signs of ongoing ischemia
2. Myocardial infarction within the past 7 to 14 days treated with thrombolytic therapy, even if patient remains stable
3. Postinfarction angina or reinfarction after thrombolytic therapy

nied by continued injury current in the surface electrocardiogram (Figs. 12–7 and 12–8), and (4) absence of contraindications to thrombolytic therapy (Table 12–3). An additional finding of note is the presence of persistent ST segment depression in the precordial leads, which is accompanied by chest pain of greater than 30 minutes' duration. Inasmuch as the majority of acute myocardial infarction interventional trials have required the presence of ST segment elevation, the distribution of the infarct-related arteries has been divided approximately equally between the left anterior descending and the right coronary arteries, which together account for 85 percent to 90 percent of cases. Recent evidence indicates that persistent ST depression in the precordial leads may also be a marker of acute posterior infarction due to left circumflex coronary artery occlusion.[36,37] Therefore, the presence of prolonged chest pain accompanied by this electrocardiographic finding also should be considered an indication for interventional therapy.

If the decision is made to attempt coronary reperfusion, a choice must be made quickly among several treatment strategies (Table 12–4):

A. The patient may be taken directly to the catheterization suite for diagnostic study and possible urgent revascularization.
B. Intravenous thrombolytic agents may be administered, and the patient may be taken for urgent catheterization to define precisely left ventricular function and coronary anatomy. Decisions regarding the method and timing of PTCA or coronary artery bypass graft surgery are made on the basis of the catheterization findings.
C. Intravenous thrombolytic agents can be administered, and a "period of observation" for clinical signs of reperfusion can be undertaken.
D. Intravenous thrombolytic agents may be administered; the patient can then be admitted to the coronary care unit and catheterization can be performed on an elective basis.

We favor option "A" for patients with contraindications to thrombolytic treatment who present to tertiary care facilities. The decision whether to perform revascularization by PTCA or coronary bypass grafting surgery is made on the basis of specific angiographic criteria. It should be pointed out that emergency PTCA in acute myocardial infarction may have certain advantages in properly equipped tertiary care facilities. For example, in a study performed by Rothbaum and colleagues,[33] 151 patients underwent PTCA as primary treatment for acute myocardial infarction. The procedure was successful in 87 percent of patients, including 18 patients with cardiogenic shock. Following urgent PTCA, the mean residual stenosis severity was reduced to 29 percent. Of note, the in-hospital mortality was 5 percent in patients with successful angioplasty versus 37 percent in

Figure 12–7. A 12-lead electrocardiogram in patient with acute anterior wall myocardial infarction. (*A*) Baseline electrocardiogram 3 hours from onset of symptoms immediately prior to intravenous r-tPA infusion. ST segment elevations were present in precordial and lateral leads. (*B*) Electrocardiogram at 90 minutes of thrombolytic therapy. Rapid resolution of ST segment elevations was evident. (*C*) Predischarge tracing showing further evolution of anterior wall myocardial infarction. Although Q waves are present in leads V1 to V3, lateral leads that previously showed ST segment elevations demonstrated no evidence of lateral wall transmural myocardial infarction.

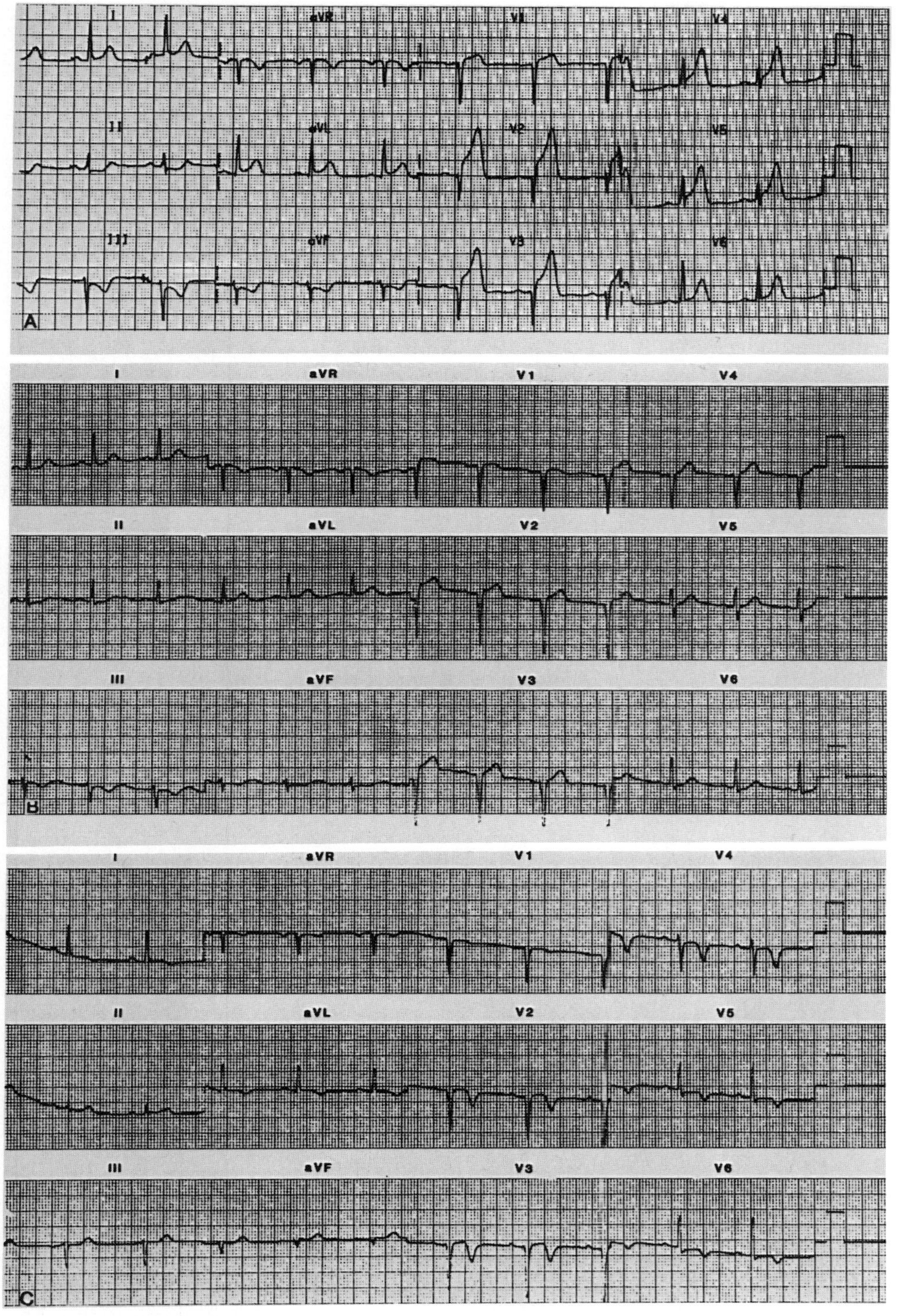

Figure 12–7. See facing page for legend.

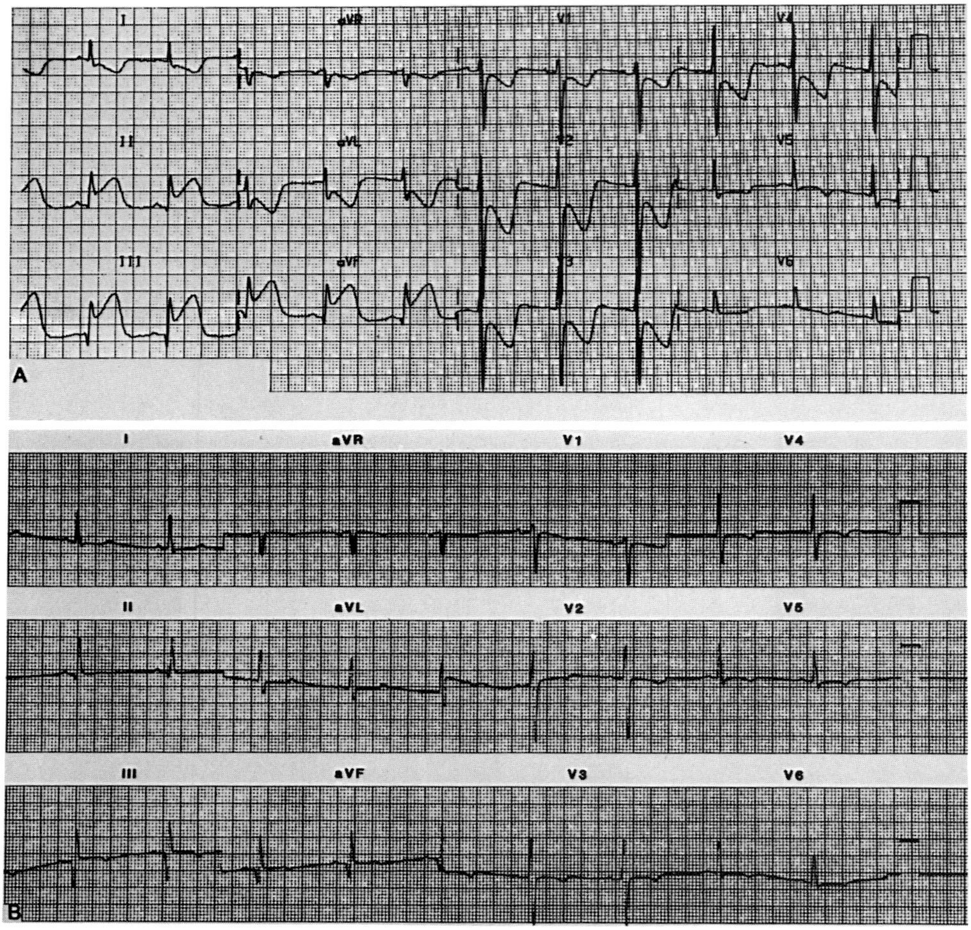

Figure 12–8. A 12-lead electrocardiogram in patient with acute inferoposterior myocardial infarction. (*A*) Baseline electrocardiogram 3 hours from onset of symptoms prior to intravenous r-tPA infusion showing significant ST segment elevations in inferior leads and reciprocal ST segment depressions in precordial leads. (*B*) Predischarge electrocardiogram showing typical development of Q waves despite successful reperfusion. Excellent preservation of R waves in inferior leads is suggestive of myocardial salvage after reperfusion.

those who had unsuccessful attempts. In addition, the posthospital cardiac mortality was only 2 percent during an average followup period of 20 months. The marked increases in arterial luminal diameter were accompanied by significant improvement in left ventricular ejection fraction. This mode of therapy, however, can be applied only in relatively few cardiac centers. Nonetheless, it has the practical advantages of a lower incidence of bleeding complications and a lower incidence of intramyocardial hemorrhage[38] attendent with thrombolytic therapy.

Option "B" is most suitable for patients without contraindication to thrombolytic therapy who present early with extensive myocardial infarction complicated by hemodynamic instability. This subgroup of patients may require urgent PTCA in conjunction with intravenous thrombolysis. Coronary arteriography will identify those high-risk patients who are candidates for urgent coronary

Table 12–3. Contraindications to Thrombolytic Therapy

1. History of bleeding diathesis or significant GI bleeding
2. Oral anticoagulant therapy
3. Left bundle branch block
4. Prosthetic heart valve
5. Dilated cardiomyopathy
6. Uncontrolled hypertension (diastolic pressure >110 mm Hg by several measurements)
7. Recent (within 2 weeks) significant surgical or biopsy procedure or cardiopulmonary resuscitation
8. Any prior cerebrovascular accident or TIA
9. Severe trauma within the last 6 months
10. Other serious advanced illnesses
11. Diabetic hemorrhagic retinopathy
12. High likelihood of left atrial thrombosis (e.g., mitral stenosis with atrial fibrillation)
13. Pregnancy, first 28 days postpartum, or childbearing potential
14. Any other condition in which bleeding would constitute a significant hazard or would be particularly difficult to manage because of its location

artery bypass surgery, for example, those with left main or severe multivessel disease. This aggressive approach to high-risk patients is limited to hospitals with active interventional programs.

Option "C" seems somewhat questionable, because the various clinical markers of reperfusion (relief of chest pain, rapid decline of ST segment elevation, and reperfusion arrhythmias) are too insensitive to predict accurately the status of the infarct-related artery.[39] If a thrombolytic agent were available that was more effective in achieving coronary recanalization and if noninvasive indices of myocardial reperfusion were more accurate, then an observation strategy could be adopted.

Option "D" seems most suitable for the vast majority of patients. Thus, intravenous thrombolytic agents are administered rapidly after evaluation of the patient in the emergency room. This treatment is supplemented by intravenous analgesics, and by intravenous nitroglycerin and a beta-blocking agent if the hemodynamic condition of the patient permits. Thrombolytic therapy is followed by intravenous heparin and oral aspirin to prevent reocclusion of the infarct-related artery. This seems to be especially important when r-tPA, with its short half-life, is used. Cardiac catheterization is usually performed within the first 7 days of myocardiac infarction. Subsequent revascularization therapy is implemented as dictated by the clinical and coronary arteriographic findings.

Angiographic Findings in Acute Myocardial Infarction

Coronary arteriography performed in the early hours of acute myocardial infarction demonstrates single-vessel disease in approximately 65 percent of patients, double-vessel involvement in 25 percent, and triple-vessel and/or left main coronary disease in 10 percent.[29] The precise incidence of triple-vessel coronary disease is probably underestimated in these figures inasmuch as most clinical trials requiring coronary arteriography have excluded patients with cardiogenic shock.

When patients are taken directly for coronary arteriography in the first 6 hours of acute myocardial infarction (without the prior administration of throm-

Table 12–4. Interventional Treatment in Myocardial Infarction—Therapeutic Options

Therapeutic Option	Indications	Limitations
Urgent cardiac catheterization with immediate revascularization by means of PTCA or surgery	Patients with contraindications to thrombolytic therapy and clinical and electrocardiographic signs of ongoing ischemia	Limited to medical facilities with cardiac catherization laboratory and CT surgery rapidly available around the clock
Intravenous thrombolytic therapy followed by urgent cardiac catheterization and necessary revascularization	Preferred option in patients with hemodynamic instability. Early cardiac catheterization allows for patient's stratification according to clinical status and coronary anatomy	Requires emergent transport from community hospital to tertiary care facility
Intravenous thrombolytic therapy followed by "period of observation" to detect clinical and electrocardiographic signs of reperfusion	Inability for rapid transfer of patient with extensive acute myocardial infarction to tertiary care facility. "Low" risk patient with acute myocardial infarction (e.g., inferior wall myocardial infarction with symptoms well controlled with routine treatment)	Low sensitivity of noninvasive markers of reperfusion prevents accurate prediction of the status of the infarct-related artery
Intravenous thrombolytic therapy with delayed cardiac catheterization	The most practical option, which can be applied to the vast majority of patients with myocardial infarction	In at least 25 percent of patients, reperfusion and myocardial salvage will not be achieved. In an additional 13 to 45 percent of patients, after initial reperfusion, reclosure of the infarct-related artery may occur. Early cardiac catheterization after thrombolytic therapy (e.g., 2 to 7 days) is indicated to prevent reinfarction

bolytic agents), the infarct-related artery is totally occluded in almost 90 percent of cases. Whereas coronary artery vasospasm may initiate coronary occlusion in some patients, the intracoronary administration of nitroglycerin only occasionally restores any degree of antegrade flow. If a patient is being treated with thrombolytic agents during the catheterization procedure, the cardiologist watches for signs of reperfusion. The patient is queried frequently about the level of discomfort. In addition, the electrocardiogram is monitored carefully for changes in the level of ST segment elevation. Both decreases in ST segment elevation (see Fig. 12–7) and abrupt increases in the degree of ST elevation have been observed in conjunction with reperfusion. Dysrhythmias that are specific for reperfusion during acute myocardial infarction include accelerated idioventricular rhythm and the development of reflex sinus bradycardia and hypotension, especially during reperfusion of the inferoposterior left ventricular wall (Bezold-Jarisch reflex).[40,41]

Table 12–5. Definitions of Perfusion in the TIMI Trial

Grade 0 (no perfusion)
No antegrade flow beyond the point of occlusion
Grade 1 (penetration without perfusion)
The contrast material passes beyond the area of obstruction but "hangs up" and fails to opacify the entire coronary bed distal to the obstruction for the duration of the cineangiographic filming sequence.
Grade 2 (partial perfusion)
The contrast material passes across the obstruction and opacifies the coronary bed distal to the obstruction. However, the rate of entry of contrast material into the vessel distal to the obstruction or its rate of clearance from the distal bed (or both) are perceptibly slower than its entry into or clearance from comparable areas not perfused by the previously occluded vessel (e.g., the opposite coronary artery or the coronary bed proximal to the obstruction).
Grade 3 (complete perfusion)
Antegrade flow into the bed distal to the obstruction occurs as promptly as antegrade flow into the bed proximal to the obstruction, and clearance of contrast material from the involved bed is as rapid as clearance from an uninvolved bed supplied by the same vessel or the opposite artery.

When these events occur, a repeat angiogram is performed to recheck the perfusion status of the infarct-related artery.

The perfusion status of the infarct-related artery is classified according to the TIMI criteria shown in Table 12–5. If TIMI grade 0 or 1 perfusion is present in a patient with signs of ongoing ischemia or hemodymanic instability, the cardiologist should consider performing "salvage" PTCA in order to acutely restore antegrade flow. In patients who exhibit grade 0 or 1 perfusion of the infarct-related artery and who have severe diffuse multivessel and/or left main coronary involvement, a strong case can be made for urgent coronary artery bypass graft surgery. If TIMI grade 2 or 3 perfusion is demonstrated in the infarct-related artery in conjunction with the stenosis greater than 70 percent in severity, several treatment options exist: If patients have left main or triple-vessel disease, we recommend semiurgent bypass grafting. Usually this procedure can be delayed until the next day. If single-vessel or double-vessel disease is present with lesions deemed suitable for PTCA, urgent PTCA of the infarct-related artery may be undertaken, or alternatively the catheterization procedure may be terminated and the patient returned to the coronary care unit with followup catheterization planned to reassess the status of the infarct-related artery several days later. The former approach has the advantage of achieving a more complete revascularization during one procdure. The latter approach has the advantage of allowing for continued clot lysis (see Fig. 12–4) and perhaps avoiding the need for PTCA as occurs in approximately 14 percent of patients.[26] In addition, acute PTCA may be associated with greater vessel reactivity and a resultant increased need for emergency coronary bypass grafting (see Fig. 12–6).[26]

PATIENTS PRESENTING IN A STABLE STATE AFTER ADMINISTRATION OF THROMBOLYTIC AGENT

With the increasing use of intravenous thrombolytic agents, a greater percentage of patients will be receiving these agents in community hospital settings. Subsequent transfer to tertiary care facilities for diagnostic and therapeutic catheterization will become more common.

The majority of such patients will demonstrate pathologic Q waves, along with enzymatic evidence of myocardial cell necrosis. Historically, we attempt to ascertain information regarding chest pain, ST segment changes (see Figs. 12–7 and 12–8), and reperfusion arrhythmias during the thrombolysis phase. In addition, we attempt to identify whether serial serum CK values reflect an early peak and washout indicating reperfusion.

The catheterization findings in these patients will most frequently demonstrate an akinetic region of myocardium supplied by the infarct-related artery. The infarct-related artery may be totally occluded, or more likely it will be patent with a high-grade residual stenosis. Stable patients with totally occluded infarct-related coronary arteries are usually treated medically. Patients with left main and triple-vessel coronary artery disease most likely should be referred for coronary artery bypass graft surgery.

We generally perform PTCA on candidates with suitable angiographic anatomy, realizing that it is difficult to ascertain the amount of salvageable myocardium supplied by the infarct-related artery. At the time of PTCA, we note whether recurrent ischemia and ST segment changes occur with balloon dilatation. These findings may indicate myocardial salvage although direct evidence for this hypothesis is lacking currently.

PATIENTS PRESENTING WITH RECURRENT INFARCTION

Patients recently treated with thrombolytic agents who do not undergo cardiac catheterization constitute a group at risk for reocclusion and reinfarction.[41] The rate of coronary reocclusion after the administration of thrombolytic agents varies between 13 percent and 45 percent[26,28–30] despite systemic anticoagulation, with the majority of reocclusions occurring in the first 48 hours after treatment. If reinfarction occurs in a tertiary care facility with an interventional program, we recommend emergent cardiac catheterization and coronary revascularization by means of PTCA or aortocoronary bypass surgery.

SUMMARY

Large multicenter trials have shown an improvement in both survival and left ventricular function in patients undergoing reperfusion therapy in acute myocardial infarction. The most practical approach in treatment of patients with acute myocardial infarction involves intravenous administration of effective thrombolytic agents as soon as possible in the course of myocardial infarction. This approach using r-tPA results in reperfusion in approximately two-thirds of patients. In patients with contraindications to thrombolytic therapy and extensive injury current or hemodynamic compromise, emergent cardiac catheterization should be performed followed by immediate PTCA or bypass surgery. In patients who have already been treated with thrombolytic agents, controversy exists as to the optimal timing of cardiac catheterization to define coronary anatomy and the need for additional revascularization.

We suggest that the most beneficial therapeutic strategy for the majority of patients is rapid administration of an effective intravenous thrombolytic agent combined with aspirin and heparin. Cardiac catheterization and PTCA or coronary artery bypass graft surgery may be deferred in stable patients. This approach is supported by evidence showing a lack of additional improvement in mortality and left ventricular function in patients treated with urgent PTCA.

The advent of new therapeutic modalities in acute myocardial infarction, such as thrombolysis, has created a new subset of patients who either will have an improved prognosis if coronary artery reperfusion is completed or will have an increased risk for recurrent myocardial ischemia if definite revascularization is delayed.

REFERENCES

1. Herrick, JB: Clinical features of sudden obstruction of the coronary arteries. JAMA 59:2015, 1912.
2. DeWood, MA, Spores, J, Notske, R, et al: Prevalence of total coronary occlusion during the early hours of transmural myocardial infarction. N Engl J Med 303:897, 1980.
3. Rentrop, KP, Blanke, H, Karsch, KR, et al: Acute myocardial infarction: Intracoronary application of nitroglycerin and streptokinase. Clin Cardiol 2:354, 1979.
4. Mathey, DG, Kuck, KH, Tilsner, V, et al: Nonsurgical coronary artery recanalization in acute transmural myocardial infarction. Circulation 63:489, 1981.
5. Ganz, W, Ninomiya, K, Hashida, J, et al: Intracoronary thrombolysis in acute myocardial infarction: Experimental background and clinical experience. Am Heart J 102:1145, 1981.
6. Anderson, JL, Marshall, HW, Bray, BE, et al: A randomized trial of intracoronary streptokinase in the treatment of acute myocardial infarction. N Engl J Med 308:1312, 1983.
7. Kennedy, JW, Ritchie, JL, Davis, KB, and Fritz, JK: Western Washington randomized trial of intracoronary streptokinase in acute myocardial infarction. N Engl J Med 309:1477, 1983.
8. Khaja, F, Walton, JA, Brymer, JF, et al: Intracoronary fibrinolytic therapy on acute myocardial infarction. N Engl J Med 308:1305, 1983.
9. Rentrop, KP, Feit, F, Blanke, H, et al: Effects of intracoronary streptokinase and intracoronary nitroglycerin infusion on coronary angiographic patterns and mortality in patients with acute myocardial infarction. N Engl J Med 311:1457, 1984.
10. Simoons, ML, van de Brand, M, DeZwaans, C, et al: Improved survival after early thrombolysis in acute myocardial infarction. Lancet 2:578, 1985.
11. Raizner, AE, Tortoledo, FA, Verani, MS, et al: Intracoronary thrombolytic therapy in acute myocardial infarction: A prospective, randomized, controlled trial. Am J Cardiol 55:301, 1985.
12. Kennedy, JW, Gensini, GG, Timmis, GC, and Maynard, C: Acute myocardial infarction treated with intracoronary streptokinase: A report of the Society for Cardiac Angiography. Am J Cardiol 55:871, 1985.
13. Weinstein, J: Treatment of myocardial infarction with intracoronary streptokinase: Efficacy and safety data from 209 United States cases in the Hoechst-Roussel registry. Am Heart J 104:894, 1982.
14. Ong, L, Reisner, P, Coromilas, J, et al: Left ventricular function and rapid release of creatinine MB in acute myocardial infarction. N Engl J Med 309:1, 1983.
15. Sheehan, FH, Mathey, DG, Schofer, J, et al: Effect of interventions in salvaging left ventricular function in acute myocardial infarction: A study of intracoronary streptokinase. Am J Cardiol 52:431, 1983.
16. Sheehan, FH, Mathey, DG, Schofer, J, et al: Factors determining recovery of left ventricular function following thrombolysis in acute myocardial infarction. Circulation 71:1121, 1985.
17. Schwartz, H, Leiboff, RL, Katz, RJ, et al: Arteriographic predictors of spontaneous improvement in left ventricular function after myocardial infarction. Circulation 71:466, 1985.
18. Kennedy, JW, Ritchie, JL, Davis, KB, et al: Western Washington intracoronary streptokinase trial follow-up. N Engl J Med 312:1073, 1985.
19. Verstraete, M, Bory, M, Collen, D, et al: Randomized trial of intravenous recombinant tissue-type plasminogen activator versus intravenous streptokinase in acute myocardial infarction. Lancet 1:842, 1985.
20. Sheehan, FH, Braunwald, E, Canner, P, et al: The effect of intravenous thrombolytic therapy on left ventricular function: A report on tissue-type plasminogen activator and streptokinase from thrombolysis in myocardial infarction (TIMI phase I) trial. Circulation 75:817, 1987.
21. White, HD, Norris, RM, Brown, MA, et al: Effect of intravenous streptokinase on left ventricular function and early survival after acute myocardial infarction. N Engl J Med 317:850, 1987.
22. ISAM Study Group. A prospective trial of intravenous streptokinase in acute myocardial infarction (ISAM). N Engl J Med 314:1465, 1986.
23. Kennedy, JW: Streptokinase for the treatment of acute myocardial infarction: A brief review of randomized trials. J Am Coll Cardiol 5:28B, 1987.

24. Gruppo Italiano Per Lo Studio Della Streptochinasi Nell' Infarto Miocardico (GISSI): Effectiveness of intravenous thrombolytic treatment in acute myocardial infarction. Lancet 1:397, 1986.
25. Van De Werf, F, Ludbrook, PA, Bergmann, SR, et al: Coronary thrombolysis with tissue-type plasminogen activator in patients with evolving myocardial infarction. N Engl J Med 310:609, 1984.
26. Topol, EJ, Califf, RM, George, BS, et al: A randomized trial of immediate versus delayed elective angioplasty after intravenous tissue plasminogen activator in acute myocardial infarction. N Engl J Med 317:581, 1987.
27. Guerci, AD, Gerstenblith, G, Brinker, JA, et al: A randomized trial of intravenous tissue plasminogen activator for acute myocardial infarction with subsequent randomization to elective coronary angioplasty. N Engl J Med 317:1613, 1987.
28. Gold, HK, Leinbach, RC, Garabedian, HD, et al: Acute coronary reocclusion after thrombolysis with recombinant human tissue-type plasminogen activator: Prevention by a maintenance infusion. Circulation 73:347, 1986.
29. Chesebro, JH, Knatterud, G, Roberts, R, et al: Thrombolysis in myocardial infarction (TIMI) trial, phase I: A comparison between intravenous tissue plasminogen activator and intravenous streptokinase. Circulation 76:142, 1987.
30. Topol, EJ, O'Neill, WW, Langburd, AB, et al: A randomized, placebo-controlled trial of intravenous recombinant tissue-type plasminogen activator and emergency coronary angioplasty in patients with acute myocardial infarction. Circulation 75:420, 1987.
31. Hartzler, GO, Rutherford, BD, McConahay, DR, et al: Percutaneous transluminal coronary angioplasty with and without thrombolytic therapy for treatment of acute myocardial infarction. Am Heart J 106:965, 1983.
32. O'Neill, W, Timmis, GC, Bourdillon, PD, et al: A prospective randomized clinical trial of intracoronary streptokinase versus coronary angioplasty for acute myocardial infarction. N Engl J Med 314:812, 1986.
33. Rothbaum, DA, Linnemeier, TJ, Landin, RJ, et al: Emergency percutaneous transluminal coronary angioplasty in acute myocardial infarction: A 3 year experience. J Am Coll Cardiol 10:264, 1987.
34. Meyer, J, Merx, W, Schmitz, H, et al: Percutaneous transluminal coronary angioplasty immediately after intracoronary streptolysis of transmural myocardial infarction. Circulation 66:905, 1982.
35. Serruys, PW, Wijns, W, van den Brand, M, et al: Is transluminal coronary angioplasty mandatory after successful thrombolysis? Br Heart J 50:257, 1983.
36. Berry, C, Zalewski, A, Kovach, R, et al: Surface electrocardiogram in the detection of transmural myocardial ischemia during percutaneous transluminal coronary angioplasty. Am J Cardiol, 1989 (in press).
37. Boden, WE, Kleiger, RE, Gibson, RS, et al: Electrocardiographic evolution of posterior acute myocardial infarction: Importance of early precordial ST-segment depression. Am J Cardiol 59:782, 1987.
38. Waller, BF, Rothbaum, DA, Pinkerton, CA, et al: Status of the myocardium and infarct-related coronary artery in 19 necropsy patients with acute recanalization using pharmacologic (streptokinase, r-tissue plasminogen activator), mechanical (percutaneous transluminal coronary angioplasty) or combined types of reperfusion therapy. J Am Coll Cardiol 9:785, 1987.
39. Miller, FC, Krucoff, MW, Satler, LF, et al: Ventricular arrhythmias during reperfusion. Am Heart J 112:928, 1986.
40. Mark, AL: The Bezold-Jarisch reflex revisited: Clinical implication of inhibitory reflexes originating in the heart. J Am Coll Cardiol 1:90, 1983.
41. Schroder, R, Neuhaus, KL, Leizorovicz, A, et al for the ISAM Study Group: A prospective placebo-controlled double-blind multicenter trial of intravenous streptokinase in acute myocardial infarction (ISAM): Long-term mortality and morbidity. J Am Coll Cardiol 9:197, 1987.
42. ISIS-2 (Second International Study of Infarct Survival) Collaborative Group: Randomized trial of intravenous streptokinase, oral aspirin, both or neither among 17,187 cases of suspected acute myocardial infarction: ISIS-2. Lancet 2:349, 1988.
43. Robertson, T, Babb, J, Baim, D, et al: Results of TIMI IIA: Immediate versus postponed PTCA during or after rt-PA thrombolysis for MI. Eur Heart J 9 (suppl 1):149, 1988.

CHAPTER 13

Beta-Adrenergic Blockers in Patients with Acute Myocardial Infarction

Curt D. Furberg, M.D., Ph.D.
Robert P. Byington, Ph.D.

In 1985, 755,000 patients in the United States alone were admitted to a hospital with the diagnosis of acute myocardial infarction (MI), and 638,000 were discharged alive. Thus, 117,000 died during the hospital stay, corresponding to an average in-hospital mortality of 15.5 percent. Of the patients with acute MI who survive the hospital phase, more than 90 percent eventually succumb to their coronary disease. Their annual mortality has been estimated to be 4 to 10 times that of a matched noncoronary population. Identifying preventive interventions to reduce this toll represents a major public health challenge. It is apparent that to be effective in improving survival, either during the acute event or in the long-term, an intervention must favorably influence one or more of the morbid mechanisms accounting for the coronary deaths.

MORBID MECHANISMS

In principle, there are five morbid mechanisms responsible for coronary deaths: (1) progressive coronary atherosclerosis, (2) coronary thrombosis, (3) electrical complications such as ventricular fibrillation, (4) mechanical complications such as heart failure, and (5) recurrent ischemia resulting from an imbalance between oxygen supply and demand. These mechanisms are related and often overlapping. Progression of the underlying coronary atherosclerosis operates only in the long-term.

Interventions with the potential for counteracting the morbid mechanisms have been evaluated in a large number of randomized clinical trials, on which extensive review articles provide detailed information.[1–6] These interventions may be summarized as follows:

1. The most fundamental cause of MI is coronary atherosclerosis, and lipid-lowering regimens with diet or drugs have been tested with the hope of retarding its rate of progression.

2. Three types of intervention have been aimed at preventing both the extension of an existing thrombus and rethrombosis or at achieving thrombolysis: conventional anticoagulants, platelet-active drugs, and thrombolytic agents.
3. Almost half of all deaths in patients with coronary disease are sudden and presumably due to ventricular arrhythmias. Various classes of antiarrhythmic agents have been tested, intravenously and orally, in the expectation of reducing the risk for ventricular fibrillation.
4. In the past, limited attention has been paid to patients with the most complicated MIs (e.g., patients with heart failure, hypotension, and shock). Most of the trial data in congestive heart failure are from non-MI populations. Of potential interest are direct-acting vasodilators and ACE inhibitors.
5. Improvement of the balance between oxygen supply and demand reduces the risk of recurrent ischemic events as well as of certain arrhythmias and mechanical failure. Three types of interventions with potential for improving the oxygen balance have been evaluated in patients with acute MI: physical exercise, beta-adrenergic blockers, and calcium channel blockers.

The presumed major mechanisms for increased cardiovascular mortality during the postinfarction period include cardiac arrhythmias, left ventricular dysfunction, and persistent myocardial ischemia. Raised levels of circulating catecholamines or enhanced sympathetic drive can increase both the severity of myocardial ischemia and the frequency of ventricular arrhythmias. After the clinical introduction of propranolol for angina pectoris and arrhythmias in 1963, it was conceived that beta-blocker administration might favorably influence the acute and long-term course of MI patients by attenuating the undesirable consequences of increased sympathetic nervous system activity. However, inasmuch as these drugs could also depress left ventricular function—the other major factor contributing to mortality after infarction—beta-blockers were avoided initially in patients with acute MI or were used in small doses for fear of causing new or aggravating existing congestive heart failure.

PROVEN AND UNPROVEN INTERVENTIONS

Acute Interventions

Conventional anticoagulants, platelet-active drugs, and thrombolytic agents, the three types of interventions in acute MI aimed at preventing the extension of an existing thrombus and rethrombosis or at achieving thrombolysis, have a well-documented favorable effect on survival.[2,5–9] It appears that their mechanisms of action are different and that the combination of a platelet-active agent (aspirin) and a thrombolytic compound (streptokinase) is most beneficial.[9]

Beta-blockers given within the first 24 hours of an acute MI, first as an intravenous bolus and followed by oral therapy, have also been shown to reduce in-hospital mortality.[4,6,10] Pooled analysis of trials evaluating nitrates in acute MI are suggestive of a beneficial effect.[6] In contrast, antiarrhythmics and calcium channel blockers have no proven benefit on short- or long-term mortality.[3,11] In fact, calcium channel blockers may even cause a slight excess of deaths when given to patients with acute MI.

Long-Term Interventions

Beta-blockers represent the most effective prophylactic long-term treatment of patients who have survived the acute phase of an MI.[1,4,12] Aspirin has a smaller but favorable effect.[8] Physical exercise[1] and angiotensin converting-enzyme-inhibitors may be beneficial to subgroups of patients with MI but belong to the category of promising but not proven interventions. Long-term treatment with oral anticoagulants, antiarrhythmics, lipid-lowering agents, and calcium channel blockers has no documented effect on all-cause mortality.[1,3,11]

The major outcome data of beta-blocker trials in acute MI and over the long-term following hospital discharge are presented below.

MATERIAL AND METHODS

We chose to consider those trials reported prior to December 1987 in which both intervention and followup were carried out during and/or beyond the time of hospital discharge. Trials were included in this review if they met the following criteria: (1) random assignment of subjects to either an intervention or a control group, and (2) a total sample size of at least 100. These criteria were chosen for two important reasons: first, to restrict this review to trials that incorporate in their design some protection (randomization) against treatment allocation bias, and, second, to focus on those trials that could possibly have had sufficient statistical power, as judged by sample size, to discern a clinically important effect or trend.

Total mortality has been used whenever possible as the primary response variable in this review, regardless of whether this was the choice in the published report. This approach minimizes potential bias inherent in end-point determination, inasmuch as total mortality relies only on a simple count without any element of judgment. To reduce the bias that may come about from the differential withdrawal of patients, all patients who were randomized have been included in the mortality estimates, if the data are available.

Because many of the studies gave only the number of deaths for each treatment group, classical survival curves could not be computed. We chose, therefore, to compare the proportion of deaths in each treatment group by a chi-square test so that there might be some consistency in the analysis between studies. We recognize that this is only an approximation to the comparison of survival curves, but in our experience the results are usually similar. When differences for end-points other than total mortality are said to be statistically significant in this review, this designation is in most instances the conclusion of the published report and usually denotes a conventional p-value of <0.05.

RESULTS

Acute (Short-Term) Trials

Oral Administration

Thirteen published and unpublished trials meeting the review criteria evaluated the effect of short-term, oral administration of beta-blockers.[4] In four of the trials, treatment continued beyond the hospital stay or for more than 4 weeks. Most of the trials were conducted or reported in the 1960s and represent the first generation of beta-blocker trials. The beta-blocking doses were generally low compared with those shown to be effective in subsequent trials. The patients were enrolled within 1 to 3 days of the onset of symptoms. Propranolol was tested in six trials, oxprenolol in four, practolol in two, and alprenolol and atenolol in one each. One trial evaluated two beta-blockers.

All trials were fairly small; the largest enrolled 454 patients. Beta-blocker therapy was not shown to be beneficial in any of the individual trials. Overall, there was a total of 156 early deaths among 1691 patients (9.2 percent) allocated to the beta-blocker groups compared with 149 deaths in 1508 control patients (9.9 percent).

Intravenous/Oral Administration

In 14 trials[4,10] that met our review criteria, an initial loading dose was given intravenously in the acute phase of the MI and was followed by oral medication for the remainder of the trial (Table 13–1). The trials were reported between 1979 and 1986 and comprise the second generation beta-blocker trials. In contrast to the previous trials that initiated treatment with an oral dose, the patients were enrolled as early as possible, usually within 6 to 8 hours. Treatment varied from 27 hours to 1 year. However, the mortality data in Table 13–2 reflect 7-day mortality. Seven different beta-blockers were tested, and most data are available for atenolol and metoprolol. The differences in drug dosages reflect varying beta-blocking potency.

One large trial, ISIS, reported a statistically significant 1-week benefit of beta-blockers (see Table 13–2). Three hundred and seventeen of the 8037 patients allocated to receive atenolol (3.9 percent) died compared with 367 of 7990 control

Table 13–1. Description of 14 Short-Term Trials of IV/Orally Administered Beta-Blockers[4,10]

Investigator/ Trial	**Year of Report**	**Initiation of tx**	**Duration of tx**	**Beta-Blocker**	**Dose (mg)**	
					IV	*Oral (Daily)*
Anderson	1979	median 6 hr	1 yr	alprenolol	5	400
Hjalmarson	1983	mean 11.3 hr	3 mo	metoprolol	15	200
Yusuf	1983	<12 hr	10 days	atenolol	5	100
UKCSG	1984	<6 hr	in-hosp	timolol	2 + 14*	10
ICSG	1984	<6 hr	in-hosp	timolol	2 + 14*	10
Federman	1984	<6 hr	28 days	timolol	5.5	20
Heber	1984	<6 hr	5 days	labetalol	**	**
PREMIS	1984	<6 hr	27 hr	propranolol	0.1/kg	320
MILIS	1984	mean 8 hr	9 days	propranolol	0.1/kg	***
Owensby	1984	<12 hr	3 days	pindolol	3	15
MIAMI	1985	<24 hr	16 days	metoprolol	15	200
Salathia	1985	<6 hr	1 yr	metoprolol	15	200
TIARA	1986	<6 hr	1 mo	timolol	5.5	20
ISIS	1986	<12 hr	7 days	atenolol	5–10	100

*Infused over 24 hours.
**Dose dependent on blood pressure.
***Dose dependent on heart rate and blood pressure.

Table 13–2. Seven-Day Mortality in 14 Randomized Trials With an Initial IV Dose of a Beta-Blocker[4,10]

	Control			Beta-Blocker			
Investigator/ Trial	**No. Randomized**	**No. Deaths**	**Rate (%)**	**No. Randomized**	**No. Deaths**	**Rate (%)**	**Relative Risk**
Anderson	242	24	9.9	238	28	11.8	1.19
Hjalmarson	697	23	3.3	698	18	2.6	0.78
Yusuf	233	16	6.9	244	6	2.5	0.36
UKCSG	52	5	9.6	56	4	7.1	0.74
ICSG	71	4	5.6	73	3	4.1	0.73
Federman	51	0	0.0	50	1	2.0	—
Heber	83	0	0.0	83	3	3.6	—
PREMIS	371	10	2.7	364	12	3.3	1.22
MILIS	135	4	3.0	134	4	3.0	1.01
Owensby	50	1	2.0	50	1	2.0	1.00
MIAMI	2,901	93	3.2	2,877	79	2.7	0.85
Salathia	384	17	4.4	416	18	4.3	0.98
TIARA	98	5	5.1	102	3	2.9	0.58
ISIS	7,990	367	4.6	8,037	317	3.9	0.86
TOTAL	13,358	569	(4.3)	13,422	497	(3.7)	0.87

patients (4.6 percent), a 15 percent relative mortality reduction. The pooled analysis (see Table 13–2) shows that in the 14 reviewed trials, 497 of 13,442 beta-blocker patients died (3.7 percent) compared with 569 of 13,358 control patients (4.3 percent). Thirteen trials that did not meet our review criteria would have added a total of approximately 700 patients to the database, and their overall mortality trend was similar to that of the reviewed trials.

Further analysis of the ISIS and of pooled trial results indicates that the benefit of beta-blocker use in acute MI patients occurs primarily within the first 24 hours when the mortality rate is the highest.[10] In addition to the reduction in early mortality, beta-blockers also reduce the risk of MI extension or reinfarction and cardiac arrest (ventricular fibrillation). The relative magnitude of these effects is similar to that for mortality (approximately 15 percent).

The low 7-day mortality rates among control patients with an acute MI are explained by the trial eligibility criteria. As many as half of the patients admitted with an acute MI had absolute or relative contraindications to beta-blocker therapy. For example, the excluded patients had more complicated infarcts.

The data do not allow a comparison of the different beta-blockers. Atenolol has a well-documented benefit. Metoprolol is probably not more effective than other beta-blockers without intrinsic sympathomimetic activity (ISA).

Long-Term Trials

Nineteen published and unpublished randomized controlled trials have evaluated the long-term effect of beta-blockers on all-cause mortality.[4,10] Long-term has arbitrarily been defined as at least 1 year of treatment, and the review was restricted to trials that had a total sample size of more than 100 patients. Thus, four trials were excluded because of duration and two because of size.

Table 13–3. Description of 19 Long-Term (1 Year or Longer) Trials of Oral Beta-Blockers[4,10]

Investigator/Trial	Year of Report	Initiation of tx Post-MI	Duration of tx	Beta-Blocker	Daily Dose (mg)
Wilhelmsson	1974	6 wk	2 yr	alprenolol*	400
Ahlmark	1974	2 wk	2 yr	alprenolol*	400
Barber	1976	median 3 hr	2 yr	practolol*	600
Multicentre Internat	1977	mean 13 days	mean 15 mo	practolol*	400
Andersen	1979	median 6 hr	1 yr	alprenolol*	400
Wilcox	1980	24 hr	1 yr	propranolol/	120
				atenolol	100
Rehnqvist	1980	discharge	1 yr	metoprolol	200
Norwegian	1981	7–28 days	mean 17 mo	timolol	20
Taylor	1982	mean 13 mo	mean 4 yr	oxprenolol*	80
Hansteen	1982	mean 5 days	1 yr	propranolol	160
BHAT	1982	mean 10 days	mean 25 mo	propranolol	180–240
Julian	1982	5 days	1 yr	sotalol	320
Australian-Swedish	1983	2–21 days	2 yr	pindolol*	15
Manger Cats	1983	mean 4 wk	1 yr	metoprolol	200
EIS	1984	median 24 days	1 yr	oxprenolol*	320
Olsson	1985	before discharge	3 yr	metoprolol	200
Salathia	1985	<6 hr	1 yr	metoprolol	200
Schwartz	1985	not available	about 4 yr	oxprenolol*	160
LIT	1987	mean 10 days	1 yr	metoprolol	200

*Beta-blocker with intrinsic sympathomimetic activity (ISA).

The 19 trials were reported between the years 1974 and 1986 (Table 13–3). Treatment was usually initiated prior to hospital discharge. Only four trials had a mean duration of treatment of more than 2 years. Nine different beta-blockers have been tested, although the largest databases exist for propranolol, metoprolol, oxprenolol, practolol, and timolol.

Four trials (Table 13–4) showed a statistically significant reduction in all-cause mortality—the Norwegian Timolol trial, the Beta-blocker Heart Attack Trial (propranolol), the trials by Schwartz and coworkers (oxprenolol) and Salathia and colleagues (metoprolol). In the last trial, treatment was initiated on hospital admission and the significance emerges only if deaths during the first week of therapy are excluded.

Overall, there were 1,008 deaths among 10,171 control patients, which corresponds to an average mortality of 9.9 percent. The mortality was 21 percent lower among the beta-blocker-treated patients—841 deaths among 10,723 patients (7.8 percent). The average mortality reduction in the trials of beta-blockers without ISA was 66 percent greater than that of the trials of beta-blockers with ISA, 24 versus 12 percent. In addition, most trials showed a very favorable trend in terms of reduction and nonfatal reinfarction. In pooled analysis with 84 percent complete data,[10] the reduction in nonfatal reinfarction was 27 percent.

DISCUSSION

The clinical trials provide overwhelming scientific evidence that beta-blockers, whether given acutely or in the long-term, reduce all-cause mortality and non-

Table 13–4. All-Cause Mortality* in 19 Long-Term Trials of Beta-Blockers in MI Patients[4,10]

Investigator/Trial	Control			Beta-Blocker			Relative Risk
	No. Randomized	No. Deaths	Rate (%)	No. Randomized	No. Deaths	Rate (%)	
Wilhelmsson	116	14	12.1	114	7	6.1	0.51
Ahlmark	93	11	11.8	69	5	7.2	0.61
Barber	213	38	17.8	207	33	15.9	0.89
Multicenter Internat	1,520	127	8.4	1,533	102	6.7	0.79
Andersen	218	40	18.3	209	32	15.3	0.83
Wilcox	122	12	9.8	251	28	11.2	1.14
Rehnqvist	52	6	11.5	59	4	6.8	0.59
Norwegian	939	152	16.2	945	98	10.4	0.64
Taylor	471	48	10.2	632	60	9.5	0.93
Hansteen	282	37	13.1	278	25	9.0	0.68
BHAT	1,921	188	9.8	1,916	138	7.2	0.74
Julian	583	52	8.9	873	64	7.3	0.82
Australian-Swedish	266	47	17.7	263	45	17.1	0.97
Manger Cats	293	16	5.5	291	9	3.1	0.56
EIS	883	45	5.1	858	57	6.6	1.30
Olsson	147	31	21.1	154	25	16.2	0.77
Salathia	364	43	11.8	391	27	6.9	0.58
Schwartz	488	39	8.0	485	17	3.5	0.44
LIT	1,200	62	5.2	1,195	65	5.4	1.05
TOTAL	10,171	1,008	(9.9)	10,723	841	(7.8)	0.79

*Mortality after day 7 for trials in which treatment was initiated upon admission.

fatal reinfarction. The trials have also raised several questions, many of which relate to the clinical care of individual MI patients.

How Do the Beta-Blockers Exert Their Favorable Effect on Survival?

As expected, the reduction in all-cause mortality is due to a reduction in atherosclerotic cardiovascular deaths. The benefit is explained particularly by a prevention of sudden cardiac deaths.[1,4,12] For example, the mortality experience of the Beta-Blocker Heart Attack Trial (BHAT) is typical of the long-term trials (Table 13–5). Also, experimental studies have shown that beta-blockers raise the threshold for ventricular fibrillation in ischemic myocardium. A reduction in the incidence of ventricular fibrillation during beta-blockade has been shown in acute trials.[4,10] MI patients with complex ventricular arrhythmias, who constitute a high-risk subgroup, respond very favorably to beta-blockers.[13] However, the observed reduction in nonsudden deaths (see Table 13–5), coupled with the observed reduction in nonfatal reinfarction with beta-blocker therapy, cannot be explained by an antiarrhythmic effect alone and suggests an "anti-ischemic" effect. This mechanism is probably separate from the antianginal effect of beta-blockers, inasmuch as other compounds with antianginal properties do not influence survival (e.g., calcium channel blockers).

Which Patients Should Be Treated?

Approximately half of all patients admitted early with an acute MI and about 20 percent of those surviving 1 to 3 weeks have relative or absolute contraindications to beta-blocker treatment, such as hypotension, bradycardia, severe congestive heart failure, AV conduction disorders, and obstructive lung disease.

Table 13–5. Cause-Specific Mortality by Treatment Group in the Beta-Blocker Heart Attack Trial (Average Length of Followup = 25 Months)

	Placebo Group (N = 1921)		Propranolol Group (N = 1916)				
Cause of Death	**No. of Deaths**	**Percent**	**No. of Deaths**	**Percent**	**Absolute Risk**	**Relative Risk**	**p-Value (Two-Sided)**
Total Mortality	188	9.8	138	7.2	−2.6/100	0.74	0.004
Noncardiovascular	17	0.9	11	0.6	−0.3/100	0.65	NS†
Cardiovascular	171	8.9	127	6.6	−2.3/100	0.74	0.009
Nonatherosclerotic	7	0.4	8	0.4	0.0/100	1.15	NS†
Atherosclerotic	164	8.5	119	6.2	−2.3/100	0.73	0.006
Nonsudden	75	3.9	55	2.9	−1.0/100	0.74	NS†
Sudden*	89	4.6	64	3.3	−1.3/100	0.72	0.04

*Death within 1 hour of symptoms.
†NS = not significant.

Post-hoc analysis[14] in the BHAT suggests that patients with uncomplicated MIs (and an already low annual mortality) only benefit to a very small degree from beta-blocker therapy (Table 13–6). The largest mortality reductions were found in patients who had had transient electrical and/or pump complications. Similar observations have been reported subsequently in other trials. The trial experience in elderly patients is limited, but there seems to be a good rationale to extrapolate the results to this population. For example, in the BHAT, a trend toward an even greater benefit was observed in patients 60 years of age or older when compared with MI patients below age 60.[15]

To the clinician and the patient, the absolute benefit of a preventive measure appears to be more important than the relative treatment benefit. In a low-risk population, a reduction of the annual mortality from 2 percent to 1.5 percent, means that 200 such patients have to be treated for 1 year to save one life. The relative benefit is 25 percent. A similar relative benefit in a high-risk population would reduce a 16 percent annual mortality to 12 percent or, in other words, one life saved per 25 such patients treated. The apparent paradox is that a 5 percent relative mortality reduction in a high-risk group (from 16.0 percent to 15.2 percent, or one life saved per 125 treated) is preferable to a 25 percent reduction in a low-risk group (2.0 percent to 1.5 percent, or one life saved per 200 treated).

If this reasoning is applied to the beta-blocker trials, one can conclude that the prime candidates for beta-blocker prevention are the high-risk patients. Analyses of the long-term trials have shown that such subgroups (i.e., patients with transient electrical and mechanical complications, and patients with complex ventricular arrhythmias on a predischarge 24-hour ambulatory ECG) benefit the most in absolute terms. In most instances, the relative benefits exceeded those of the corresponding low-risk populations. The elderly, as a group, also seem to be prime candidates inasmuch as the proportion of complicated MIs increases with age. The early fear of treating type II diabetics appears unfounded. In fact, diabetic MI patients are prime candidates for prophylactic beta-blockers. In deciding who to treat prophylactically, one should be reminded that there are other indications for long-term beta-blocker use (e.g., angina pectoris and hypertension).

When Should Beta-Blocker Therapy Be Initiated?

The reviews of the acute (short-term) trials clearly show that if beta-blockers are contemplated, therapy should be initiated with an intravenous bolus within 6 to 8 hours of onset of pain. The relatively low 7-day mortality among patients without contraindications to beta-blockers (approximately 4 percent, see Table 13–2) and the small relative benefit (approximately 15 percent) raise issues related to cost–benefit. In light of the larger benefit associated with thrombolytic therapy and aspirin,[7,9] the role of beta-blockers in the very early phase of an MI is debatable. However, it is possible that beta-blocker therapy, particularly on the first day of the infarct, can provide added benefit to a thrombolysis-aspirin regimen.

For the long-term, the choices are limited inasmuch as no intervention besides beta-blocker therapy has a documented effect on survival and risk of reinfarction. In most of the long-term trials, beta-blocker therapy was started 1 to 3 weeks after the infarction while the patients were still hospitalized. It was a clear advantage to initiate treatment by the time the patients had begun to recover,

Table 13–6. All-Cause Mortality (%) by Treatment Group and Risk Group in the Beta-Blocker Heart Attack Trial

	Placebo		Propranolol					
Risk Group	**No. of Patients**	**Mortality (p1)**	**No. of Patients**	**Mortality (p2)**	**Z-Value of Diff**	**Absolute Risk**	**Relative Risk p1/p2**	**Adjusted Relative Risk***
None	1079	6.6	1047	6.2	−0.35	−0.4	0.94	0.96
Electrical only	423	10.9	443	5.2	−3.09	−5.7	0.48	0.43
Mechanical only	202	16.8	201	10.4	−1.87	−6.4	0.62	0.57
Both	217	17.1	225	12.9	−1.23	−4.2	0.76	0.70

*Adjusted for 13 baseline factors predictive of mortality.

were in a stable condition, and could be observed. It seems prudent to recommend that oral beta-blockers be started 6 to 9 days after the acute event in patients who are hemodynamically stable, have no contraindications to this treatment, and are at increased risk of mortality and reinfarction. These patients are prime candidates for beta-blocker therapy. No trials have compared the value of acute and delayed initiation of beta-blocker treatment. Because both approaches work, the clinician can choose either option.

How Long Should Treatment Be Continued?

If therapy is initiated within a few hours of an acute MI, it seems reasonable to continue it after hospital discharge. The long-term trials provide a substantial database for the assessment of treatment benefit up to 2 years. Beyond this time point the data are limited, and a recommendation for continued treatment has to be based on an extrapolation of the 2-year results. Because the cumulative mortality curves for the propranolol and placebo groups for the complicated MI patients in BHAT (Fig. 13–1) continue to diverge for 36 months and most post-MI patients have angina or ventricular arrhythmias, it seem prudent, in the absence of any troublesome adverse reaction, not to time-limit beta-blocker therapy.

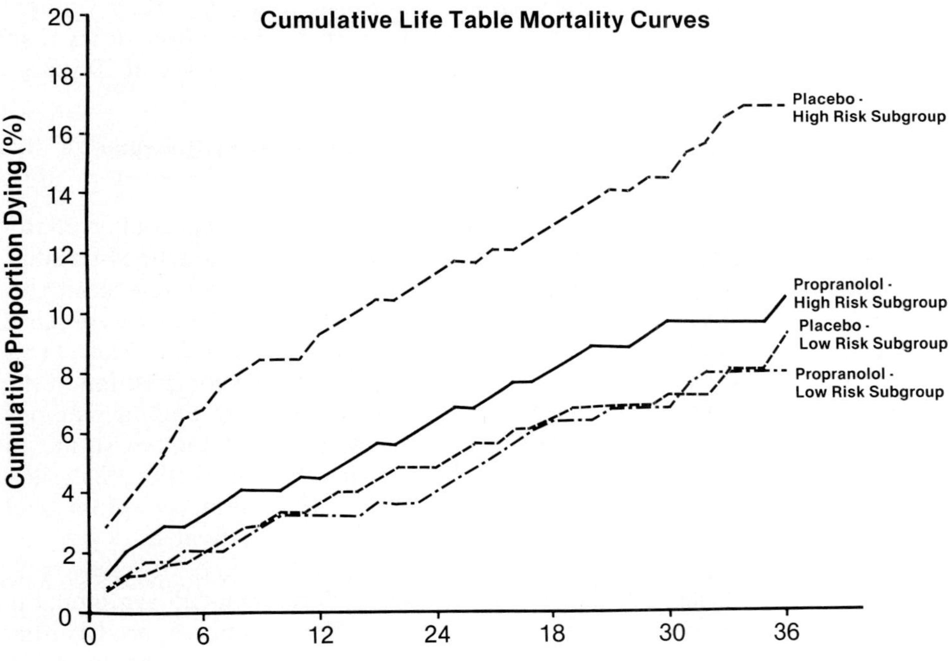

Figure 13–1. Cumulative life table mortality curves by treatment group and risk group. Beta-Blocker Heart Attack Trial. High risk = having at least one of the following at baseline: complete or incomplete AV block, ventricular fibrillation or tachycardia, atrial fibrillation, pulmonary edema, cardiogenic shock, persistent hypotension, congestive heart failure, or basilar rales.

Are All Beta-Blockers Equally Effective and What Dosage Should Be Used?

No clinical trial has compared the preventive and adverse effect of two different beta-blockers. Several factors can explain numerical differences in treatment effect across trials. The inclusion of a high proportion of low-risk, uncomplicated MI patients would tend to dilute the benefit in the high-risk groups. Equipotency is difficult to determine and it is possible that for some beta-blockers and trials, particularly the early ones, a less than optimal dosage was tested. Chance is a powerful factor to consider. However, there may be ancillary pharmacological properties, which could also be important. It appears that beta-blockers with ISA (see Table 13–3) are less effective than those without ISA (see Table 13–4). There is no scientific evidence that the cardioselective beta-1 blockers, atenolol and metoprolol, are more effective than the nonselective. In fact, the strongest data on the favorable long-term mortality effect come from trials of propranolol and timolol. There are some speculatons that the beta-2 blockade may enhance the antiarrhythmic action of beta-1 blockade.

Overviews of the kind presented here can offer more unbiased insights into how these drugs work and how they compare than individual trial reports. The beta-blockers recommended in the preventive treatment of MI are timolol, propranolol, metoprolol, and atenolol. The side-effect profile may be most favorable for atenolol. The recommended daily doses are those evaluated in the clinical trials—timolol 20 mg, propranolol 180 to 240 mg, metoprolol 200 mg, and atenolol 100 mg. Elderly patients often require lower drug doses than their younger counterparts. Unfortunately, there is no evidence that much lower doses than those cited above provide a preventive effect in people over the age of 70 years.

What Are the Potential Negative Effects of Beta-Blocker Treatment?

In deciding whether or not to treat patients with beta-blockers after infarction, the risks of therapy must be weighed against the potential benefits. In studies of patients with no absolute or relative contraindications to beta-blocker treatment, severe adverse reactions leading to discontinuation of therapy were fairly infrequent. The proportion of patients taken off active treatment for medical reasons ranged from approximately 5 percent to 20 percent. The composition of the patient populations, the drug dosages and duration of treatment, and the methods of ascertaining and reporting adverse effects are factors that need to be considered in comparing these numbers. A notable finding was the observation that side-effects were common with placebo treatment. Often we attribute symptoms and signs to a patient's treatment rather than the condition being treated.

Cardiovascular problems accounted for the greatest number of severe reactions in the beta-blocker groups. These untoward effects included symptomatic congestive heart failure, hypotension with and without dizziness, bradycardia, and atrioventricular block. Heart failure was much less common than expected, perhaps because most of the trials excluded from participation patients with even moderate heart failure.

The trials also showed a high frequency of minor side-effects with beta-blockers, which did not lead to discontinuation of the treatment. These effects included cold extremities, nausea, constipation, asthma, fatigue, mental depression, impotence, and dry eyes.

If we accept that high-risk patients are the prime candidates for preventive therapy, we have to be prepared to pay a price—a greater incidence of adverse effects. Regarding adverse effects by risk group in the BHAT,[14] the incidence of congestive heart failure in the uncomplicated group and the group with the electrical complications only was about 5 percent to 6 percent over 25 months, whether or not they received beta-blockers. If the patients had a history of transient mechanical complications and were given placebo, their risk was twice that (10 percent) and if propranolol was added, the risk of developing congestive heart failure increased by another 5 percent.

SUMMARY

Beta-blockers given within the first 24 hours of an acute MI, first as an intravenous bolus followed by oral therapy, have been shown to reduce in-hospital mortality following a myocardial infarction. For the long-term, beta-blockers represent the only documented effective prophylactic treatment for MI patients.

The reduction in all-cause mortality is due primarily to a reduction in atherosclerotic cardiovascular deaths, particularly sudden cardiac deaths. This finding is consistent with the experimental observation that beta-blockers raise the threshold for ventricular fibrillation. Indeed, MI patients with complex ventricular arrhythmias respond very favorably to beta-blockers. However, reductions in nonsudden deaths and nonfatal reinfarctions have also been observed, suggesting that the beneficial effects of beta-blockers are not limited to antiarrhythmic effects alone and that these drugs may also have anti-ischemic effects.

The prime candidates for beta-blocker therapy are the high-risk MI patients with transient electrical and/or pump complications during the acute phase. If therapy is initiated within hours of an acute infarction, it seems reasonable to continue it after hospital discharge. Evidence from the large, long-term trials suggest that, in the absence of any troublesome adverse reaction and given that most post-MI patients experience ventricular arrhythmias and angina, it seems reasonable not to limit the duration of treatment.

REFERENCES

1. May, GS, Eberlein, KA, Furberg, CD, et al: Secondary prevention after myocardial infarction: A review of long-term trials. Prog Cardiovasc Dis 24:331, 1982.
2. May, GS, Furberg, CD, Eberlein, KA, and Geraci, B: Secondary prevention after myocardial infarction: A review of short-term acute phase trials. Prog Cardiovasc Dis 25:335, 1983.
3. Furberg, CD: Effect of antiarrhythmic drugs on mortality after myocardial infarction. Am J Cardiol 52:32C, 1983.
4. Yusuf, S, Peto, R, Lewis, J, et al: Beta blockade during and after myocardial infarction: An overview of the randomized trials. Prog Cardiovasc Dis 27:335, 1985.
5. Yusuf, S, Collins, R, Peto, R, et al: Intravenous and intracoronary fibrinolytic therapy in acute myocardial infarction: Overview of result on mortality, reinfarction and side-effects from 33 randomized controlled trials. Eur Heart J 6:556, 1985.
6. Yusuf, S: Interventions that potentially limit myocardial infarct size: Overview of clinical trials. Am J Cardiol 60:11A, 1987.
7. Gruppo Italiano Per Lo Studio Della Streptochinasi Nell' Infarto Miscardico (GISSI): Effectiveness of intravenous thrombolytic treatment in acute myocardial infarction. Lancet 1:397, 1986.

8. Antiplatelet Trialists' Collaboration: Secondary prevention of vascular disease by prolonged antiplatelet treatment. Br Med J 296:320, 1988.
9. ISIS Collaborative Group: Results of a large randomized trial of intravenous streptokinase and oral aspirin in acute myocardial infarction (abstr). J Am Coll Cardiol 11:232A, 1988.
10. ISIS-1 (First International Study of Infarct Survival) Collaborative Group: Randomised trial of intravenous atenolol among 16,027 cases of suspected acute myocardial infarction: ISIS 1. Lancet 2:57, 1986.
11. Yusuf, S and Furberg, C: Effect of acute or chronic administration of calcium antagonists on mortality following myocardial infarction (abstr). J Am Coll Cardiol 9:24A, 1987.
12. Frishman, WH, Furberg, CD, and Friedewald, WT: Beta-adrenergic blockade for survivors of acute myocardial infarction. N Engl J Med 310:830, 1984.
13. Friedman, LM, Byington, RP, Capone, RJ, et al: Effect of propranolol in patients with myocardial infarction and ventricular arrhythmia. J Am Coll Cardiol 7:1, 1986.
14. Furberg, CD, Hawkins, CM, and Lichstein, E: Effect of propranolol in post-infarction patients with mechanical or electrical complications. Circulation 69:761, 1984.
15. Hawkins, CM, Richardson, DW, and Vokonas, PS: Effect of propranolol in reducing mortality in older myocardial infarction patients. The Beta-Blocker Heart Attack Trial experience. Circulation 67:I–94, 1983.

CHAPTER 14

Conventional Drug Therapy of Patients with Acute Myocardial Infarction

C. Richard Conti, M.D.

Presently, all patients with an evolving myocardial infarction should be "considered" for thrombolytic therapy. The evidence is strong that lytic therapy, at least with streptokinase, decreases mortality. Thus, one must consider the use of "conventional" drugs in the context of patients who do or do not receive thrombolytic therapy. Perhaps some of these conventional drugs will broaden the opportunity and make lytic therapy effective for a longer period of time after the infarction. In other instances, some of these drugs may prevent the complications of lytic therapy, such as reperfusion injury and arrhythmias, and in still other instances a few of these drugs may prevent thrombus reformation.

GENERAL APPROACH

One must develop a rationale for treating the individual patient with acute myocardial infarction. The obvious pathogenetic mechanisms responsible for acute myocardial infarction include (1) severe coronary artery stenosis in most instances, (2) thrombotic occlusion of the artery supplying the ischemic myocardium, and (3) a possible contribution of coronary artery spasm to initiate the thrombus formation or prolong the occlusion once the thrombus is formed.

It seems clear that one should decrease myocardial oxygen consumption if coronary artery disease is limiting flow, should dilate the coronary artery if coronary artery spasm has decreased flow, and should lyse the thrombus-occluded coronary artery that has stopped coronary flow.

Current practice emphasizes the reduction of myocardial oxygen demand. This is accomplished by the use of oxygen, analgesia (morphine sulfate), beta-blockers (intravenous metoprolol), vasodilators (nitrates), anticoagulants (heparin), antiplatelet agents (aspirin), antiarrhythmics (lidocaine), diuretics (furosemide), and inotropes (digitalis, dopamine, dobutamine, and so on). With this combination of drugs, blood pressure is generally maintained at an optimal level, anxiety states are calmed, venous return is reduced (thus decreasing the filling pressure and ventricular volume), tachyarrhythmias are controlled, and cardiac output is maintained. Using one or more of these therapies, it is reasonable to expect that infarction size will be limited.

Obviously, not all of these drugs will be required in any one patient, especially if the patient has an uncomplicated myocardial infarction. However, intravenous nitrates can be used safely in most patients in the early stages of infarction (unless the patient is hypovolemic).

SPECIFIC THERAPY

Oxygen

For some reason, oxygen is used routinely in most patients with any acute cardiac event. It is used whether the patient is hypoxemic or not. This is not only economically wasteful but a potential hazard. In my view, oxygen should be administered only if there is evidence of hypoxemia, for example, pulmonary edema and cyanosis. In the acutely ill cardiac patient, when there is doubt, it is worthwhile obtaining an arterial oxygen saturation to document the need for this type of therapy. However, if thrombolytic therapy is contemplated, an arterial puncture is contraindicated and it may be best to give oxygen to the patient without objective evidence for hypoxia,[1] if there is doubt about the patient's oxygen saturation.

Analgesia

The major indication for using analgesia, for example, morphine sulphate intravenously, in patients with an evolving acute myocardial infarction is to sedate and calm the patient. Admittedly, morphine sulfate does have vasodilator properties and may decrease myocardial oxygen consumption by lowering blood pressure, and perhaps by slowing heart rate and decreasing venous return. However, in my view, it is not the best drug for this purpose. My own approach is to reserve the use of small doses of intravenous morphine for patients who continue to have pain despite other therapies directed at decreasing myocardial oxygen consumption or increasing myocardial oxygenation.

Beta-Blockers

The role of beta-blockers in the management of an evolving myocardial infarction is controversial. Many are concerned, and I share that concern, that one can do harm by administering a negative chronotropic and negative inotropic agent in the early phases of an acute myocardial infarction. However, clinical trials have shown otherwise. One such example is the clinical trial in which the beta-blocker timolol was administered intravenously within 4 hours of the onset of chest pain and compared with placebo.[2] The International Collaborative Study Group published their results in 1984 and showed a reduction in myocardial ischemia and infarction size, as judged clinically in the following manner. The timolol-treated patients had a prompt fall in ST segment amplitude and CK release, chest pain, and requirements for analgesic medication. In this study, timolol was administered intravenously for the first 24 hours and then orally for the remainder of the hospital stay. Other beta-blocker heart attack trials have shown a decreased mortality in patients receiving beta-blockers compared with placebo.[3] However, beta-blockers were not administered in the early phases of acute myocardial infarction in most of these trials.

From the standpoint of safety, I prefer to use short-acting beta-blockers. The only ultra short-acting beta-blocker currently available is esmolol. The advantage of this beta-blocker is that its onset is rapid and if the patient has any adverse reactions, the effects will disappear within 15 or 20 minutes.

The decision to use a beta-blocker in the early phase of acute myocardial infarction must be individualized. Guidelines from clinical trials suggest that they are beneficial.[3] However, if there are contraindications to their use, such as bronchospasm, significant bradycardia or hypotension, they should not be employed. In contrast, if the patient has significant systemic hypertension, ventricular ectopy, recurrent ischemia, or rapid atrial fibrillation, treatment with beta-blockers seems logical.

Beta-blockers undoubtedly work by reducing myocardial oxygen demand inasmuch as they decrease heart rate and blood pressure. They probably alter platelet aggregation and may contribute to the prevention of arrythmias. In addition, data from animal studies indicate that there is a shift in blood flow from normal areas to ischemic zones. The mechanism for this shift is unknown, but one can speculate that slowing the heart rate provides longer diastolic filling time, thus augmenting blood flow in a heart whose oxygen demand is reduced. In addition, a beta-blocker may make the ventricle less stiff and allow better perfusion of subendocardial tissues on a mechanical basis by decreasing left ventricular end-diastolic pressure.

In the United States the most commonly used intravenous beta-blocker in acute myocardial infarction is metoprolol. The drug is given in a dose of 5 mg intravenously at 2- to 5-minute intervals up to a dose of 15 mg and then followed by 50 mg orally, three to four times a day, then 100 mg twice a day. Obviously if hypotension or severe bradycardia ensues, the drug dose should be decreased or discontinued.

Therapy of Myocardial Infarction With Nitrates[4]

Until recently it was recommended that nitrates be avoided in patients with acute myocardial infarction. The rationale was that nitrate-induced hypotension reduced coronary perfusion pressure and perhaps extended the infarction. Perhaps the lack of hemodynamic monitoring in the past contributed to this concern. In those patients who become hypotensive, hemodynamic monitoring might have shown a normal systemic blood pressure and a low or normal left ventricular filling pressure. Many patients who responded in this manner may have been hypovolemic.

Symptom Relief

The use of nitrates in patients with acute myocardial infarction can be grouped into two major headings: (1) treatment of symptoms of myocardial ischemia during the initial presentation and (2) treatment of pulmonary congestion.

When nitrates are used to treat the symptoms of cardiac pain in the early stages of acute myocardial infarction, many patients obtain relief or at least have diminished morphine requirements. If the decision to use nitrates is made, the intravenous form of the drug should be used.

Although it seems reasonable to expect that nitrates might limit infarction size, studies have not conclusively proved that hypothesis. In contrast, intravenous nitrates are effective treatment for pulmonary edema secondary to acute myocardial infarction. Intravenous nitrates rapidly reduce left ventricular end-diastolic pressure, which, in turn, decreases pulmonary venous pressure and relieves pulmonary congestion. In addition, lowering left ventricular end-diastolic pressure allows better perfusion of subendocardium, probabaly decreases peri-infarction ischemic zones, and may improve systolic function of the ventricle, thereby increasing cardiac output.

Four major prospective randomized studies have been reported in patients with acute myocardial infarction receiving intravenous nitroglycerin.

Flaherty and coworkers[5] reported on 104 patients randomly assigned to intravenous nitrate (56 patients) and placebo (48 patients) within 18 hours of infarction. The infusion lasted 48 hours. When intravenous nitrate was given within 10 hours after infarction, ejection fraction increased and thallium defect score was less than in patients who were given placebo or who received nitrates later than 10 hours after onset of infarction.

Bussmann[6] compared 31 patients with acute myocardial infarction receiving intravenous nitroglycerin for 48 hours with 29 patients not receiving nitroglycerin. Only patients with pulmonary wedge pressures greater than 12 mm Hg were included in this study. There were two groups—those receiving early treatment (less than 8 hours) and those receiving late treatment (greater than 8 hours) after the onset of chest pain. All patients had transmural myocardial infarction. Treatment was initiated 10.2 hours (mean) after the onset of the myocardial infarction. The mean infusion rate of nitroglycerin was 47 mcg/min. The study showed that mean creatine kinase was 23 percent lower in the nitroglycerin-treated patients compared with controls. There was no difference between early and late treatment when CK or CKMB enzymes were used as end-points.

Jaffe and associates[7] randomized 85 patients to nitroglycerin and placebo infusion for 24 hours. The infusion was initiated within 10 hours after the acute infarction (mean 6 hours). The goal of the infusion was to lower blood pressure by 10 percent or a maximum dose of 200 mcg/min. In these patients creatine kinase was 37 percent lower with nitroglycerin treatment but only in the subgroup of patients with inferior transmural myocardial infarction (p less than 0.05).

In another prospective trial Derrida and colleagues[8] randomized 74 patients with acute myocardial infarction to either nitroglycerin or control. They noted a significant reduction of hospital mortality from 23 percent to 5 percent in those receiving nitroglycerin. In this study blood pressure was lowered by 20 mm Hg, and the infusion was maintained for 1 to 7 days. Mean nitroglycerin dose was 51 mcg/min. Patients received this dose 10 hours (mean) after the onset of the infarction.

Prognosis of Patients with Acute Myocardial Infarction Treated with Intravenous Nitroglycerin

Flaherty and associates [9] reported a 10-day mortality of 4 percent in patients treated with intravenous nitrates compared with 7 percent in patients treated with placebo. Mortality increased to 15 percent in 3 months in the early treated nitrate group and 22 percent to 27 percent in the other subgroups, but these differences were not statistically significant.

Bussmann and Haler[10] reported that sudden death and reinfarction was reduced at 18 months in those treated with nitrates (11 percent) compared with the control group (39 percent).

Safety/Adverse Effects of Nitrates In Patients with Acute Myocardial Infarction

Although it is clear that intravenous nitrates can have beneficial effects in many patients with myocardial infarction, adverse effects such as hypotension and bradycardia also can occur. Thus, the intravenous drug should be given only to patients who are continuously monitored in a coronary care unit.

Nitrates should not be given to patients who are hypotensive for unknown reasons or who have uncorrected hypovolemia. The problem of hypovolemia is best illustrated in the patient with a recent myocardial infarction who has been sweating profusely for a prolonged period of time prior to hospital admission. In this type of patient, pooling of blood in the periphery after nitroglycerin administration may have disastrous results. However, it can be corrected by raising the legs and infusing intravenous fluids.

Intravenous nitroglycerin should be started in a low dose, for example, 10 mcg/min, and increased every 2 to 5 minutes by 10 mcg. Once symptoms are controlled and hemodynamics are optimized, one can maintain a steady state infusion of this drug. However, it must be recognized that most patients will become tolerant to the drug and increasing doses of the drug will be required. In my experience, doses exceeding 200 mcg per minute are rarely needed. If the patient stabilizes and nitrate therapy is to be continued, one can easily switch to oral preparations by slowly withdrawing the intravenous nitroglycerin.

Nitroprusside

Evidence supporting the use of intravenous nitroprusside in the early phases of acute myocardial infarction is lacking. Cohn and colleagues[11] reported the effect of short-term infusion of sodium nitroprusside on mortality rate in acute myocardial infarction complicated by left ventricular failure. Those who received early treatment (less than 7 hours from the onset of symptoms) had an almost twofold increase in mortality compared with a placebo control group. This was in contrast to the reverse finding in patients who received late treatment (greater than 7 hours after the onset of symptoms). Despite this gloomy result, nitroprusside still has a place in the management of patients with acute myocardial infarction, particularly in those with ventricular septal defect or papillary muscle dysfunction with resultant mitral regurgitation. This drug should be used with the same cautions as intravenous nitroglycerin. In addition, prolonged use of the drug may result in nitroprusside toxicity, although this is a rare occurrence.

Calcium Antagonists

In 1984, the Norwegian Nifedipine Multicenter Trial was published.[12] Nifedipine was given to patients within 12 hours of the onset of symptoms. On clinical assessment there was no reduction in infarct size nor was there any reduction in short- or long-term mortality compared with placebo-treated patients. Muller and coworkers[13] reported a similar disappointing result with this drug. Unfortunately, in both trials, the drug was not used in a time frame less than 4 hours from onset of symptoms, and, therefore, it may not be relevant to the acute management of patients with myocardial infarction.

In 1984, the Danish study group on verapamil in myocardial infarction published the results of a large multicenter Danish study.[14] They showed no reduction in 6-month or 12-month mortality rates in patients treated with conventional doses of verapamil compared with placebo-treated patients. However, the incidence of AV block and heart failure was significantly higher in the verapamil-treated group and in the control group.

A recent study was published by the diltiazem reinfarction group.[15] They treated patients with "non-Q-wave" myocardial infarction with diltiazem. Therapy was begun with 30 mg and increased by 30 mg every 6 hours to 90 mg every 6 hours for up to 14 days. The results indicated a 50 percent reduction of recurrent acute myocardial infarction and refractory post-infarction angina in those who received diltiazem. There was no difference in mortality between those patients who received diltiazem or placebo. Once again, this study may not have relevance to the acute management of myocardial infarction inasmuch as therapy was implemented between 24 and 72 hours after the onset of non-Q-wave myocardial infarction.

Based on the reported studies with calcium antagonists, I draw the following conclusions: (1) Mortality is not decreased when calcium antagonists are administered. Unfortunately, there are no data to indicate what would happen if they were administered within the early hours of a myocardial infarction. (2) Nifedipine and verapamil do have a role in the management of patients with acute myocardial infarction, but there should be clear indications for their use, for example, treatment of rapid atrial fibrillation with verapamil or treatment of severe hypertension with nifedipine. (3) Diltiazem is an effective drug to decrease the incidence of reinfarction in patients with non-Q-wave infarction, but one should not be lulled into thinking that short-term results can be applied to long-term outcome. My own approach in these patients with non-Q-wave myocardial infarction is to investigate their coronary anatomy and make decisions about subsequent diagnostic studies and therapy based on those findings.

Anticoagulants

In 1977, Chalmers and colleagues[16] reviewed six randomized trials and found a 15.4 percent mortality rate for anticoagulated patients versus 19.6 percent rate for those patients not anticoagulated.

As a single agent, there is no evidence to support the hypothesis that intravenous heparin in full anticoagulation doses reduces infarct size or increases survival in patients with acute myocardial infarction. However, this lack of efficacy may have no relevance to current clinical practice. In the patient who is treated with thrombolytic therapy or angioplasty, full anticoagulation with heparin and long-term anticoagulation with coumarin may have a beneficial effect. However, this hypothesis needs to be tested. One concern that I share with many others is the use of intravenous heparin in patients who have received thrombolytic therapy. It seems as though these patients may be more prone to hemorrhagic complications requiring transfusion.

I do not believe there is any question that the use of anticoagulation reduces thromboembolic complications associated with acute myocardial infarction. Handley and Wray and their colleagues[17–19] showed that low-dose heparin reduced the incidence of deep vein thrombosis in patients with acute myocardial infarction from 23 percent to 4 percent. In these patients, heparin was started within 12 to 18 hours after the onset of symptoms and continued for 10 days. There was no increased incidence of bleeding complications compared with the placebo-treated patients.

The use of anticoagulation with heparin in patients with acute myocardial infarction is not universally accepted. However, on balance, the decreased incidence of systemic pulmonary and cerebral emboli makes the use of anticoagulation in the early phases of acute myocardial infarction a reasonable therapeutic strategy.

Anti-Platelet Therapy[20,21]

The Persantine-Aspirin Re-infarction Study (Paris II) revealed beneficial effects of Persantine and aspirin compared with placebo in patients who had a non-Q-wave infarction, those not taking digitalis, those receiving beta blockade at the initiation of the study, those in New York Heart Association Functional Class I, those with their first myocardial infarction, and those receiving Persantine and aspirin within 85 days of the acute myocardial infarction. Other trials comparing aspirin alone, aspirin plus dypyridamole, or sulfinpyrazone demonstrated a trend toward reduction in nonfatal myocardial infarction and death from all causes in the drug-treated group compared with the placebo-treated group. However, none was statistically significant. In addition, the variability of medication dose, timing of intervention, and followup period were such that most of these trials are not comparable. Unfortunately, all of these results have very little relevance to the early management of patients with myocardial infarction. As far as I can determine no one has tested the hypothesis that using antiplatelet agents within the first few hours of myocardial infarction will show benefit. Nonetheless, it seems logical to me that inasmuch as the pathogenesis of myocardial infarction is related to thrombus formation and platelet aggregation, the use of an agent such as aspirin might decrease platelet aggregation and subsequent thrombus formation in patients undergoing lytic therapy or balloon angioplasty or even in patients who spontaneously lyse clot.

My own practice is that unless there is a contraindication to its use, I recommend aspirin early in the management of acute myocardial infarction.

Antiarrhythmic Therapy

The prototype antiarrhythmic drug in the patient with an acute myocardial infarction is lidocaine.[22] I have not advocated the routine use of lidocaine in patients as a prophylaxis against arrhythmias. However, in patients receiving thrombolytic therapy or early balloon angioplasty, it is sensible to use intravenous lidocaine to prevent the reperfusion arrhythmias that are bound to occur in many of these patients. Intravenous infusion of 1 to 2 mg/min should be sufficient to prevent significant arrhythmias in these patients. If the patient has received a beta-blocker, it may be unnecessary to use lidocaine. Ryden and colleagues,[23] in 1983, published results of a double-blind trial of metoprolol in acute myocardial infarction and showed that beta-adrenergic blocking drugs decreased the incidence of ventricular fibrillation.

Diuretics

The routine use of a diuretic such as furosemide cannot be condoned in patients with uncomplicated acute myocardial infarctions. However, in the setting of acute pulmonary edema, there is clearcut indication for their use, although one should be careful about the loss of potassium and magnesium in such patients. The dose response of intravenous furosemide or other loop diuretics is variable. My practice is to begin with a low dose, for example, 20 mg of furosemide intravenously, and observe the effect over the next hour.

Inotropic Agents

In my view, there must be clearcut indication for the use of any inotropic agent, including digoxin, in patients with acute myocardial infarction. A major indication for digoxin is the patient with atrial fibrillation with a rapid ventricular rate. Studies have been published, including MILIS, in which the cumulative mortality was higher for digoxin-treated patients compared with those who did not receive digoxin.[24] The MILIS study was not a randomized trial. The decision to use digoxin was made by the patient's personal physician on the basis of the usual clinical indications. Some have been tempted to interpret these results as indicating that digoxin increased mortality in patients receiving it. I do not interpret it that way but believe instead the data indicate that those who received digoxin had more predictors of mortality than did those who did not receive the drug.

In addition to using digoxin in patients with atrial fibrillation or atrial flutter, I usually administer the drug to patients who have symptoms of persistent heart failure and cardiomegaly on chest x-ray or a large ventricular aneurysm on two-dimensional echocardiography or ventriculography.

Atropine

Atropine sulfate in a dose of 0.5 to 1.0 mg intravenously can be given to patients with acute myocardial infarction who have symptomatic bradycardia or heart block. When symptoms persist despite adequate doses of this drug, temporary transvenous pacing should be instituted.

SUMMARY

In medicine and in cardiology one must be aware that there is no "standard" management for any condition. However, some guidelines can be offered for the management of myocardial infarction in the early stages. The following can be considered an aggressive but stepwise approach to therapy of patients with suspected myocardial infarction using conventional drugs with or without thrombolytic therapy or coronary angioplasty.

Any patient presenting with prolonged chest pain occurring at rest should have an electrocardiogram. If the ECG is abnormal, an evolving myocardial infarction can be suspected. In this setting, oxygen should be administered if the patient is dyspneic, cyanotic, or has rales in the chest, intravenous nitroglycerin should be given, and the patient's response should be assessed. Caution should be observed at this point if the patient is sweating or hypotensive. Administration of a vasodilator in a dehydrated patient may drop the blood pressure further. If pain is relieved and the ECG returns to normal, the working diagnosis is severe angina. However, acute myocardial infarction should not be dismissed. A strong case for the use of intravenous heparin can be made to prevent the redevelopment of intracoronary clot inasmuch as thrombosis probably occurs in most patients presenting with unstable and severe angina, as it most surely does in patients with an evolving acute myocardial infarction.

If nitrates and oxygen relieve chest pain but the ECG remains abnormal, for example, ST segment elevation, the diagnosis of acute evolving myocardial infarction must be considered and intravenous nitrates should be continued. If the patient has no relief of pain from nitrates and oxygen and the ECG remains abnormal, morphine sulfate should be administered intravenously in sufficient dosage to relieve the chest pain but not produce hypotension or hypoventilation.

Once the diagnosis of myocardial infarction has been made, some would begin administering intravenous lidocaine as prophylaxis against the ventricular arrhythmias commonly encountered in the earlier stages of myocardial infarction. It has not been my practice to use prophylactic lidocaine, but I believe it is prudent to have a low threshold for the use of this drug in patients with frequent PVCs, especially if they are multifocal.

If the patient exhibits symptomatic bradycardia or heart block, a trial with intravenous atropine is warranted.

Additionally, while all of this is going on, one should contemplate using betablockers if there is good indication, and thrombolytic therapy if there are no contraindications to its use.

REFERENCES

1. Maroko, PR, Radvany, P, Braunwald, E, et al: Reduction of infarction size by oxygen inhalation following acute coronary occlusion. Circulation 2:360, 1975.
2. The International Collaborative Study Group: Reduction of infarct size with the early use of timolol in acute myocardial infarction. N Eng J Med 301:9, 1984.
3. Hjalmarson, A, Herlitz, J, Malek, I, et al: Effect on mortality of metoprolol in acute myocardial infarction. Lancet 2(8251):823, 1981.
4. Conti, CR: Nitrate therapy for ischaemic heart disease. Eur Heart J 6(Suppl A):3, 1985.
5. Flaherty, JT, Becker, LC, Bulkley, BH, et al: A randomized prospective trial of intravenous nitroglycerin in patients with acute myocardial infarction. Circulation 68:576, 1983.
6. Bussmann, W-D: The role of nitroglycerin in acute myocardial infarction. In Lictlen, PR, Engel, H-J, Schrey, A, and Swan, HJC (eds): Nitrates III. Cardiovascular Effects. Springer-Verlag, Berlin, 1981, pp 329–340.
7. Jaffe, AS, Geltman, EM, Triefenbrunn, AJ, et al: Reduction of the extent of inferior myocardial infarction with intravenous nitroglycerin: A randomized prospective study. Circulation 64 (Suppl 4):IV–195, 1981.
8. Derrida, JP, Sal, R, and Chiche, P. Nitroglycerin infusion in acute myocardial infarction. N Engl J Med 297, 1977.
9. Flaherty, JT, Becker, LC, Weisfeldt, ML, et al: Results of a prospective randomized clinical trial of intravenous nitroglycerin in acute myocardial infarction. Circulation 62(Suppl 3):III–82, 1980.
10. Bussmann, W-D and Haller, M: Possible evidence for a reduction of early and late mortality during nitroglycerin therapy in acute myocardial infarction. Klin Wochenschr 61:417, 1983 (in German, English summary).

11. Cohn, JH, Franciosa, JA, Francis, GS, et al: Effect of short-term infusion of sodium nitroprusside on mortality rate in acute myocardial infarction complicated by left ventricular failure. N Engl J Med 306:1129, 1982.
12. The Norwegian Multicenter Study Group: Timolol-induced reduction in mortality and reinfarction in patients surviving acute myocardial infarction. N Engl J Med 304:801, 1981.
13. Muller, JE, Morrison, J, Stone, PH, et al: Nifedipine therapy for patients with threatened and acute myocardial infarction: A randomized, double-blind, placebo-controlled comparison. Circulation 69(4):740, 1984.
14. The Danish Study Group on Verapamil in Myocardial Infarction: Verapamil in acute myocardial infarction. Eur Heart J 5:516, 1984.
15. Gibson, RS, Boden, WE, Theroux, P, et al: Diltiazem and reinfarction in patients with non-Q-wave myocardial infarction. N Engl J Med 315(7):423, 1986.
16. Chalmers, TC, Matta, RJ, Smith, H Jr, et al: Evidence favoring the use of anticoagulants in the hospital phase of acute myocardial infarction. N Engl J Med 297(20):1091–1096, 1977.
17. Handley, AJ: Low-dose heparin after myocardial infarction. Lancet 2(778):623, 1972.
18. Handley, AJ, Emerson, PA, and Fleming, PR: Heparin in the prevention of deep vein thrombosis after myocardial infarction. Br Med J 2(811):436, 1972.
19. Wray, R, Maurer, B, and Shillingford, J: Prophylactic anticoagulant therapy in the prevention of calf-vein thrombosis after myocardial infarction. N Engl J Med 288(16):815, 1973.
20. Frishman, WH and Miller, KP: Platelets and antiplatelet therapy in ischemic heart disease. Curr Prob Cardiol 11(2):73, 1986.
21. Friedewald, WT, Furberg, CD, and May, GS: Aspirin and myocardial infarction. Cardiovasc Rev Rep 5(12):1285, 1984.
22. DeSilva, RA, Hennekens, CH, Lown, B, et al: Lidocaine prophylaxis in acute myocardial infarction: An evaluation of randomized trials. Lancet 2:855, 1981.
23. Ryden, L, Ariniego, R, Arnman, J, et al: A double blind trial of metoprolol in acute myocardial infarction: Effects on ventricular tachyarrhythmias. N Engl J Med 308:614, 1983.
24. Muller, J, Turi, Z, Stone, P, et al: Digoxin therapy and mortality following MI: Experience in the MILIS Study. N Engl J Med 314:265, 1986.

CHAPTER 15

New Approaches to Management of Arrhythmias after Myocardial Infarction

Anne B. Curtis, M.D.
Michael Mansour, M.D.

Arrhythmias are common in the setting of myocardial infarction, and they are an important cause of morbidity and mortality. Disturbances of cardiac electrical activity such as atrioventricular (AV) block and atrial tachyarrhythmias are often transient. Although they may contribute to aggravation of ischemic injury or heart failure, therapy is generally successful. On the other hand, sustained ventricular tachycardia and ventricular fibrillation occurring postinfarction are ominous findings that necessitate immediate therapy and intensive investigation. Newer techniques for evaluation, as well as therapy with new antiarrhythmic drugs, devices, and surgery are being developed to improve outcome in postinfarction patients with important arrhythmias. The purpose of this chapter is to review the current understanding of these arrhythmias and their management in patients with acute myocardial infarction. Special emphasis will focus upon the newer opportunities for recognition and management of arrhythmias in this clinical setting.

DETECTION OF ARRHYTHMIAS IN THE MYOCARDIAL INFARCTION PATIENT

Before addressing specific arrhythmias and their management, it is important to discuss methods to identify and follow these electrical disorders of the heart beat in the patient after myocardial infarction. Because the presence of ventricular arrhythmias is clearly a risk factor for sudden death after myocardial infarction, their detection is central to any attempt to treat them. Some demographic factors such as age, history of heart failure or previous myocardial infarction, and status of left ventricular function are associated with a higher probability of ventricular arrhythmias.[1-3] Although patients with left ventricular dysfunction and ventricular arrhythmias are at higher risk for sudden death than patients without these clinical findings, it is a difficult task to determine who among these patients will actually develop lethal arrhythmias.

Specific Methods

Resting ECG (12 Lead)

The resting electrocardiogram displays the electrical activation of the heart at a point in time. It is used widely for diagnosis of myocardial infarction, but it is relatively insensitive for detection of arrhythmias and conduction disturbances that may be transient. However, the presence of ventricular ectopic beats on a routine ECG in the patient after myocardial infarction has been correlated with an increased risk of sudden death over a 2- to 5-year followup.[4,5]

CCU Monitoring

With the introduction of the coronary care unit, mortality from myocardial infarction declined, due in large part to the detection of potentially lethal ventricular arrhythmias by continuous monitoring of cardiac rhythm.[6] The onset of supraventricular arrhythmias and conduction disturbances can also be determined rapidly and appropriate therapy can be begun. Analysis of heart rhythms in this setting can be done visually or automatically by computer. Quantitation of arrhythmia frequency can be accomplished quite accurately by computer analysis to within 3 percent of actual arrhythmia frequency, although the importance of such accuracy in a monitored setting is unclear.[7] Monitoring of cardiac rhythm in the CCU setting is most valuable for detecting changes in cardiac rhythm promptly in the first hours to days of a myocardial infarction, when patients are relatively unstable and changes such as reperfusion or ischemia occur abruptly.

Ambulatory ECG Monitoring

Ambulatory (Holter) ECG monitors have been very useful in identifying arrhythmias in the postinfarction patient. The specific type of monitor required and the duration have not been resolved. They have been used for as briefly as 1 hour[8] and 6 hours[9] but are more commonly used for 24-hour periods to assess which patients are at increased risk of sudden death.[10] The frequency of ventricular arrhythmias, however, is known to undergo a marked degree of variability. Some patients who have no ventricular ectopy during 1 hour or day may have a substantially higher frequency of arrhythmias during another recorded hour or day.[11] While all the factors controlling this variability are not known, sympathetic activation contributes to a characteristic circadian pattern. PVCs in post-MI patients are known to increase in frequency in the hours after waking, peak about noon, and reach a low frequency around midnight to 6 AM.[12] Thus, monitoring should be scheduled to include these early morning periods.

Several studies have demonstrated that predischarge ambulatory ECG monitoring is a relatively inadequate method for detecting patients who will subsequently experience sudden death.[1,8,9] Although the presence of ventricular arrhythmias on a 24-hour ambulatory ECG in the postinfarction patient is correlated with an increased risk of sudden death, the majority of patients with this finding will not die suddenly.[13] No arrhythmia can be identified in an asymptomatic patient that reliably predicts sudden cardiac death, and to our knowledge no studies yet published have demonstrated an increase in sudden death without a comparable increase in total mortality.[13,14]

Ambulatory ECG monitoring can be extremely valuable in patients with symptomatic arrhythmias, both supraventricular and ventricular, for diagnosis and to guide therapy. When symptomatic arrhythmias occur infrequently, monitors that are patient-activated can be used to detect arrhythmias, with transmission of the information transtelephonically for analysis.

Signal-Averaged ECG

The "signal-averaged" electrocardiogram is a noninvasive method to assess the presence or absence of an electrophysiologic abnormality that identifies patients at risk for development of sustained ventricular tachycardia (VT) or fibrillation (VF). Inasmuch as the surface ECG consists of actual cardiac electrical signals together with "noise," the ability to detect information contained in the recorded ECG will depend upon the signal-to-noise ratio. Signal averaging is a standard technique used to maximize this signal-to-noise ratio. In some patients, signal-averaged ECGs obtained during sinus rhythm show low-amplitude oscillatory potentials. Known as "late potentials," these signals are thought to represent diseased myocardial zones with delayed activation capable of providing the substrate for reentrant rhythms. Several studies indicate that the signal-averaged ECG may be a useful method for screening patients with and without spontaneous nonsustained VT through identification of late potentials. These patients may be at risk for developing sustained VT as demonstrated by electrophysiologic study, particularly in the setting of ventricular dysfunction. Patients with no late potentials may be at such low risk for development of sustained VT that they may not require invasive evaluation.[15–21] Late potentials detected by the signal-averaged ECG have been shown to persist despite administration of antiarrhythmic drugs that prevent inducibility of ventricular tachycardia during electrophysiologic study.[22]

Exercise ECG

Low-level exercise tolerance testing is valuable in the postinfarction patient to assess prognosis. Predischarge low-level exercise testing may detect ischemia or arrhythmias as an early screening technique. Exercise-induced ventricular arrhythmias in the post-MI patient have been strongly correlated with mortality on short-term followup, particularly in patients with resting left ventricular dysfunction.[23] Although ventricular arrhythmias may become manifest with stress, there is often a lack of reproducibility from one stress test to another. This limits the usefulness of the technique for evaluation and management of arrhythmias. Exercise-induced ventricular arrhythmias may be associated with a higher cardiovascular risk,[24] and exercise testing may be valuable in conjuction with ambulatory ECG monitoring in selected patients, although the latter technique is more sensitive in detecting ventricular ectopy.[25] Such a noninvasive approach to management of arrhythmias may be sufficient in symptomatic patients without life-threatening symptoms, especially if results with exercise testing are reproducible. An example of such a patient is one with palpitations or dizziness from PVCs who has not experienced a sustained arrhythmia. On the other hand, whereas these noninvasive tests can identify patients at higher risk for sudden death, their low positive predictive value remains a problem in deciding on appropriate management of asymptomatic patients with abnormal tests.[23]

Programmed Ventricular Stimulation

Use of programmed ventricular stimulation during an electrophysiologic study has received attention as a means to predict risk of sudden death in patients following myocardial infarction. In a series of 62 patients with coronary artery disease and asymptomatic nonsustained ventricular tachycardia, 45 percent were found to have sustained ventricular tachycardia inducible by programmed stimulation.[26] Therapy was guided by results of the electrophysiologic study in 44 patients, with 19 noninducible patients receiving no therapy and 25 patients receiving antiarrhythmic drugs that appeared effective at electrophysiologic study. After a mean followup of 28 months, 11 patients died suddenly. Only 1 of 19 patients who were noninducible died suddenly. Three of 44 patients who received therapy based on results of programmed stimulation died suddenly. Sudden death occurred in 8 of 18 who received "empiric" therapy. However, at least 40 percent of patients who have had a myocardial infarction have inducible, sustained ventricular tachycardia even in the absence of symptoms or suspected clinical arrhythmias.[27] Inasmuch as the majority of these patients are not destined for sudden death, routine electrophysiologic studies in such asymptomatic patients must still be considered investigational.

On the other hand, results of programmed stimulation are widely valuable in the management of patients with sustained ventricular tachycardia or ventricular fibrillation. Patients who have had a myocardial infarction and develop sustained ventricular tachycardia are almost always inducible with programmed stimulation.[28] Long-term prognosis in these inducible patients is improved when the arrhythmias are suppressed by antiarrhythmic drugs guided by results of repeat programmed stimulation.[26,29]

Comparison of Invasive with Noninvasive Studies

Because electrophysiologic studies (EPS) are invasive procedures, there has been interest in comparing results of this approach with results of noninvasive evaluation. In patients with coronary artery disease who had sustained ventricular arrhythmias, ambulatory ECG monitoring detected arrhythmias suitable for antiarrhythmic drug assessment in 50 percent of patients compared with EPS, in which monomorphic ventricular tachycardia suitable for electropharmacologic testing was induced in 82 percent of patients.[30] For patients with very frequent nonsustained tachycardias, especially when associated with symptoms, ambulatory ECG monitoring can be used for evaluation of antiarrhythmic efficacy with the goal of abolishing prolonged symptomatic tachycardias.[31] In asymptomatic patients in whom the goal is prevention of sudden death, a commonly defined end-point of therapy is at least a 75 percent reduction in frequency of PVCs (ideally up to 90 percent reduction) as well as total abolition of nonsustained ventricular tachycardia.[32] This definition of efficacy recognizes the known day-to-day variability in frequency of ventricular arrhythmias. In patients with primary ventricular fibrillation or recurrent ventricular tachycardia treated with antiarrhythmic drugs, EPS is superior in predicting the response to antiarrhythmic drugs over at least 18 months when compared with Holter monitoring.[33]

The advantage of an invasive approach over a noninvasive approach to guide drug therapy in preventing recurrences of ventricular tachycardia has been supported in a controlled clinical trial by Mitchell and coworkers.[29] Patients suitable for evaluation by either invasive or noninvasive testing were randomized to either approach. Invasive EPS required more drug trials than therapy guided by ambulatory ECG monitoring (5.5 versus 3.1) to identify effective therapy and necessitated a longer hospital stay. However, the probability of remaining free of arrhythmia at 2 years was 80 percent with the invasive approach versus only 50 percent with noninvasive evaluation. Some other investigations, as pointed out by Greenspan,[34] were not aggressive enough in their stimulation protocols to be valuable for assessing predictive value of EPS.

No convincing evidence has been presented to suggest that induction of nonsustained VT, polymorphic VT, or VF is a reliable indicator of risk of arrhythmic death.[28,34] Patients with a history of symptomatic ventricular arrhythmias and inducible sustained monomorphic VT are at an increased risk for sudden cardiac death. In this group, therapy that prevents induction of sustained VT is associated with a lower rate of sudden cardiac death than empiric therapy.[26,35]

Antiarrhythmic drugs can be tested serially during EPS to determine their efficacy in preventing induction of ventricular tachycardia. The technique can be performed rapidly and safely and can evaluate drugs serially both for their antiarrhythmic and proarrhythmic effects.[32,35,36] Evaluation of ventricular arrhythmias by EPS is more expensive, at least in the short-term, because of the length of the hospital stay and the cost of the invasive procedure, which often must be repeated several times. It is possible, however, that with better identification of effective therapy, fewer hospitalizations for recurrent arrhythmias will be necessary with the invasive approach, thus reducing the cost differential.[29] Patients who have had sustained ventricular tachycardia or ventricular fibrillation should be evaluated by invasive EPS to optimize therapy. "Empiric" therapy is not adequate in these high-risk patients. Patients with symptomatic nonsustained ventricular tachycardia may be evaluated either noninvasively or invasively. Infrequent symptomatic ventricular arrhythmias may require invasive evaluation if prolonged monitoring is inadequate to guide therapy. The advantages and disadvantages of the techniques for evaluating arrhythmias are summarized in Table 15–1.

ATRIOVENTRICULAR CONDUCTION DISTURBANCES

Mechanisms, Acute Management, Chronic Management

The incidence of atrioventricular conduction disturbances in the setting of myocardial infarction varies between 12 percent and 25 percent, and the incidence of complete AV block varies from 2 percent to 10 percent.[37] AV conduction disturbances associated with inferior infarction are transient in most cases and have a good prognosis. Those associated with anterior infarction, however, usually indicate a poorer prognosis.[38,39] The site of AV block with inferior infarction is generally in the proximal part of the conduction system. In a series of 37 patients[40] who had second- or third-degree AV block within the first 6 hours of inferior infarction, the conduction disturbance usually responded to atropine and disappeared within 24 hours. In these patients, advanced AV block typically appeared suddenly. In contrast, in patients with inferior infarction and second- or third-degree AV block developing after the first 6 hours, a characteristic pro-

Table 15–1. Techniques for Evaluating Arrhythmias in the Post-MI Patient

Technique	Indications	Advantages	Disadvantages
12-lead ECG	Immedate diagnosis of persistent arrhythmias and heart block; precise measurements	Inexpensive; may be repeated frequently	Insensitive for detecting transient arrhythmias
CCU ECG monitoring	Monitoring for cardiac arrhythmias in peri-infarction period	Rapid detection of heart block and arrhythmias	Sustained ventricular arrhythmias often not preceded by ventricular ectopy
Ambulatory ECG monitoring	Diagnosis of arrhythmias; quantitation of arrhythmia frequency; evaluation of therapy	Detection of transient arrhythmias; correlation of arrhythmias with symptoms or activities	Day-to-day variability of arrhythmia frequency; may not detect infrequent arrhythmias
Signal-averaged ECG	Identify late potentials which may predict risk of sustained VT	Noninvasive; negative result may negate need for electrophysiologic study	Role in management of arrhythmias not clear
Exercise ECG	Identify exercise-induced arrhythmias	Noninvasive; assessment of effect of catecholamines on arrhythmias	Lack of reproducibility
Electrophysiologic study	Sustained VT; VF; infrequent symptomatic ventricular arrhythmias; differential diagnosis of wide-complex tachycardia	Detection of potentially lethal arrhythmias when there is little baseline ectopy; evaluation of response to therapy	Invasive; expensive

Table 15–2. Atrioventricular Block in Acute MI

Location of Infarct	Involved Artery	Location of AV Block	Type of AV Block	Prognosis	Rx
Inferior	RCA (circumflex)	Intranodal	1st degree AV block Mobitz I (Wenckebach) AV Block	Good	Atropine Temporary pacer Permanent pacer generally not necessary
Anterior	LAD	Infranodal	Bundle branch block Mobitz II AV block	Poor	Temporary pacer Permanent pacer

drome was often seen. This began with gradual prolongation of the PR interval, with normal QRS morphology, followed by progressive progression to type 1 second-degree block. AV block in this group tended to last more than 40 hours and was less responsive to atropine. The conduction disturbance in these patients probably was due to direct effects of ischemia rather than enhanced vagal tone. In most of these patients, AV block resolves and permanent pacing is not necessary.

In anterior infarction, normal conduction and intraventricular conduction disturbances may progress suddenly to high-degree AV block with little or no warning. The incidence of high-degree AV block is highest in patients with new bilateral bundle branch block (right bundle branch block associated with either left anterior or left posterior fascicular block, or alternating bundle branch block) in the setting of acute myocardial infarction. These patients would most benefit from prophylactic temporary pacemakers.[41] These findings are summarized in Table 15–2.

Patients who survive acute myocardial infarction complicated by bundle branch block and transient high-degree AV block are at high risk of sudden death in the year following myocardial infarction. In the first year after infarction, such patients who are continuously paced have a 10 percent risk of sudden death or recurrent high-grade AV block versus 65 percent in those who do not receive permanent pacemakers.[41] Patients with bundle branch block without high-degree AV block during acute MI have a higher mortality than patients with MI and no bundle branch block, but the value of permanent pacing in this group of patients is not clear.[41,42]

SUPRAVENTRICULAR TACHYCARDIA

Mechanisms, Acute Management, Chronic Management

Atrial arrhythmias occur in about 10 percent of patients with acute myocardial infarctions.[43,44] The most common of these arrhythmias is atrial fibrillation.[44] The presence of atrial flutter or fibrillation in the setting of acute infarction is associated with increased mortality.[43,45] Atrial flutter is both a less common and less stable rhythm than atrial fibrillation. When the diagnosis of atrial flutter is unclear, vagal maneuvers or verapamil may slow a rapid ventricular response and make the diagnosis more obvious.

Atrial fibrillation usually occurs *later than 24 hours after* the onset of infarction and is most often a consequence of either pericarditis or heart failure. Occasionally, pneumonia or pulmonary embolism may be the cause. In contrast, atrial fibrillation occurring during the *early hours* of myocardial infarction is relatively rare, and its pathogenesis is poorly understood. In a recent study, 3 percent of 214 patients developed atrial fibrillation within 3 hours of the onset of chest pain.[46] It was demonstrated that these patients all had inferior infarctions with coexistent occlusion of the left circumflex artery proximal to the origin of its left atrial circumflex branch and impaired perfusion of the AV nodal artery. Because these two arteries both contribute to left atrial perfusion, the hypothesis was formed that acute left atrial ischemia is the pathophysiologic mechanism of early atrial fibrillation.

Recent onset atrial fibrillation with a rapid ventricular rate in a patient who is not hemodynamically stable should be treated urgently (within minutes) with electrical cardioversion. Electrical cardioversion, however, is not without risks, and, before it is used, an assessment of the probability of maintenance of sinus rhythm should be made. Hemodynamically stable patients with rapid ventricular rates who are symptomatic (angina, shortness of breath, or lightheadedness) can usually be managed over minutes to hours with agents that slow AV conduction. Intravenous verapamil, digoxin, or beta-blockers are usually successful. Many of these patients will revert to normal sinus rhythm once the ventricular response is controlled. Long-term prophylaxis against recurrence of atrial fibrillation can be achieved with antiarrhythmic drugs such as procainamide or quinidine. If these agents are not tolerated, a class 1C agent (encainide or flecainide) may be helpful.

VENTRICULAR ARRHYTHMIAS

Mechanisms

One of the most important causes for sudden cardiac death after myocardial infarction is ventricular tachycardia.[14,31,32,47] In an effort to treat ventricular tachycardia in the patient with ischemic myocardium more successfully, investigators have attempted to define better the mechanisms of these arrhythmias. Ventricular ectopy occurring during the acute ischemic event may be due primarily to reentry rather than increased automaticity. Convincing evidence has been obtained to support the occurrence of *reentry* in acute and chronic ischemic myocardium, and it is a mechanism for generation of arrhythmias by ischemic tissue.[48–51] On the other hand, *abnormal automaticity* has been demonstrated in ischemic Purkinje fibers. The relative importance of these two phenomena during acute infarction is controversial. There is also evidence that *reflection* might operate in the first few minutes of ischemia when injury currents are intense. Reflection is a form of reentry in which impulse propagation proceeds in a retrograde fashion along a pathway previously traveled to enter a site of conduction block, or impulse propagation occurs that is dependent on subthreshold potentials.[52] Several investigators have described *afterdepolarizations* in Purkinje fibers in the infarct zone in dogs up to several days after coronary occlusion,[50] but this may not be an important mechanism of arrhythmogenesis in vivo. Reentry as a primary mechanism for the generation of arrhythmias in patients with ischemia and infarction has been implicated convincingly by investigators, but supporting evidence for the roles of abnormal automaticity, afterdepolarizations, and reflection is less secure.[49–53].

Reperfusion of myocardium during acute myocardial infarction is a common occurrence with the use of thrombolytic agents and angioplasty in an effort to salvage injured myocardium. The electrophysiologic mechanisms associated with reperfusion arrhythmias are unknown.[54] Reperfusion has been associated with *accelerated idioventricular* and *ventricular arrhythmias.*[55,56]

The electrophysiologic properties of the ischemic myocardium, such as a shift in the threshold for activation, inhomogeneous recovery of excitability, and decreased conduction velocity provide a suitable substrate for the initiation and perpetuation of ventricular fibrillation.[54] The electrophysiologic disparity between normal and ischemic tissue suggests that a potential site of action for an antiarrhythmic drug could be either the normal or the ischemic tissue. A drug may act to decrease the difference in the electrophysiologic properties between ischemic and normal areas of the myocardium and reduce the opportunity for reentrant activity.

Acute Management

Goals

The primary goals for acute management of ventricular arrhythmias are to prevent the occurrence of sustained ventricular tachycardia or ventricular fibrillation to limit further injury to ischemic myocardium, and to terminate these arrhythmias immediately if they occur. These goals may be achieved by continuous monitoring of cardiac rhythm, prophylactic and therapeutic use of antiarrhythmic drugs, and cardioversion.

Approaches

To manage ventricular arrhythmias occurring in post-MI patients, the clinician must have an understanding of their clinical course and outcome. In the initial 4 to 6 hours after infarction, ventricular fibrillation may occur in up to 15 percent of patients.[57] Frequent and complex ventricular arrhythmias occur in up to 40 percent of patients in the subsequent 6 to 72 hours and then decrease to reach a nadir by 3 to 5 days following infarction.[58] Although complex PVCs, such as frequent or multiform PVCs, couplets, salvos, or the R-on-T phenomenon, have been termed "warning arrhythmias" and felt to herald the onset of ventricular tachycardia and ventricular fibrillation, sustained ventricular tachyarrhythmias may occur in the absence of antecedent ventricular ectopy. In addition, prevention of PVCs does not necessarily prevent the development of VT or VF, and complex ventricular ectopy may be observed in patients who do not develop VF.[31]

The MILIS (Multicenter Investigation of the Limitation of Infarct Size) study showed that primary ventricular fibrillation occurring in patients without left ventricular failure did not have a negative effect on prognosis.[59] However, a more recent study demonstrated that primary ventricular fibrillation was indeed associated with an increased risk of in-hospital death.[60] Patients with out-of-hospital VF who do not evolve evidence for large myocardial infarctions are also at high risk of sudden death.[61]

Many drugs have been shown to control ventricular ectopy, but lidocaine remains the only antiarrhythmic agent that has been conclusively demonstrated to reduce the incidence of ventricular fibrillation after acute MI.[47,62] Higher doses than those often utilized clinically may be necessary to demonstrate this effect, and in older patients the risk of toxicity may outweigh the benefit of prophylactic use of lidocaine.[63,64] Lidocaine is a membrane-stabilizing agent producing little change in conductivity while shortening the action potential. Lidocaine, as with other drugs in Vaughan class 1,[65] exhibits its major electrophysiologic effects by interference with rapid sodium conductance into the myocardial cell.[60] Lidocaine does not usually have a significant effect on cardiac output or other hemodynamic parameters, but cardiac conduction abnormalities and decreased contractility can occur in patients with preexisting conduction defects or high plasma concentrations. Its plasma half-life is prolonged in patients with decreased hepatic function such as occurs in those with heart failure and in patients more than 70 years old.[63]

Procainamide can be used intravenously in acute myocardial infarction to treat serious ventricular arrhythmias rapidly when lidocaine cannot be used or is ineffective.[32,60] It is a class 1A antiarrhythmic and causes moderate reduction in conduction velocity with prolongation of action potential duration; this produces electrocardiographic findings of QRS and QT prolongation.[60] Procainamide has mild ganglionic blocking properties causing peripheral vasodilation. This decrease in afterload may negate its negative inotropic effect and, thus, cause little hemodynamic change in patients with low cardiac output states after acute myocardial infarction.[32,60]

Beta-receptor blocking agents such as metoprolol have not been found to affect the occurrence of premature ventricular contractions or short bursts of ventricular tachycardia.[66] However, metoprolol has been demonstrated to have a prophylactic effect against ventricular fibrillation in acute myocardial infarction, and early intervention with metoprolol appears well tolerated generally.[67] Propranolol was investigated in the BHAT trial and found to lower the incidence of sudden death and reinfarction in postinfarction patients as well as reduce the number of patients with morning ventricular arrhythmias.[68]

Bretylium may be effective in treating ventricular tachycardia that has been unresponsive to lidocaine or procainamide.[32,60] A derivative of guanethidine, it exerts an antisympathetic response by depleting catecholamines.[60] The beneficial effects of bretylium are in part due to a direct electrophysiologic effect that equalizes the duration of effective refractory periods and ventricular action potentials in normal and ischemic myocardium, and, therefore, it creates conditions capable of blocking reentrant pathways.[69] Bretylium has been found to be effective in treating recurrent ventricular tachycardia and ventricular fibrillation.[54] Bretylium plus defibrillation may combine to allow successful resuscitation from cardiac arrest when either alone has failed. Bretylium may also produce spontaneous defibrillation.[32,54,60,69] Bretylium has a low incidence of mostly well-tolerated side effects. These include hypotension, which is usually responsive to intravenous fluids and may be ameliorated by tricyclic antidepressant drugs such as protriptyline.[69,70]

Atrioventricular sequential or ventricular demand pacemakers have also been used on occasion in the acute management of ventricular tachycardia to eliminate bradycardia or atrioventricular block that predispose to ventricular tachycardia.[31]

CHRONIC VENTRICULAR ARRHYTHMIAS

Goals

Sustained ventricular tachycardia and ventricular fibrillation require aggressive management to reduce the incidence of recurrent arrhythmias and sudden death. The goal of therapy for symptomatic nonsustained ventricular arrhythmias is to ameliorate symptoms, usually through the use of antiarrhythmic drugs. Although asymptomatic ventricular arrhythmias are associated with an increased risk of sudden death in postinfarction patients, therapy has not yet been shown to alter prognosis. The appropriate management of these patients is therefore controversial.

Approaches

Ventricular arrhythmias have been identified as an independent risk factor for sudden death in patients with coronary artery disease.[1,2,8,9,32,59,71,72] The probability of sudden death within 1 to 5 years following a myocardial infarction has been directly related to the incidence of premature ventricular contractions.[8,9] Patients with three or more consecutive ventricular premature contractions have been shown to have an incidence of sudden death up to 22 percent within 1 year after myocardial infarction.[1,59] Equally important is myocardial dysfunction as a marker of high risk for sudden death following recent myocardial infarction.[2,3,8] A low ejection fraction combined with frequent ectopy ($\geq$10 PVCs/hr) places the patient at highest risk for sudden cardiac death.[3]

Antiarrhythmic drugs can protect against recurrence of life-threatening ventricular fibrillation or ventricular tachycardia.[71,72] However, it is still unknown whether treatment of asymptomatic ventricular arrhythmias can reduce the incidence of sudden death following infarction. To attempt to address this issue the Cardiac Arrhythmia Pilot Study (CAPS) was undertaken. Its purpose was to determine whether postinfarction ventricular arrhythmias could be recognized satisfactorily and treated after acute myocardial infarction.[73,74] The CAPS study enrolled patients $<$75 years of age with $\geq$10 premature ventricular complexes per hour in a 24-hour electrocardiographic recording and a left ventricular ejection fraction $>$20 percent. Patients were randomized to receive encainide, flecainide, imipramine, moricizine,[75,76] or placebo and followed for 1 year. Ventricular arrhythmias were suppressed successfully and the drugs were sufficiently well-tolerated to suggest that a large clinical trial to address the question of morbidity was feasible. Whether adequate suppression of ventricular arrhythmias prevents sudden cardiac death is currently being evaluated by the Cardiac Arrhythmia Suppression Trial of the National Institutes of Health. The results are expected in the mid-1990s.

One other study of prophylactic antiarrhythmic therapy in survivors of acute MI showed that aprindine, a tertiary amine with properties similar to quinidine and procainamide, lowered mortality at 1 month but not at 1 year.[77]

When patients present with sustained ventricular tachycardia or ventricular fibrillation in the setting of acute MI, intensive evaluation and treatment are necessary if one is to attempt to reduce the risk of sudden death. The approaches to management of ventricular arrhythmias are summarized in Table 15–3. Pharmacotherapy is generally attempted first, optimally with evaluation of drug efficacy by electrophysiologic testing.

Table 15–3. Approaches to Treatment of Ventricular Arrhythmias in the Post-MI Patient

Treatment	Indications	Advantages	Disadvantages
Pharmacologic			
Quinidine Procainamide Disopyramide Mexiletine Tocainide Lidocaine Flecainide Encainide	Initial treatment of ventricular arrhythmias	Therapy easily discontinued if it fails	Most drugs have side effects that limit use
Amiodarone	Treatment of ventricular arrhythmias when other drug therapy has failed	Most effective antiarrhythmic drug for life-threatening ventricular arrhythmias	Many serious potential side effects, especially pneumonitis
Nonpharmacologic			
Antitachycardia devices	Rarely indicated; termination of VT when pharmacologic treatment fails and repeated evaluation ensures safety	Avoids need for surgery in drug-refractory patients; automatic; painless	Risk of acceleration of arrhythmia a major problem
AICD	VT/VF when other treatment fails, cardiac arrest without precipitating cause and negative EP study	Greatly reduces risk of sudden death	Requires surgery; cannot prevent arrhythmias
Subendocardial resection	Coronary artery disease and/or aneurysm; VT resistant to drugs	Often curative	Requires major surgery, expertise in mapping VT
Catheter ablation	Experimental; nonoperative candidates or when other therapy fails	May cure VT without need for surgery	May cause death from ventricular arrhythmias or low output syndrome

Pharmacotherapy. Quinidine and procainamide are two of the most commonly used antiarrhythmics, with broad efficacy for treating supraventricular and ventricular arrhythmias. Both drugs act to block sodium channels in the heart and produce moderate reduction in conductivity and prolongation of action potential duration;[78] they are, thus, classified as type 1A antiarrhythmics.

Quinidine causes mild depression of myocardial contractility. The most common side effects of quinidine therapy are gastrointestinal. Serious ventricular tachyarrhythmias associated with excessive QT prolongation are the likely cause of "quinidine syncope," a syndrome potentiated by hypokalemia.[63]

Procainamide is commonly tested in the electrophysiologic laboratory for suppression of ventricular tachycardia, because it is conveniently given intravenously. When procainamide has no effect on VT, other type 1A antiarrhythmics are also unlikely to be effective.[79] The majority of patients develop antinuclear antibodies after 3 to 6 months of therapy, and 15 percent to 20 percent develop a lupus-like syndrome that usually disappears when the drug is discontinued.[63]

In patients with symptomatic ventricular arrhythmias, Class 1A antiarrhythmic drugs will suppress inducible VT in about one-third of patients.[80,81] Success rates are lower when significant left ventricular dysfunction is present. Flecainide, a newer antiarrhythmic drug, has been shown to be effective in patients with nonsustained ventricular tachycardia[82] and for control of resistant VT.[83–85] Flecainide produces marked slowing of conduction but no change in action potential duration, and, thus, it produces prolonged PR and QRS intervals on ECG with little effect on the QT interval.[63,84,86] Provocation of potentially lethal ventricular arrhythmias can occur, particularly in patients with a history of sustained ventricular tachycardia and left ventricular dysfunction.[82,83,85,87,88]

Encainide has been shown to be a potent suppressor of ventricular ectopic activity. Like flecainide, it is a class 1C agent that causes marked slowing of conduction with no change in action potential duration. It has only mild negative inotropic activity.[89] It can aggravate arrhythmias and does so more frequently in patients with a history of congestive heart failure and intraventricular conduction delay on ECG.[84,89] Proarrhythmic effects from type 1C antiarrhythmic drugs may be encountered in approximately 10 percent of treated patients. However, this problem is not unique to these drugs, and proarrhythmia may occur with any antiarrhythmic agent. With the conventional antiarrhythmic agents, monitoring of serum levels is useful in evaluating therapy. Encainide is an exception, because it is extensively metabolized to active metabolites after absorption.

Mexiletine and tocainide both depress the maximal rate of depolarization of the action potential while decreasing its duration. They are, thus, similar to lidocaine in action.[80,87,90] Untoward cardiovascular effects are relatively rare with these drugs. However, extracardiac side effects can be troublesome, with up to 40 percent of patients requiring discontinuation of therapy. The most common side effects are gastrointestinal and neurological (tremor, diplopia). In addition, granulocytopenia and pulmonary fibrosis have been reported with tocainide. The incidence of arrhythmia aggravation when mexiletine is used to treat refractory ventricular arrhythmias is generally lower than that reported when other drugs are employed.[87]

In patients with latent sinus node dysfunction, the use of class 1 agents in association with a beta-blocker or amiodarone may be associated with marked bradycardia.[91]

Amiodarone is well established as a highly effective antiarrhythmic agent, but there are many serious potential side effects that mandate caution in its use. Amiodarone has unusual pharmacokinetics in that it is absorbed slowly, has low bioavailability, binds extensively to tissues, and has an elimination half-life as long as 107 days.[92] Loading doses are, therefore, necessary to achieve control of arrhythmias more quickly. Amiodarone is the most effective currently available antiarrhythmic agent, but its toxic side effects limit its use to those patients refractory to conventional agents.[93–96] The adverse effects of greatest concern are the potentially fatal ones: hepatitis, exacerbation of arrhythmias, exacerbation of congestive heart failure, and pulmonary fibrosis.[92,97] Emergent use of intravenous amiodarone is a significant advance in the management of critically ill patients with recurrent ventricular tachycardia or ventricular fibrillation refractory to conventional agents.[96]

The medically treated patients of DiMarco and associates[98] generally had antiarrhythmic drug therapy directed by results of electropharmacologic studies. Of these, 75 percent were discharged from the hospital with no inducible arrhythmias. A major factor in the improved outcome with medical treatment compared with that in prior series is the use of amiodarone as directed by electropharmacologic studies.[48,99,100]

The role of EPS after loading with amiodarone has been controversial, because the majority of patients remain inducible and yet may remain free of recurrent arrhythmias in followup. Most variables such as change in ease of inducibility of ventricular tachycardia or change in refractory periods have not been of value in assessing prognosis. However, hemodynamic instability of ventricular arrhythmias on amiodarone may predict that recurrences of arrhythmias may present as sudden death.[101]

There have been a small number of reports of using amiodarone in combination with class 1 antiarrhythmics to control refractory ventricular arrhythmias. The combined use of antiarrhythmic agents that increase the duration of the action potential may result in marked QT prolongation and torsades de pointes. This hazard may be associated with the use of amiodarone in association with a class 1A agent.[91]

Drug combinations may be useful for treatment of ventricular arrhythmias when monotherapy fails.[10,102] Class 2 (beta-blockers) agents have also been shown to be useful in some cases alone[81,103,104] and in combination with Class 1A drugs for treating ventricular ectopy. Class 1B agents such as mexiletine or tocainide may also be combined successfully with other agents. Their lack of effect on the QT interval is an important consideration when therapy in combination with 1A agents or amiodarone is contemplated.

Sotalol is a nonselective β-adrenergic receptor blocking drug with class 3 antiarrhythmic drug activity. Its main electrophysiologic effect is to prolong repolarization and refractoriness in Purkinje fibers and ventricular muscle. Sotalol is effective in the treatment of supraventricular tachycardia, in suppression of premature ventricular contractions and nonsustained ventricular tachycardia, and in the treatment of inducible sustained ventricular tachycardia. Sotalol has been effective in controlling patients with ventricular tachycardia refractory to class 1 agents, with an acceptable side effect profile.[105] It has been demonstrated to be effective by both the oral and intravenous routes with similar electrophysiologic effects.

Recainam is a new propylurea antiarrhythmic compound displaying potent class 1 activity and favorable pharmacologic properties. It has been effective in intravenous and oral trials for suppressing ventricular arrhythmias and increasing ventricular fibrillation thresholds. Recainam has demonstrated an acceptable adverse effect profile and hemodynamically it has demonstrated only modest negative inotropic effects.[106]

NONPHARMACOLOGIC METHODS. When pharmacologic therapy for ventricular arrhythmias fails, nonpharmacologic techniques have been developed for management of these potentially fatal arrhythmias. Such techniques include antitachycardia pacemakers, the automatic implantable cardioverter-defibrillator (AICD), surgery, and catheter ablation.

Antitachycardia Devices. Antitachycardia pacemakers have been successful in highly selected patients.[107] Overdrive pacing has been used for long QT syndromes or bradycardia-related VT. For termination of VT, available modalities include introduction of extrastimuli, scanning, and burst pacing. The induced extrastimuli enter the reentrant circuit, thus terminating the arrhythmia by making the pathway refractory.[108] There is a risk of accelerating ventricular tachycardia with this method, and, therefore, use of this technique requires meticulous evaluation, including repetitive in-hospital termination of ventricular tachycardia to prove safety. Successful antitachycardia pacing may necessitate concurrent administration of antiarrhythmic drugs. Because of the risk of accelerating ventricular tachycardia, many antitachycardia devices are implanted in conjunction with an AICD. Combination antitachycardia/defibrillator devices are being developed and will enter clinical testing soon.

Automatic Implantable Cardioverter-Defibrillator. Prevention of sudden cardiac death by the automatic implantable cardioverter-defibrillator (AICD)[108-114] has been well documented. One-year mortality rates from sudden death have been reported at approximately 2 percent[110,115,116] in patients who have been refractory to conventional antiarrhythmic drug therapy.[114] These results compare quite favorably with 1-year sudden death rates of up to 15 percent for patients with EPS or ambulatory ECG monitoring guided medical therapy, 15 percent to 24 percent for patients treated with amiodarone, and 20 percent to 50 percent for patients receiving empiric drug therapy.

Because the present AICD does not prevent VT or VF, patients remain subject to recurrences. Patients with frequent episodes of VF or VT are poor candidates for the device owing to the limited number of discharges that the device is able to deliver.[108]

Many centers routinely implant the patch electrodes for the AICD in patients undergoing antitachycardia surgery, with implantation of the active unit should VT or VF remain inducible. Some centers have implanted the AICD in most postoperative VT patients whether or not VT has remained inducible, but experienced investigators[113] have noted that only 4 percent of their patients who survived the arrhythmia surgery for VT died suddenly in a period of followup of 42 $\pm$ 22 months. Of all their patients, 25 percent had inducible arrhythmia postoperatively and 4 percent had spontaneous arrhythmia during the followup period, excluding the 4 percent who experienced sudden death. The cost of the device as well as reported complications of coronary artery erosion, patch or generator infection, lead migration, venous thrombosis, inappropiate discharges, and failure to sense or terminate arrhythmias make discriminate use of the AICD in selected patients a more practical approach.[108,110,113]

The current AICD requires thoracotomy or sternotomy for implantation of the patches. Previously, a nonepicardial catheter electrode system in conjunction with an AICD had not produced reliable VT/VF termination.[116] Recently, the development of a reproducible, effective, and reliable[117] AICD device with a triple nonepicardial electrode system using two transvenous catheter electrodes and a submuscular patch electrode in the midaxillary line (avoiding the need for thoracotomy) has been developed and is undergoing clinical trials.

Although the AICD and antitachycardia pacemakers can terminate ventricular arrhythmias, they cannot prevent their initiation. A potentially curative approach to management of ventricular arrhythmias is surgery, most commonly subendocardial resection.

Subendocardial Resection. Initial attempts to abolish ventricular tachycardia by aneurysmectomy alone or in conjunction with coronary artery bypass grafting met with only limited success.[118] Subsequently, subendocardial resection guided by electrophysiogically guided mapping of sites of origin of ventricular tachycardia has been shown to produce superior results. In one study, 50 percent of patients who had blind aneurysmectomy for ventricular tachycardia had recurrent arrhythmias versus 11 percent who had map-guided resection.[119] The role of the border zone of the endocardium between normal and diseased myocardium has been emphasized in the genesis of arrhythmias.[120] Preoperative endocardial mapping to localize the site of origin of VT is important, particularly because some patients will be noninducible at surgery.[121] Intraoperatively, epicardial and endocardial mapping is performed during VT to confirm the site of origin of the arrhythmia, and subendocardial resection is performed in addition to aneurysmectomy if the latter is present. Early subendocardial resection 1 to 4 months following MI has been reported[98,122] to have the same operative mortality as surgery performed at 1 year. Operative mortality has improved to approximately 10 percent, depending on the general stability of the patient.[98,121] Long-term followup of 36 patients who underwent ventricular aneurysmectomy and electrophysiologically directed subendocardial resection for treatment of recurrent refractory VT has shown that all patients discharged from the hospital were alive at the end of a followup period of 6 to 54 months. In this group, poor systolic function of the nonaneurysmal ventricular segments was the strongest and the only independent predictor of operative mortality.[122]

Localized subendocardial resection for VT related to inferior wall infarction has been associated with a higher rate of recurrence of the tachycardia when compared with similar surgery after anterior myocardial infarction.[123] Cryosurgery alone or in combination with localized subendocardial resection has been reported to be highly effective for VT due to inferior MI, because ablation of tissue near the posterior papillary muscle can be accomplished with preservation of mitral valve function.[124] Map-guided subendocardial resection during normothermic cardiopulmonary bypass allows repeated induction of VT during the operation and immediate assessment of the efficacy of the resection. At postoperative electrophysiologic study, 85 percent of patients were no longer inducible, and overall 91 percent of patients survived surgery.[125]

Lasers have been used for intraoperative ablation of VT.[126–128] The extent of the laser ablation can be both visually and electrically guided. Both argon and Nd:YAG lasers delivered directly to the surface of ventricular myocardium produce a vaporized crater with a coagulated tissue base.[129] The feasibility and safety of laser photoablation in patients with ventricular tachycardia have been demonstrated. In normal ventricle, argon laser discharge energies below 100 J are unlikely to produce perforation, whereas this becomes extremely likely over 300 J. By comparison, diseased human ventricle requires substantially higher laser discharge energies. This is probably related to the presence of excessive fibrosis in infarcted tissue and in the transitional zones.[130] In a series of 17 patients, intraoperative laser photocoagulation was performed on the normothermic heart during VT. Surgical mortality was 11.7 percent. There were 55 VT morphologies with successful laser ablation in 52 of 55; cryoblation was required in 2 of 55, and one VT was not ablated but was controlled postoperatively with procainamide. Intraoperative mapping is an integral part of the reported success with laser ablation techniques. In the 17 patients noted above, 6 additional VT morphologies were induced in 5 individuals after ablation of the initial mapped sites. None of the survivors with VT associated with coronary artery disease had inducible VT postoperatively.[127]

Intraoperative map-guided successful ablation has also been demonstrated in another small series of patients deemed unresectable by routine surgery techniques and would be expected to be surgical failures.[126]

Catheter Ablation. Catheter ablation of ventricular tachycardia[131–133] has been less efficacious than intraoperative mapping and ablation with lasers[126] or cryosurgery.[124] In one series of 33 patients, catheter ablation of VT was successful in 15 patients (45 percent) who became noninducible or were controlled on previously ineffective drugs.

There has been interest in the use of lasers for transcatheter ablation of VT, and the effects of lasers on myocardium have been compared with electric shock. Electric shock can produce lesions comparable in size and morphology, but it is associated with more ventricular tachycardia and left ventricular dysfunction than is the laser technique.[129,134] Laser injury to the left ventricle can be produced without significant hemodynamic changes[128] and an acceptably low incidence of laser-induced sustained ventricular arrhythmias. When Nd:YAG laser radiation is delivered by the transcatheter technique, lesion sizes are significantly larger than those produced in isolated muscle. This is an enhanced laser effect likely due to the presence of blood with transarterial delivery. Nd:YAG laser has been found to be efficacious in ablating the focus or foci in an experimental preparation of pacing-induced simulated VT[135,136] and in patients with drug-resistant VT.[127]

Transplantation. *Cardiac transplantation* has been reported as a last resort in patients with refractory life-threatening arrhythmias but has been limited to those with poor ventricular function precluding other corrective procedures.[120]

SUMMARY AND CONCLUSIONS

More effective modalities for the evaluation and management of arrhythmias in the postinfarction patient continue to evolve. They offer the hope of significantly ameliorating the morbidity and mortality associated with these arrhythmias. Although arrhythmias and disturbances of conduction are among the most important and potentially lethal consequences of myocardial infarction, advances in evaluation and management of these problems have helped to improve prognosis for these patients. Greater long-term arrhythmia-free survival can be achieved when therapy is guided by programmed electrical stimulation. Pacemakers, newer antiarrhythmic drugs, the automatic implantable cardioverter-defibrillator, catheter ablation, and surgery are all important tools in the management of ventricular arrhythmias and the prevention of sudden death.

REFERENCES

1. Bigger, JT, Weld, FM, and Rolnitzky, LM: Prevalence, characteristics and significance of ventricular tachycardia (three or more complexes) detected with ambulatory electrocardiographic recording in the late hospital phase of acute myocardial infarction. Am J Cardiol 48:815, 1981.
2. Mukharji, J, Rude, RE, Poole, WK, et al: Risk factors for sudden death after acute myocardial infarction: Two-year follow-up. Am J Cardiol 54:31, 1984.
3. The Multicenter Postinfarction Research Group: Risk stratification and survival after myocardial infarction. N Engl J Med 309:331, 1983.
4. Chiang, B, Perlman, L, Ostrander, L, et al: Relationship of premature systoles to coronary heart disease and sudden death in the Tecumseh epidemiologic study. Ann Intern Med 79:1159, 1969.
5. Coronary Drug Project Research Group: Prognostic importance of premature beats following myocardial infarction. JAMA 223:116, 1973.
6. Goldman, L: Coronary care units: A perspective on their epidemiologic impact. Int J Cardiol 2:284, 1982.
7. Zipes, DP: Genesis of cardiac arrhythmias: Electrophysiological considerations. In Braunwald, E (ed): Heart Disease. WB Saunders Company, Philadelphia, 1988, pp 610–611.
8. Ruberman, W, Weinblatt, E, Goldberg, JD, et al: Ventricular premature complexes and sudden death after myocardial infarction. Circulation 64:297, 1981.
9. Moss, AJ, Davis, HT, DeCamilla, J, et al: Ventricular ectopic beats and their relation to sudden and nonsudden cardiac death after myocardial infarction. Circulation 50:998, 1979.
10. Lown, B and Graboys, TB: Management of patients with malignant ventricular arrhythmias. Am J Cardiol 39:910, 1977.
11. Morganroth, J, Michelson, EL, Horowitz, LN, et al: Limitations of routine long-term electrocardiographic monitoring to assess ventricular ectopic frequency. Circulation 58:408, 1978.
12. Lichtstein, E, Morganroth, J, Harrist, R, et al: Effect of propranolol on ventricular arrhythmia: The Beta-Blocker Heart Attack Trial experience. Circulation 67 (Suppl I):5, 1983.
13. Josephson, ME: Treatment of ventricular arrhythmias after myocardial infarction. Circulation 74:653, 1980.
14. Cain, ME: Management of ventricular arrhythmias occurring in patients after myocardial infarction. Angiology 39:307, 1988.
15. Denniss, AR, Ross, DL, Richards, DA, et al: Changes in ventricular activation time on the signal-averaged electrocardiogram in the first year after acute myocardial infarction. Am J Cardiol 60:580, 1987.
16. Buxton, AE, Simson, MB, Falcone, RA, et al: Results of signal-averaged electrocardiography and electrophysiologic study in patients with nonsustained ventricular tachycardia after healing of acute myocardial infarction. Am J Cardiol 60:80, 1987.
17. Kienzle, MG, Falcone, RA, and Simson, MB: Alterations in the initial portion of the signal-averaged QRS complex in acute myocardial infarction with ventricular tachycardia. Am J Cardiol 61:99, 1988.
18. Denniss, AR, Richards, DA, Cody, DV, et al: Correlation between signal-averaged electrocardiogram and programmed stimulation in patients with and without spontaneous ventricular tachyarrhythmias. Am J Cardiol 59:586, 1987.
19. Buckingham, TA, Ghosh, S, Homan, SM, et al: Independent value of signal-averaged electrocardiography and left ventricular function in identifying patients with sustained ventricular tachycardia with coronary artery disease. Am J Cardiol 59:568, 1987.
20. Turitto, G, Fontaine, JM, Ursell, SN, et al: Value of the signal averaged electrocardiogram as a predictor of the results of programmed stimulation in nonsustained ventricular tachycardia. Am J Cardiol 61:1272, 1988.
21. Lindsay, BD, Markham, J, Schechtman, KB, et al: Identification of patients with sustained ventricular tachycardia by frequency analysis of signal-averaged electrocardiograms despite the presence of bundle branch block. Circulation 77:122, 1988.
22. Denniss, AR, Ross, DL, Richards, DA, et al: Effect of antiarrhythmic therapy on delayed potentials detected by the signal-averaged electrocardiogram in patients with ventricular tachycardia after acute myocardial infarction. Am J Cardiol 58:261, 1986.

23. Weld, FM, Chu, KL, Bigger, JT, et al: Risk stratification with low-level exercise testing 2 weeks after acute myocardial infarction. Circulation 64:306, 1981.
24. Califf, RM, McKinnis, RA, McNeer, JF, et al: Prognostic value of ventricular arrhythmias associated with treadmill exercise testing in patients studied with cardiac catheterization for suspected ischemic heart disease. J Am Coll Cardiol 1:1060, 1983.
25. Rauscha, F, Glogar, D, Weber, H, et al: Diagnostic value of exercise testing versus long-term ECG in evaluation of arrhythmias in old age. Eur Heart J 5:79, 1984.
26. Buxton, AE, Marchlinski, FE, Flores, BT, et al: Nonsustained ventricular tachycardia in patients with coronary artery disease: Role of electrophysiologic study. Circulation 75:1178, 1987.
27. Brugada, P, Waldecker, B, Kersschot, Y, et al: Ventricular arrhythmias initiated by programmed stimulation in four groups of patients with healed myocardial infarction. J Am Coll Cardiol 8:1035, 1986.
28. Wellens, HJJ, Brugada, P, and Stevenson, WG: Programmed electrical stimulation of the heart in patients with life-threatening ventricular arrhythmias: What is the significance of induced arrhythmias and what is the correct stimulation protocol? Circulation 72:1, 1985.
29. Mitchell, LB, Duff, JH, Manyari, DE, et al: A randomized clinical trial of the noninvasive and invasive approaches to drug therapy of ventricular tachycardia. N Engl J Med 317:1681, 1987.
30. Swerdlow, CD and Peterson, J: Prospective comparison of Holter monitoring and electrophysiologic study in patients with coronary artery disease and sustained ventricular tachyarrhythmias. Am J Cardiol 56:577, 1985.
31. Josephson, ME: Treatment of ventricular arrhythmias after myocardial infarction. Circulation 74:653, 1986.
32. Somberg, JC, Miura, D, and Keefe, DL: The treatment of ventricular rhythm disturbances. Am Heart J 111:1162, 1986.
33. Platia, EV and Reid, PR: Comparison of programmed electrical stimulation and ambulatory electrocardiographic (Holter) monitoring in the management of ventricular tachycardia and ventricular fibrillation. J Am Coll Cardiol 4:493, 1984.
34. Greenspan, AM: Can electrophysiologic testing predict mortality after myocardial infarction? J Am Coll Cardiol 7:1243, 1986.
35. Anderson, JL and Mason, JW: Testing the efficacy of antiarrhythmic drugs. N Engl J Med 315:391, 1986.
36. Mason, JW and Winkle, RA: Electrode-catheter arrhythmia induction in the selection and assessment of antiarrhythmic drug therapy for recurrent ventricular tachycardia. Circulation 58:971, 1978.
37. Rotman, M, Wagner, GS, and Wallace, AG: Bradyarrhythmias in acute myocardial infarction. Circulation 55:703, 1972.
38. Davies, MJ, Anderson, RH, and Becker, AE: The Conduction System of the Heart. Butterworth and Co., London, 307–227, 1983.
39. George, M, Edin, B, and Greenwood, TW: Relation between bradycardia and the site of myocardial infarction. Lancet 2:739, 1967.
40. Feigl, D, Ashkenazy, J, and Kishon, Y: Early and late atrioventricular block in acute inferior myocardial infarction. J Am Coll Cardiol 4:35, 1984.
41. Hindman, MC, Wagner, GS, Marlene, J, et al: The clinical significance of bundle branch block complicating acute myocardial infarction. Circulation 58:689, 1978
42. Hindman, MC, Wagner, GS, Marlene, J, et al: The clinical significance of bundle branch block complicating acute myocardial infarction 1. Clinical characteristics, hospital mortality, and one-year follow-up. Circulation 58:679, 1978.
43. Jewitt, DE, Balcon, R, Raftery, EB, et al: Incidence and management of supraventricular arrhythmias after acute myocardial infarction. Lancet 2:734, 1967.
44. James, TN: Myocardial infarction and atrial arrhythmias. Circulation 24:761, 1961.
45. Keefe, DL, Miura, D, and Somberg, JC: Supraventricular tachyarrhythmias: Their evaluation and therapy. Am Heart J 111:1150, 1986.
46. Hod, H, Lew, AS, Keltai, M, et al: Early atrial fibrillation during evolving myocardial infarction: A consequence of impaired left atrial perfusion. Circulation 75:146, 1987.
47. Wyman, MG, Slaughter, RL, Farolina, DA, et al: Multiple bolus technique for lidocaine administration in acute ischemic heart disease. II. Treatment of refractory ventricular arrhythmias and the pharmacokinetic significance of severe left ventricular failure. J Am Coll Cardiol 2:764, 1983.
48. Miller, JM and Josephson, ME: Malignant ventricular arrhythmias early after myocardial infarction: Brighter prospects. J Am Coll Cardiol 6:769, 1985.

49. Akhtar, M, Tchou, PJ, and Jazayeri, M: Mechanisms of clinical tachycardias. Am J Cardiol 61:9A, 1988.
50. Lazzara, R and Scherlag, BJ: Generation of arrhythmias in myocardial ischemia and infarction. Am J Cardiol 61:20A, 1988.
51. deBakker, JMT, vanCapelle, FJL, Janse, MJ, et al: Reentry as a cause of ventricular tachycardia in patients with chronic ischemic heart disease: Electrophysiologic and anatomic correlation. Circulation 77:589, 1988.
52. Rosen, MR: Mechanisms for arrhythmias. Am J Cardiol 61:2A, 1988.
53. Belhassen, B, Chalwani, M, and Laniado, S: Reentry and cyclic AMP-mediated triggered activity: Dual mechanisms of ventricular tachycardia in healed myocardial infarction. Am J Cardiol 61:1153, 1988.
54. Lucchesi, BR: Rationale of therapy in the patient with acute myocardial infarction and life-threatening arrhythmias: A focus on bretylium. Am J Cardiol 54:14A, 1984.
55. Bigger, JT, Dresdale, RJ, Heissenbuttel, RH, et al: Ventricular arrhythmias in ischemic heart disease: Mechanism, prevalence, significance and management. Prog Cardiovasc Dis 19:255, 1977.
56. Lang, TW, Corday, E, Gold, H, et al: Consequence of reperfusion after coronary occlusion: Effects of hemodynamic and regional myocardial metabolic function. Am J Cardiol 33:69, 1974.
57. Pantridge, JF, Webb, SW, and Adgey, AAJ: Arrhythmias in the first hours of acute myocardial infarction. Prog Cardiovasc Dis 23:265, 1981.
58. Lie, KI, Wellens, HJJ, Downar, E, et al: Observations on patients with primary ventricular fibrillation complicating acute myocardial infarction. Circulation 52:755, 1975.
59. Tofler, GH, Stone, PH, Muller, JE, et al: Prognosis after myocardial infarction complicated by ventricular fibrillation (abstract). Circulation 74:II-304, 1986.
60. Volpi, A, Maggioni, A, Franzosi, MG, et al: In-hospital prognosis of patients with acute myocardial infarction complicated by primary ventricular fibrillation. N Engl J Med 317:257, 1987
61. Wilber, DJ, Garan, H, Finkelstein, D, et al: Out-of-hospital cardiac arrest: Use of electrophysiologic testing in the prediction of long-term outcome. N Engl J Med 318:19, 1988.
62. Lie, KI, Wellens, JH, vanCapelle, FJ, et al: Lidocaine in the prevention of primary ventricular fibrillation. N Engl J Med 291:1325, 1974.
63. The Medical Letter on Drugs and Therapeutics: Drugs for cardiac arrhythmias. 28:111, 1986.
64. Dunn, HM, McComb, JM, Kinney, CD, et al: Prophylactic lidocaine in the early phase of suspected myocardial infarction. Am Heart J 110:353, 1985.
65. Classification of antiarrhythmic drugs. In Sandoe, E, Flensted-Jensen, E, and Olsen, KH, (eds): Symposium on Cardiac Arrhythmias (Elsinore, Denmark, 1970), pp449–472. Sodertalje, Sweden, AB Astra, 1970.
66. Ryden, L, Ariniego, R, Arnman, K, et al: A double-blind trial of metoprolol in acute myocardial infarction. N Engl J Med 308:614, 1983.
67. The Miami Trial Research Group: Other clinical findings and tolerability. Am J Cardiol 56:39G, 1985.
68. Beta Blocker Heart Attack Study Group: The beta-blocker heart attack trial. JAMA 246:2073, 1981.
69. Torresani, J: Bretylium tosylate in patients with acute myocardial infarction. Am J Cardiol 54:21A, 1984.
70. Chatterjee, K, Mandel, WJ, Vyden, JK, et al: Cardiovascular effects of bretylium tosylate in acute myocardial infarction. JAMA 1223:757, 1983.
71. Bigger, JT, Fleiss, JL, Kleiger, R, et al: The relationships among ventricular arrhythmias, left ventricular dysfunction, and mortality in the 2 years after myocardial infarction. Circulation 69:250, 1984.
72. Graboys, TB, Lown, B, Podrid, PJ, et al: Long-term survival of patients with malignant ventricular arrhythmia treated with antiarrhythmic drugs. Am J Cardiol 50:437, 1982.
73. The CAPS Investigators: The cardiac arrhythmia pilot study. Am J Cardiol 57:91, 1986.
74. The CAPS Investigators: Effects of encainide, flecainide, imipramine and moricizine on ventricular arrhythmias during the year after acute myocardial infarction. Am J Cardiol 61:501, 1988.
75. Hession, MJ, Lampert, S, Podrid, PJ, et al: Ethmozine (moricizine HCI) therapy for complex ventricular arrhythmias. Am J Cardiol 60:59F, 1987.
76. Wyndham, CRC, Pratt, CM, Mann, DE, et al: Electrophysiology of Ethmozine (moricizine HCL) for ventricular tachycardia. Am J Cardiol 60:67F, 1987.

77. Gottlieb, SH, Achuff, SC, Mellits, ED, et al: Prophylactic antiarrhythmic therapy of high-risk survivors of myocardial infarction: Lower mortality at 1 month but not at 1 year. Circulation 975:792, 1987.
78. Rosen, MR and Wit, AL: Electropharmacology of antiarrhythmic drugs. Am Heart J 106:829, 1983.
79. Waxman, HL, Buxton, AE, Sadowski, LM, et al: The response to procainamide during electrophysiologic study for sustained ventricular tachyarrhythmias predicts the response to other medications. Circulation 67:30, 1983.
80. Whitford, EC, McGovern, B, Schoenfeld, MH, et al: Long-term efficacy of mexiletine alone and in combination with class IA antiarrhythmic drugs for refractory ventricular arrhythmias. Am Heart J 115:360, 1988.
81. Greenspan, AM, Spielman, SC, and Horowitz, LN: Combination antiarrhythmic drug therapy for ventricular tachyarrhythmias. PACE 9:565, 1986.
82. LaL, R, Chapman, PD, Naccarelli, GV, et al: Flecainide in the treatment of nonsustained ventricular tachycardia. Ann Intern Med 105:493, 1986.
83. Flecainide Ventricular Tachycardia Study Group: Treatment of resistant ventricular tachycardia with flecainide acetate. Am J Cardiol 57:1299, 1986.
84. Webb, CR, Morganroth J, Senior, S, et al: Flecainide: Steady state electrophysiologic effects in patients with remote myocardial infarction and inducible sustained ventricular arrhythmia. J Am Coll Cardiol 8:214, 1986.
85. LaL, R, Chapman, PD, Naccarrelli, GV, et al: Short- and long-term experience with flecainide acetate in the management of refractory life-threatening ventricular arrhythmias. J Am Coll Cardiol 6:772, 1985.
86. Roden, DM and Woosley, RL: Drug therapy: Flecainide. N Engl J Med 315:37, 1986.
87. Campbell, RWF: Drug therapy: Mexiletine. N Engl J Med 316:29, 1987.
88. Johansson, BW: Effect of beta blockade on ventricular fibrillation and ventricular tachycardia-induced circulatory arrest in acute myocardial infarction. Am J Cardiol 57:34F, 1986.
89. Winkle, RA, Peters, F, Kates, RE, et al: Clinical pharmacology and antiarrhythmic efficacy of encainide in patients with chronic ventricular arrhythmias. Circulation 64:290, 1981.
90. Roden, DM and Woosley, RL: Tocainide. N Engl J Med 315:41, 1986.
91. Levy, S: Combination therapy for cardiac arrhythmias. Am J Cardiol 61:95A, 1988.
92. Mason, JW: Drug therapy: Amiodarone. N Engl J Med 316:455, 1987.
93. DiCarlo, LA, Morady, F, Sauve, MJ, et al: Cardiac arrest and sudden death in patients treated with amiodarone for sustained ventricular tachycardia or ventricular fibrillation: Risk stratification based on clinical variables. Am J Cardiol 55:372, 1985.
94. Morady, F, Sauve, MJ, Malone, P, et al: Long-term efficacy and toxicity of high-dose amiodarone therapy for ventricular tachycardia or ventricular fibrillation. Am J Cardiol 52:975, 1983.
95. Fogoros, RN, Anderson, KP, Winkle, RA, et al: Amiodarone: Clinical efficacy and toxicity in 96 patients with recurrent, drug-refractory arrhythmias. Circulation 68:88, 1983.
96. Scheinman, MM: Indications for the use of amiodarone: A personal perspective. Clin Cardiol 10:11, 1987.
97. Kennedy, JI, Myers, JL, Plumb, VJ, et al: Amiodarone pulmonary toxicity. Arch Intern Med 147:50, 1987.
98. DiMarco, JP, Lerman, BB, Kron, IL, et al: Sustained ventricular tachyarrhythmias within 2 months of acute myocardial infarction: Results of medical and surgical therapy in patients resuscitated from the initial episode. J Am Coll Cardiol 6:759, 1985.
99. Yazaki, Y, Haffajee, CI, Gold, RL, et al: Electrophysiologic predictors of long-term clinical outcome with amiodarone for refractory ventricular tachycardia secondary to coronary artery disease. Am J Cardiol 60:293, 1987.
100. McGovern, B, Garran, H, Malacoff, RF, et al: Long-term clinical outcome of ventricular tachycardia or fibrillation treated with amiodarone. Am J Cardiol 53:1558, 1984.
101. Horowitz, LN, Greenspan, AM, Spielman, SR, et al: Usefulness of electrophysiologic testing in evaluation of amiodarone therapy for sustained ventricular tachyarrhythmias. Am J Cardiol 55:367, 1985.
102. DiBianco, R: Chronic ventricular arrhythmias: Which drug for which patient? Am J Cardiol 61:83A, 1988.
103. Deedwania, PC, Olukotun, AY, Kupersmith, J, et al: Beta blockers in combination with class I antiarrhythmic agents. Am J Cardiol 60:21D, 1987.

104. Morganroth, J: Antiarrhythmic effects of beta-adrenergic blocking agents in benign or potentially lethal ventricular arrhythmias. Am J Cardiol 60:10D, 1987.
105. Kopelman, HA, Woosley, RL, Lee, JT, et al: Electrophysiologic effects of intravenous and oral sotalol for sustained ventricular tachycardia secondary to coronary artery disease. Am J Cardiol 61:1006, 1988.
106. Anderson, JL, Anastasiou-Nana, MI, Heath, BM, et al: Efficacy of recainam, a new antiarrhythmic drug, for control of ventricular arrhythmias. Am J Cardiol 60:281, 1987.
107. Fisher, JD, Johnston, DR, Furman, S, et al: Long-term efficacy of antitachycardia pacing for supraventricular and ventricular tachycardias. Am J Cardiol 60:1311, 1987.
108. Fisher, JD, Kim, SG, and Mercando, AD: Electrical devices for treatment of arrhythmias. Am J Cardiol 61:45A, 1988.
109. Saksena, S, Lindsay, BD, and Parsonnet, V: Developments for future implantable cardioverters and defibrillators. PACE 10:1342, 1987.
110. Marchlinski, FE, Flores, BT, Buxton, AE, et al: The automatic implantable cardioverter-defibrillator: Efficacy, complications, and device failures. Ann Intern Med 104:481, 1986.
111. Mirowski, M, Reid, PR, Winkle, RA, et al: Mortality in patients with implanted automatic defibrillators. Ann Intern Med 98:585, 1983.
112. Reid, PR, Mirowski, M, Mower, MM, et al: Clinical evaluation of the internal automatic cardioverter-defibrillator in survivors of sudden cardiac death. Am J Cardiol 51:1608, 1983.
113. Hargrove, WC, Miller, JM, and Josephson, ME: Use of the automatic implantable cardioverter-defibrillator. N Engl J Med 315:63, 1986.
114. Fogoros, RN, Fiedler, SB, and Elson, JJ: The automatic implantable cardioverter-defibrillator in drug-refractory ventricular tachyarrhythmias. Ann Intern Med 107:635, 1987.
115. Mirowski, M: The automatic implantable cardioverter-defibrillator: An overview. J Am Coll Cardiol 6:461, 1985.
116. Echt, DS, Armstrong, K, Schmidt, P, et al: Clinical experience, complications, and survival in 70 patients with the automatic implantable cardioverter/defibrillator. Circulation 71:289, 1985.
117. Saksena, S and Parsonnet, V: Implantation of a cardioverter/defibrillator without thoracotomy using a triple electrode system. JAMA 259:69, 1988.
118. Harken, AH, Horowitz, LN, and Josephson, ME: Comparison of standard aneurysmectomy and aneurysmectomy with directed endocardial resection for the treatment of recurrent sustained ventricular tachycardia. J Thorac Cardiovasc Surg 4:572, 1980.
119. Mason, JW, Stinson, EB, Winkle, RA, et al: Relative efficacy of blind left ventricular aneurysm resection for the treatment of recurrent ventricular tachycardia. Am J Cardiol 49:241, 1982.
120. Gallagher, JJ, Selle, JG, Svenson, RH, et al: Surgical treatment of arrhythmias. Am J Cardiol 61:27A, 1988.
121. Miller, JM, Marchlinski, FE, Harken, AH, et al: Subendocardial resection for sustained ventricular tachycardia in the early period after acute myocardial infarction. Am J Cardiol 55:980, 1985.
122. Josephson, ME, Horowitz, LN, Spielman, SR, et al: Role of catheter mapping in the preoperative evaluation of ventricular tachycardia. Am J Cardiol 49:207, 1982.
123. Garan, H, Nguyen, K, McGovern, B, et al: Perioperative and long-term results after electrophysiologically directed ventricular surgery for recurrent ventricular tachycardia. J Am Coll Cardiol 8:201, 1986.
124. Miller, JM, Kienzle, MG, Harken, AH, et al: Subendocardial resection for ventricular tachycardia: Predictors of surgical success. Circulation 70:624, 1984.
125. Caceres, J, Werner, P, Jazayeri, M, et al: Efficacy of cryosurgery alone for refractory monomorphic sustained ventricular tachycardia due to inferior wall infarction. J Am Coll Cardiol 11:1254, 1988.
126. Haines, DE, Lerman, BB, Kron, JL, et al: Surgical ablation of ventricular tachycardia with sequential map-guided subendocardial resection: Electrophysiologic assessment and long-term follow-up. Circulation 77:131, 1988.
127. Saksena, S, Hussain, SM, Gielchinsky, I, et al: Intraoperative mapping-guided argon laser ablation of malignant ventricular tachycardia. Am J Cardiol 59:78, 1987.
128. Svenson, RH, Gallagher, JJ, Selle, JG, et al: Neodymium: YAG laser photocoagulation: A successful new map-guided technique for the intraoperative ablation of ventricular tachycardia. Circulation 76:1319, 1987.
129. Fox, J and Vincent, GM: Hemodynamic and hematologic effects of neodymium:YAG laser injury of the left ventricle. Clin Res 33:7A, 1985.

130. Saksena, S and Gadhoke, A: Laser therapy for tachyarrhythmias: A new frontier. PACE 9:531, 1986.
131. Saksena, S, Ciccone, JM, Chandran, P, et al: Laser ablation of normal and diseased human ventricle. Am Heart J 112:52, 1986.
132. Morady, F, Scheinman, MM, DiCarlo, LA, et al: Catheter ablation of ventricular tachycardia with intracardiac shocks: Results in 33 patients. Circulation 5:1037, 1987.
133. Vincent, GM, Fox, J, Benedick, BA, et al: Laser catheter ablation of simulated ventricular tachycardia. Lasers Surg Med 7:421, 1987.
134. Josephson, ME: Catheter ablation of arrhythmias. Ann Intern Med 101:234, 1984.
135. Curtis, A and Vincent, GM: Laser Catheter Ablation of Arrhythmias. In Abela G (ed): Klewer Publishing Company, London, in press.
136. Vincent, GM, Fox, J, and Benedick, BA: Laser catheter ablation of simulated ventricular tachycardia. Lasers Surg Med 7:421, 1987.

CHAPTER 16

Risk Profiling the Patient after Acute Myocardial Infarction

Scott E. Hessen, M.D.
Albert N. Brest, M.D.

Risk stratification after myocardial infarction has become a process of increasing sophistication and clinical utility. The identification of patients at high risk of sudden death, recurrent myocardial infarction, or unstable angina pectoris after myocardial infarction allows application of diagnostic and therapeutic interventions to those patients most likely to benefit. Likewise, patients at low risk may be spared the morbidity and expense of unnecessary testing and may at the same time be reassured that their prognosis is favorable. As pressures for cost-containment grow, risk stratification, by effectively focusing application of limited resources, assumes increased importance.

The risk of recurrent cardiac morbidity and mortality after myocardial infarction is influenced by many factors (Table 16–1). In this chapter, we will examine a patient's fundamental outlook as determined by the intrinsic characteristics of the patient (i.e., the natural history of the disease). Thus, although prognosis may be affected by a variety of therapeutic interventions (e.g., coronary thrombolysis, beta-blockers, aspirin, and so on), the effect of these factors will not be examined. Because the overall long-term mortality for patients recovering from acute myocardial infarction appears to be steadily decreasing,[1] specific mortality figures presented in this chapter may not be strictly applicable to current patients. Nonetheless, relative risks are still valid and may be used to estimate a patient's prognosis after acute myocardial infarction.

Information relevant to long-term prognosis becomes available throughout a patient's hospitalization for myocardial infarction. Many factors are available during the first 24 hours, whereas others must be sought prior to discharge. Thus, risk stratification is an ongoing process; a patient's prognosis is refined throughout the hospitalization. We will examine those factors that are available during a patient's stay in the intensive care unit, and those factors that are determined predischarge. It will become evident that fundamental factors defining prognosis include left ventricular function, electrical instability, and residual ischemia. In

Table 16–1. Adverse Risk Factors After Acute Myocardial Infarction

1. Congestive heart failure (clinical, hemodynamic, or radiographic)
2. Left ventricular ejection fraction less than 0.40
3. Large infarct size (estimated by enzymes, ^{99m}technetium radionuclide scan, electrocardiographic QRS mapping, or echocardiographic techniques)
4. New bundle branch block (any type, including fascicular blocks)
5. Mobitz II second-degree or third-degree heart block
6. Anterior infarction
7. Reinfarction or infarct extension
8. Ventricular fibrillation or ventricular tachycardia
9. Ventricular premature beats (especially if frequent or complex)
10. Supraventricular arrhythmias (other than sinus bradycardia)
11. Abnormal signal-averaged electrocardiogram
12. Inducible sustained monomorphic ventricular tachycardia during electrophysiologic study
13. Postinfarction angina
14. Inability to perform exercise testing
15. Angina pectoris, ST segment elevation or depression, abnormal blood pressure response, or ventricular ectopy induced by exercise testing
16. Diabetes mellitus
17. Hypertension or loss of preexisting hypertension
18. Age greater than 70 years
19. Female gender

addition, comorbid factors, such as diabetes, and intrinsic factors, such as age and gender, are prognostically important.

EARLY HOSPITALIZATION

Demographic Considerations

Several demographic characteristics partially define a patient's ultimate prognosis after myocardial infarction. *Gender* and *race* appear to be consistently linked to prognosis in most studies.[2,3] In the Framingham study, the 12-month mortality rate after acute myocardial infarction for women was 34 percent versus 19 percent for men.[2] The poorer prognosis of women was due to increased early mortality; after the first 12 months, the mortality trends of both sexes were essentially parallel. Women also had a higher rate of reinfarction compared with men (11 percent versus 4 percent in the first year, 39 percent versus 13 percent at 5 years). Analysis of the data from the 816 patients with confirmed myocardial infarction enrolled in the Multicenter Investigation of the Limitation of Infarct Size (MILIS) showed that the cumulative mortality rate at 48 months was 36 percent for women versus 21 percent for men ($p < 0.001$).[4] In this study, blacks had a 34 percent mortality rate compared with 24 percent for whites ($p < 0.005$). Although both women and blacks had a higher baseline frequency of characteristics predictive of mortality than their male and white counterparts, statistically significant differences remained after correction for those characteristics. Whereas mortality differences for black and white men were similar (23 percent and 21 percent, respectively), black women had a significantly higher mortality than white women (48 percent versus 32 percent, respectively). Thus, women in general, and black women in particular, have increased risk of mortality after acute myocardial infarction, independent of other baseline characteristics.

The presence of *diabetes mellitus* has long been recognized as a risk factor for atherosclerotic cardiovascular disease. Diabetes also appears to contribute independently to mortality and to reinfarction.[5–7] In one large study, 1306 men who survived their first infarction were followed for a mean of 6.5 years.[6] The cumulative survival rate at 1, 2, and 5 years was 82 percent, 78 percent, and 58 percent among diabetic subjects and 94 percent, 92 percent, and 82 percent among the nondiabetic subjects ($p < 0.001$). Correction for other baseline risk factors did not affect the significance of this relationship. Mortality was similar among patients with type I and type II diabetes. Also, prognosis was not influenced by the mode of diabetic treatment (diet alone, sulfonylurea agents, or insulin); however, these subgroups contained small numbers of patients. The cumulative rate of reinfarction after 1, 2, and 5 years was 18 percent, 28 percent, and 46 percent in diabetic subjects and 12 percent, 17 percent, and 27 percent in nondiabetic subjects ($p < 0.004$).

The in-hospital and postdischarge mortality for patients *over the age of 70 years* is clearly increased.[8–12] Latting and Silverman reported that the in-hospital mortality of patients with acute myocardial infarction equal to or over the age of 70 years was 32 percent compared with 8.2 percent in younger patients.[12] This difference could not be explained by increased comorbidity of elderly patients and remained significant after baseline differences were adjusted. Other studies in the elderly indicate a poor survival after acute myocardial infarction, with mortality rates of approximately 30 percent to 40 percent at 1 year, and 60 percent at 5 years.[8–11] In one study, however, increased mortality from all causes but not cardiovascular mortality was associated with advanced age by univariate analysis; when multivariate analysis was used to adjust for baseline differences, only Killip class was an independent predictor of survival.[13] Thus, most studies have shown that elderly patients with myocardial infarction have a significantly higher in-hospital and postdischarge mortality independent of other risk factors.

Systolic or diastolic arterial hypertension after acute myocardial infarction results in increased mortality from all causes, in major coronary events, and in combined cerebrovascular events.[7,14] Hypertension emerged as a predictor of late (3- to 6-year) mortality in a study by Norris and associates, and was most marked in those patients whose other prognostic factors were favorable.[8] In contradistinction, *disappearance of preexisting arterial hypertension* after myocardial infarction results in a twofold increase in mortality, presumably because it reflects pump dysfunction.[15]

Several *hematologic parameters,* notably an increased white blood cell count 6 to 20 months after myocardial infarction,[16] depressed activity of euglobulin tissue plasminogen activator,[17] and the presence of antibodies to cardiolipin in young patients,[18] have been associated with an increased risk of reinfarction.

ARRHYTHMIAS AND CONDUCTION

The prognostic importance of the *admission electrocardiogram* to in-hospital complications was studied by Brush and coworkers.[19] The initial electrocardiogram was reviewed in 469 patients suspected of having acute myocardial infarction. An electrocardiogram was classified as positive if one or more of the following patterns were present: evidence of infarction, ischemia, or strain; left ventricular hypertrophy; left bundle branch block; or paced rhythm. Approximately 15 percent of patients with negative initial electrocardiograms were subsequently shown to have acute myocardial infarction whereas 57 percent of patients with positive initial electrocardiograms developed acute myocardial infarction. Life-threatening complications (ventricular fibrillation, sustained ventricular tachycardia, or heart block) were 23 times more likely in the group with positive electrocardiograms (14 percent versus 0.6 percent, $p < 0.001$). Among patients subsequently shown to have acute myocardial infarction, life-threatening complications occurred in 25 percent of the positive electrocardiogram group compared with only 4 percent of the negative group ($p < 0.05$). Other complications (such as recurrent chest pain, pump failure or atrial arrhythmias) were 3 to 10 times more likely in the group with positive initial electrocardiograms ($p < 0.01$). Similarly, patients with positive electrocardiograms were 17 times more likely to die than patients with negative initial electrocardiograms ($p < 0.001$).

The development of *new bundle branch block* complicating myocardial infarction has been recognized since 1938 as an adverse prognostic sign.[20] Overall, conduction blocks are reported to occur in approximately 20 percent of patients with acute myocardial infarction[21] (range 6 percent to 21 percent).[22–27] Left bundle branch block, left anterior fascicular block, and right bundle branch block with left anterior fascicular block each occur in approximately 4 percent to 5 percent of infarctions.[21,28] Isolated right bundle branch block complicates approximately 2 percent to 5 percent of myocardial infarctions whereas left posterior fascicular block and right bundle branch block with left posterior fascicular block each occur in about 1 percent of infarctions.[21,27]

Approximately 5 percent to 6 percent of patients with acute myocardial infarction without intraventricular conduction defects will develop complete AV block, often due to AV nodal ischemia.[24,29] Patients with isolated left anterior or posterior fascicular block infrequently progress to complete AV block (range 0 to 10 percent).[28,29] Patients with right bundle branch block, either alone or in combination with block of either left fascicle progress to complete AV block at a rate of 14 percent to 46 percent.[28,30–32] Patients with left bundle branch block develop complete AV block in approximately 10 percent to 20 percent of cases.[28,29,31] Patients who develop left anterior fascicular block have approximately twice the mortality of patients who do not develop any fascicular block (27 percent versus 15 percent, respectively).[23,24,28] Patients with all other forms of bundle branch block have mortality rates over 40 percent.[28]

Nimetz and coworkers found hospital mortality was not associated with development of bundle branch block per se, but correlated well with the development of *complete AV block.*[26] Patients who developed second- or third-degree AV block had a hospital mortality of 57 percent versus 12 percent without ($p < 0.0005$). Hindman and colleagues retrospectively identified 432 patients who developed bundle branch block during acute myocardial infarction.[31] Patients who progressed to second- or third-degree AV block via a type II pattern had an increased hospital mortality (47 percent versus 23 percent, $p < 0.001$). Significant differences remained when only patients without pulmonary edema or shock were considered (47 percent versus 2 percent, $p < 0.005$). Most of these deaths were related directly to the development of advanced degree AV block, suggesting that prophylactic temporary pacing may be beneficial in this group. Overall, however, temporary pacing in patients at high risk for development of complete AV block has been reported to produce little change in prognosis in most studies, probably due to the large amount of mycardial necrosis associated with bundle branch block and the subsequent pump failure that often ensues.[32] In a large multicenter retrospective review, Hindman and coworkers identified patients with new onset right bundle branch block and left anterior hemiblock, right bundle branch block and left posterior hemiblock, or alternating bundle branch block as being at high risk for development of complete heart block and recommended that these patients receive temporary prophylactic pacing.[31]

Patients with right bundle branch block with associated left anterior or posterior fascicular block who subsequently develop transient complete AV block have been shown to have a high late mortality due to sudden death, which was reduced by permanent pacing.[28,31] Thus, the presence of even transient bundle branch block or fascicular block during acute myocardial infarction is associated with a significantly increased mortality. Patients who develop transient complete AV block associated with bundle branch block (especially bifascicular block) are at high risk for sudden death after discharge.

Ventricular fibrillation (VF) or *sustained ventricular tachycardia* (VT) is a common complication of acute myocardial infarction. The frequency of ventricular arrhythmias, including ventricular premature depolarizations (VPD), VT, or VF has been shown to be related to the patient's age[33] and to infarct size,[34–36] and inversely related to the admission serum potassium concentration.[33]

The effect of VF or VT on mortality was investigated in 849 patients enrolled in the MILIS study.[37] The overall hospital mortality of patients with VT or VF was 27 percent versus 7 percent for patients without ($p < 0.001$). Patients with secondary VT or VF, that is, ventricular tachyarrhythmias associated with hypotension or heart failure, had a significantly higher mortality (51 percent versus 7 percent, $p < 0.001$). Patients with VT/VF not associated with hypotension or heart failure (primary VT/VF) did not have increased mortality (8 percent versus 7 percent). Patients in whom VT or VF occurred more than 72 hours after hospital admission had significantly more in-hosptial mortality (57 percent versus 20 percent, $p < 0.05$). The long-term mortality (mean followup 32 months) of hospital survivors with VT/VF was identical to patients whose infarctions were not complicated by VT/VF (19 percent versus 21 percent).

Schwartz and associates studied the *site of infarction* and its relationship to prognosis in patients with ventricular fibrillation during acute myocardial infarction.[38] Using a retrospective case control method, 125 patients with acute myocardial infarction complicated by ventricular fibrillation who were subsequently discharged were compared with 125 matched infarction patients without VF. Patients with anterior myocardial infarctions with VF had a significantly increased incidence of sudden death (71 percent), especially in the first year after infarction. Patients with anterior infarcts and VF had a higher incidence of left ventricular dysfunction (Killip class II or III) than their matched controls, a factor that decreases the significance of their results. Patients with inferior infarctions and VF did not have an increased mortality after discharge.

The significance of *primary ventricular fibrillation* during acute myocardial infarction was investigated in the Gruppo Italiano per lo Studio della Streptochinasi nell'Infarto (GISSI) study, which was designed primarily to assess the efficacy of streptokinase in acute myocardial infarction.[39] Primary ventricular fibrillation occurred in 332 of 11,712 patients with acute myocardial infarction (2.8 percent). Patients with primary ventricular fibrillation had almost twice the in-hospital mortality of patients without VF (10.8 percent versus 5.9 percent).[39] The relative risk of in-hospital mortality was similar for both anterior and inferior-posterior infarction groups. Treatment with streptokinase did not affect the incidence of ventricular fibrillation.

The effect of *cardiac arrest* of any etiology (VF, VT, asystole, or electromechanical dissociation) during acute myocardial infarction was investigated by Goldberg and coworkers.[40] Approximately 21 percent of patients suffered a cardiac arrest, and, of these, 48 percent occurred within the first 2 days of admission. Patients with cardiac arrest were more likely to be older, to have Q-wave infarcts, and to have more extensive infarcts based on CK measurements ($p < 0.01$). Thirty-four percent of patients with cardiac arrest during the first 2 days of hospitalization survived to be discharged compared with only 12 percent whose cardiac arrest occurred later during their hospitalization. Patients with an early cardiac arrest who were subsequently discharged from the hospital had a better long-term prognosis than late-arrest patients, but the overall prognosis for both groups was worse than for the group of patients without cardiac arrest. Thus, even in survivors of the acute arrhythmia, the occurrence of cardiac arrest was associated with an increased in-hospital mortality and may be associated with an increased mortality after hospital discharge.

Supraventricular arrhythmias are encountered commonly during acute myocardial infarction. Sinus bradycardia is a common arrhythmia in the early hours of acute myocardial infarction, particularly inferior wall infarctions, and occurs in approximately 11 percent to 26 percent of infarctions.[41,42] It is frequently a manifestation of the Bezold-Jarish reflex, and often occurs immediately after thrombolytic reperfusion of the right coronary artery. Sinus bradycardia may be associated with a better prognosis,[43] perhaps by limiting myocardial oxygen utilization and, hence, limiting infarct size. However, when the sinus rate becomes excessively slow, hypotension and frequent ventricular premature depolarizations may develop.

Sinus tachycardia is a common arrhythmia in the first few days of acute myocardial infarction, and has many diverse causes.[42] Pain, anxiety, anemia, left ventricular dysfunction, fever, atrial infarction, and exogenous catecholamines or atropine may all produce sinus tachycardia. By increasing myocardial oxygen utilization and decreasing coronary blood flow, sinus tachycardia may increase infarct size. The presence of sinus tachycardia conferred a significantly increased mortality (39 percent versus 20 percent) in the Multicenter Postinfarction Research Group study.[44]

Paroxysmal atrial tachycardia and *atrial flutter* are uncommon in acute myocardial infarctions, but have been associated with increased mortality.[42,45,46] *Atrial fibrillation* occurs in approximately 10 percent to 15 percent of patients with acute infarction. It is encountered commonly in patients with left ventricular dysfunction, atrial infarction, or pericarditis. The loss of the atrial component of ventricular filling, along with the rapid ventricular rate may result in a significant reduction in cardiac output. Like other atrial tachyarrhythmias, atrial fibrillation is associated with an increased mortality.

Rapid junctional arrhythmias are also uncommon in acute myocardial infarction.[47] The hemodynamic and prognostic implications of paroxysmal junctional tachycardia are similar to paroxysmal atrial tachycardia.

Left Ventricular Function

Infarct Size

Current animal research and human thrombolysis trials have shown that the extent of tissue necrosis during a myocardial infarction is not fixed. Time-dependent dynamic factors such as reperfusion of the infarct-related artery, collateral supply, and cardiac workload during infarction have all been shown to influence infarct size. Overall cardiac pump function is related primarily to the extent of myocardial infarction.[48] Therefore, estimation of infarct size would be expected to be predictive of prognosis after acute myocardial infarction. Infarct size, as measured as risk area (i.e., the amount of myocardium subserved by the infarct-related coronary artery) using intracoronary injection of ^{99m}Tc-macroaggregated albumin, was significantly related to left ventricular ejection fraction and subsequent mortality.[49] In this study of risk area, all cardiogenic deaths occurred in patients with risk areas greater than 33 percent of the left ventricular area. Direct measurements of infarct size are not available at hospitals without catheterization laboratories, and as such are not universally available for risk stratification. Indirect methods have been studied extensively, however, and the findings correlate well with prognosis.

Enzymatic estimation of infarct size became available in 1971 via serial measurement of plasma creatine kinase (CK)[50,51] and, subsequently, the cardiac isoenzyme of creatine kinase MB (CK-MB).[52,53] Accurate estimation of infarct size by enzymatic indices requires frequent sampling of plasma creatine kinase levels at intervals of at most 4 hours over several days. Infarct size is estimated by integration of the rate of release of CK (or CK-MB) into the blood. Using this method, infarct size index (ISI) is expressed as CK-MB gram-equivalents per square meter (g-Eq/m^2). In patients without prior myocardial infarction, enzymatically estimated infarct size using CK-MB has been correlated with left ventricular ejection fraction as determined by biplane ventriculography ($r = -0.078$) and with the percentage of normally contracting left ventricular segments ($r = 0.84$).[54] Two patients with inferior infarctions had disproportionately large estimated infarct sizes; both patients had occlusions of the right coronary artery proximal to the origin of the right ventricular blood supply, suggesting combined left and right ventricular infarction.

Using enzymatic methods, several investigators demonstrated a significant correlation between infarct size and short- and long-term survival. Geltman and colleagues prospectively studied 173 patients under age 66 after their first myocardial infarction.[34] Infarct size index among patients who died was significantly larger than those who survived (46.5 ± 5.8 [SEM] versus 21.1 ± 1.4 CK-g-Eq/m^2, $p < 0.001$). In addition, prognosis was worse for those patients with larger (ISI >30) than moderate ($15 < \text{ISI} < 30$) or smaller (ISI <15) infarcts. Patients with anterior infarcts had a higher mortality than those with inferior infarcts but also had significantly higher ISI values. When infarcts were stratified according to ISI, the mortality from anterior and inferior infarcts was similar. Patients with non-Q-wave infarctions had a mortality similar to patients with Q-wave infarctions despite significantly smaller ISI values (10.5 versus 27.7, $p < 0.001$). The authors concluded that the similar mortality despite the disparity in ISI resulted from the small number of patients with non-Q-wave infarction ($n = 31$). Patients with moderate or large infarcts (ISI >15 units) were also more likely to have frequent ventricular ectopic depolarizations, regardless of infarct location.

Sobel and associates studied 33 patients with acute myocardial infarction and calculated infarct size from serial serum CK measurements.[55] Surviving patients in New York Heart Association class I or II had significantly smaller infarcts (31 ± 4 CK-g-Eq) than those in class III or IV (91 ± 8 CK-g-Eq) or those patients who died (103 ± 14 CK-g-Eq). The authors were also able to use cumulative CK curves to help differentiate clinical reinfarction, with its secondary rise in CK, from pericarditis or noncardiac chest pain.

Estimation of infarct size by frequent sampling of plasma creatine kinase levels is impractical in most clinical settings. In addition, cost and patient discomfort make such an approach inconvenient. To evaluate the hypothesis that less frequent enzyme sampling can accurately estimate infarct size, Thompson and associates prospectively studied 580 patients with documented myocardial infarction.[56] All patients had serum CK and aspartate aminotransferase (AST) levels measured daily for 5 days. A subgroup of 54 patients had CK and AST levels measured every 2 hours for 24 to 48 hours. In this subgroup, infarct size was estimated by calculation of enzyme units released per liter of plasma rather than gram-equivalents. Both peak and the sum of the first five daily CK levels correlated well with total CK release ($r = 0.90$ and $r = 0.91$, respectively.) The peak and sum of the first five daily AST levels correlated less well with total CK release ($r = 0.74$ and $r = 0.86$). Thus peak CK measured as infrequently as once daily can provide meaningful estimates of infarct size. Peak AST is a less accurate reflection of infarct size. In the 560 patients surviving the first hospital day, the peak CK level was associated significantly with 1-year mortality. Patients surviving the first hospital day with a peak CK level less than eight times the upper limit of normal had a total mortality of 15.5 percent compared with 31.2 percent in those with higher peak CK levels ($p < 0.0001$). Peak CK was also able to predict in-hospital but not total posthospital mortality. In the year following hospital discharge, patients with high peak CK levels had a higher rate of cardiac decompensation but not of sudden cardiac death. Peak AST levels were significantly associated with total, in-hospital, and posthospital mortality. For all levels of peak CK, patients with prior infarctions had higher mortality than those patients without. Thus, peak CK levels correlate with infarct size and may be used clinically to predict which patients are at increased risk for in-hospital and posthospital mortality due to cardiac decompensation but not sudden death.

Electrocardiographic techniques for estimating infarct size, such as summing the magnitude of R or Q waves or ST segments of standard 12-lead electrocardiograms or of specialized multilead precordial mapping systems have been proposed and evaluated. Although such methods correlate reasonably well with infarct size,[57] these methods have not achieved clinical usefulness.

Echocardiographic techniques using two-dimensional cross-sectional echocardiography during acute myocardial infarction have demonstrated a significantly worse wall motion index in patients with complicated infarcts (pulmonary congestion and/or hypoperfusion) compared with uncomplicated infarcts.[58]

Myocardial infarct scintigraphy using ^{99m}Tc-pyrophosphate has been shown to provide qualitative estimates of infarct size and location. In addition, the pattern of myocardial uptake was correlated with both in-hospital complication rate and mortality.[59] The mortality associated with massive uptake was significantly greater than that for focal uptake ($p < 0.02$). Magnetic resonance imaging, cine-computed tomography, positron emission computerized tomography, and antimyosin imaging all have potential use in determining infarct size, but, as yet, have unproven clinical value.

Infarct Location

Hands and associates studied 398 patients with anterior wall myocardial infarction and 391 patients with inferior wall myocardial infarction.[60] Patients with prior infarction, true posterior infarction, those who died within the first day of hospitalization, and those patients in whom the location of infarction could not be determined electrocardiographically were excluded. Patients with anterior infarction had a higher incidence of pulmonary edema (8.0 percent versus 3.5 percent, $p = 0.01$) and of cardiac failure (30.6 percent versus 17.6 percent, $p = 0.0001$) but second- or third-degree AV block was less common (3.5 percent versus 9.4 percent, $p = 0.0003$) than in patients with inferior infarction. The 1-year mortality for anterior infarctions was 18.3 percent versus 10.5 percent for inferior infarctions ($p = 0.002$). After controlling for infarct size by assessing peak CK levels, multivariate analysis with a proportional-hazards model demonstrated a significantly increased relative risk of death in the first year after anterior myocardial infarction (relative risk = 1.89) compared with inferior infarction.

The presence of *anterior infarction* was a significant univariate predictor of mortality in the Multicenter Postinfarction Research Group study ($p < 0.05$).[44] In the multivariate model, however, only radionuclide left ventricular ejection fraction, ventricular ectopy greater than 10 beats per hour, and the presence of rales in the upper two-thirds of the lung fields remained as independent predictors of mortality. In the Western Washington Intracoronary Streptokinase Trial, infarct location remained a significant predictor of mortality ($p < 0.04$) after variables of ejection fraction and treatment with streptokinase were assessed.[61] Thus, patients with anterior wall myocardial infarction have a worse prognosis predominantly due to the larger infarct size of anterior infarctions, but some studies have also demonstrated a slightly worse prognosis due to location alone.

Among patients with acute inferior wall myocardial infarctions, the presence of precordial (V1 to V4) electrocardiographic ST segment depression lasting at least 24 hours after hospital admission portends a poorer prognosis.[62] The presence of precordial ST segment depression during inferior wall myocardial infarction was associated with larger infarctions, older age, higher Killip classification and a lower left ventricular ejection fraction.[62] Patients with inferior wall myocardial infarction and persistent precordial ST segment depression had a higher rate of reinfarction (30 percent versus 0 percent, $p < 0.01$) and a higher 1-year mortality (60 percent versus 0 percent, $p < 0.001$) than patients without precordial ST depression.

Infarct Type

Overall, in-hospital and 1-year mortality from Q-wave and non-Q-wave infarctions is similar.[63–66] In-hospital mortality for patients with non-Q-wave infarction (13 percent) was not significantly different from mortality of patients with Q-wave infarction (22 percent) in a study of 159 patients.[65] During a mean followup of 20.2 months, mortality rates were similar again when patients with Q-wave and non-Q-wave infarction were compared (18 percent versus 19 percent, respectively). Thanavaro and coworkers, studying 745 patients during their first acute myocardial infarction, showed that patients with non-Q-wave infarction had significantly decreased in-hospital mortality compared with patients with Q-wave infarcts (3 percent versus 11 percent, $p < 0.01$); however, when patients were stratified into subgroups based on enzymatically determined infarct size, mortality was similar among groups.[64]

Madias and colleagues, compared Q-wave and non-Q-wave myocardial infarction in 104 patients.[66] Fifty-nine percent of patients had a Q-wave infarct. The in-hospital mortality for non-Q-wave infarction (9.3 percent) was similar to that for Q-wave infarction (9.8 percent). However, the incidence of congestive heart failure was higher in the Q-wave infarction group (33 percent versus 9 percent). All patients who developed congestive heart failure as a result of non-Q-wave infarction had a history of previous myocardial infarction. No such correlation between congestive heart failure and prior myocardial infarction was noted in the Q-wave infarct group.

Krone and associates studied 593 patients with initial myocardial infarction, of whom 15.8 percent had non-Q-wave infarcts.[67] The 3-year mortality was 20 percent in the group with Q-wave infarction and 17 percent for non-Q-wave infarction (p = NS). Patients with Q-wave infarcts had significantly higher peak AST and LDH levels than patients with non-Q-wave infarcts ($p < 0.0001$). Patients with Q-wave infarcts and peak AST levels greater that 240 IU/liter had significantly higher mortality during the first 6 months of followup (12.2 percent) compared with patients with Q-wave infarcts and peak AST levels less than or equal to 240 IU/liter (3.9 percent) and patients with non-Q-wave infarcts (2.1 percent). All groups had similar mortality for the next 18 months. Interestingly, the group of patients with non-Q-wave infarcts had significantly higher total mortality (12.3 percent) and cardiac mortality (11.2 percent) from 24 to 36 months, which could not be accounted for by repeated myocardial infarction. This relationship was especially strong for patients over the age of 60 years. Patients with non-Q-wave myocardial infarction were also significantly more likely to have recurrent infarction within 60 days after the index infarction than patients with initial Q-wave infarctions (7.4 percent versus 1.8 percent, $p = 0.0136$). The authors concluded that early mortality (less than 6 months) was most strongly associated with the extent of myocardial damage whereas late mortality (24 to 48 months) was associated with infarct type (Q-wave versus non-Q-wave) and age.

Patients with non-Q-wave myocardial infarctions are at risk for infarct extension and reinfarction.[68–70] Madigan, Rutherford, and Frye studied 50 consecutive patients with non-Q-wave myocardial infarction.[70] Sixty percent of these patients were found to have significant (greater than 75 percent narrowing) coronary artery stenoses involving two or three major coronary vessels by coronary arteriography. Forty-six percent of patients developed unstable angina whereas only 24 percent remained angina-free. Of the medically treated group, 21 percent developed recurrent Q-wave infarction during a mean followup of 10.8 months. Reinfarction occurred in 18 percent of patients at a median time of 16 days after non-Q-wave infarction in a study by Hollander and coworkers.[68] Reinfarction was predicted by predominant ST segment depression associated with the index non-Q-wave infarction and by a history of prior angina. In this study, reinfarction was associated uniformly with death within 24 hours. In a larger study, Maisel and associates studied 1253 patients prospectively after acute myocardial infarction; 277 patients had non-Q-wave infarction.[69] Rates of reinfarction were similar between groups with non-Q-wave infarction (8 percent) and Q-wave infarction (6 percent); however, hospital mortality with extension was 43 percent in the non-Q-wave group compared with 15 percent in the group with Q-wave infarction ($p < 0.01$). The 1-year survival rates for patients with extension were 66 percent for the group with initial Q-wave infarction compared with 35 percent for those with initial non-Q-wave infarction ($p < 0.01$). Extension of infarction was the strongest univariate and multivariate variable predictive of mortality in the non-Q-wave infarction group.

Thus, although non-Q-wave myocardial infarcts tend to be smaller, overall mortality is similar compared with patients with Q-wave infarctions. Patients with non-Q-wave infarcts often have significant multivessel coronary artery disease, and are at risk to develop unstable angina and infarct extension. If reinfarction occurs, the in-hospital and 1-year mortality is significantly increased.

Reinfarction

The prognostic importance of infarct extension was studied by Fraker and associates.[71] Fifty-eight episodes of definite or suspected extension occurred in the course of 458 episodes of myocardial infarction. Patients with heart failure (Killip class III or IV) were excluded. Hospital mortality was 36 percent in patients with extension versus 9 percent in those without ($p < 0.001$). Of patients in both groups who survived hospitalization, the 1-year survival was 76 percent in patients with definite or suspected extension and 91 percent in those without extension. Of those patients surviving to leave the hospital, 19 percent of those with extension had moderate heart failure (Killip class III) after the extension. Extension of myocardial infarction occurred an average of 3.4 days after admission (range 30 hours to 11 days).

Marmor and colleagues, studying 200 patients with myocardial infarction, found that patients with Q-wave infarctions had significantly greater myocardial damage (25 CK-MB units) than patients with non-Q-wave infarcts (11 CK-MB units).[72] Reinfarction occurred in 43 percent of non-Q-wave compared with 8 percent of Q-wave infarcts. Reinfarction was usually accompanied by a secondary rise in CK more than 48 hours after the initial elevation. The in-hospital mortality of patients with non-Q-wave infarction who developed recurrent infarction was 16 percent compared with 7 percent in those without recurrent infarction. Left ventricular ejection fraction in patients with recurrent myocardial infarction significantly decreased from a mean initial value of 56 ± 11 percent to 34 ± 10 percent ten days later.

Infarct extension, defined as a significant reelevation of the CK-MB versus time curve, was studied in 848 patients with enzymatic documentation of acute myocardial infarction enrolled in the MILIS study.[73] Infarct extension occurred in 71 patients (8.4 percent). Interestingly, only 43 percent of patients identified by the central MILIS CK-MB core laboratory as having infarct extension were recognized clinically (based on recurrent ischemic pain, electrocardiographic changes, or reelevation of locally determined creatine kinase levels in their respective hospitals) as having infarct extension. This finding suggests that many episodes of infarct extension are missed or are clinically silent. In-hospital mortality was more than four times greater in the subgroup with extension compared with patients without enzymatic evidence of extension (30 percent versus 7 percent, $p < 0.01$); however, patients with extension who survived hospitalization did not have a statistically increased mortality after discharge (12 percent versus

4 percent, $p = NS$). Multivariate analysis identified the presence of angina on the second hospital day and a history of previous myocardial infarction as significant predictors of infarct extension. The presence of ST segment depression on the admission electrocardiogram was of borderline significance ($p < 0.06$) in the multivariate model. The presence of any two of these factors identified a subgroup of patients with more than twice the incidence of infarct extension (15.1 percent versus 5.8 percent). Patients with all three risk factors had a 50 percent risk of infarct extension, but the number of patients in this group was small. Thus, reinfarction or extension of myocardial infarction is common, is associated with increased in-hospital and 1-year mortality, occurs more frequently in patients with non-Q-wave infarctions, and can result in development of heart failure and depressed ejection fraction. Risk factors predicting its occurrence include the presence of angina following infarction, a history of previous myocardial infarction, and ST segment depression on the initial electrocardiogram.

Spontaneous Reperfusion

The time course of serum CK elevation after acute myocardial infarction is variable, with both rapid and slow release patterns noted. The rapid release (early time to peak CK) pattern has been shown in animal models of coronary occlusion[74] and in patients with coronary thrombolysis[75] to be associated with early reperfusion of infarcted tissue. The effects of differing times to peak CK values was studied by Ong and coworkers in 52 patients with acute Q-wave myocardial infarction.[76] Patients underwent radionuclide ventriculography within 24 hours of the onset of their symptoms and again immediately before discharge. The mean time to peak CK was 8.8 ± 2.5 hours in the rapid release group and 19.0 ± 4.9 hours in the slow release group. Peak CK levels, initial global left ventricular ejection fraction, and regional ejection fraction were similar. When the initial and final ejection fractions were compared in the two groups, the rapid release group had a significant rise in both global ejection fraction (0.38 ± 0.09 to 0.48 ± 0.08, $p < 0.001$) and regional ejection fraction of Q-wave regions (0.33 ± 0.11 to 0.43 ± 0.13, $p < 0.001$). Patients with slow CK release had no significant change of global or regional ejection fraction from hospital admission to discharge.

The prognostic importance of early peaking CK-MB levels was determined retrospectively in 342 patients with acute myocardial infarction who were randomized to receive placebo as part of the MILIS study.[77] Patients were classified as having an early peak CK-MB if the peak level occurred within 15 hours of the onset of symptoms. Patients with early peak CK-MB more frequently presented with ST segment depression (23 percent versus 11 percent, $p < 0.01$) and a lower mean left ventricular ejection fraction (41.4 percent versus 47.4 percent, $p < 0.01$). Patients with an early peak CK-MB had a smaller mean CK infarct size index (12.6 versus 18.9 g-Eq/m^2, $p < 0.01$), despite a lower mean ejection fraction at initial presentation. Patients with early peak CK-MB also had a 4.5 percent increase in global ejection fraction, whereas those with later peaking CK-MB did not. Early peaking CK-MB patients had a higher incidence of ST segment depression and a decrement in ejection fraction with exercise, suggesting residual myocardium still in jeopardy. The 4-year mortality in 314 hospital survivors was significantly higher in patients with an early CK-MB peak (47 percent versus 19 percent, $p < 0.0001$) and remained significant after adjustment for baseline differences between the two groups ($p < 0.02$). A significant difference in mortality was noted at 12 months, with increasing differences noted throughout 4 years of followup. Similarly, the 4-year life table estimates for the rate of recurrent myocardial infarction (33 percent versus 22 percent, $p < 0.05$) and fatal recurrent infarction (20 percent versus 8 percent, $p < 0.001$) were significantly higher in the group of patients with early peaking CK-MB.

Using multivariate analysis, Nidorf and coworkers have shown that an early peaking creatine kinase curve is an independent predictor of both recurrent cardiac ischemic events and mortality.[78] After 10 years of followup, the survival was 65 percent in the late-peaking group compared with 42 percent in the early-peaking group ($p < 0.05$).[78] Thus, patients with early-peaking CK or CK-MB enzyme levels probably are those patients with reperfusion of the infarct-related coronary artery. These patients have a hospital course similar to those with late-peaking CK-MB levels and are likely to have modest increases in both regional and global left ventricular ejection fraction; however, they will often have significant residual myocardium at jeopardy and will have a significantly increased risk of recurrent myocardial infarction and mortality.

Left Ventricular Function Immediately Postinfarction

Left ventricular function measured during the early hours of acute myocardial infarction is strongly related to the risk of subsequent mortality.[79] Left ventricular function was determined by contrast angiography a mean of 4.6 hours after acute myocardial infarction in 245 patients as part of the Western Washington Intracoronary Streptokinase Trial.[61] Left ventricular ejection fraction was the strongest determinant of 1-year mortality ($p < 0.0001$), followed by treatment with streptokinase and infarct location.

Left ventricular function, as manifested on initial chest x-ray, was studied in 273 patients with acute myocardial infarction by Battler and coworkers.[80] The presence of pulmonary congestion, increased left-heart dimension, and enlarged cardiothoracic ratio on initial chest x-ray were found to identify patients at increased risk of dying within the first month or first year after acute myocardial infarction. In the absence of pulmonary congestion, 94 percent and 88 percent of patients survived the first month and first year, respectively. When diffuse alveolar edema was present, only 18 percent of patients survived 1 month, and no patients survived the first year. Patients with an enlarged cardiothoracic ratio or left-heart dimension but without pulmonary congestion had a 24 percent 1-year mortality compared with 9 percent with an initial normal cardiothoracic ratio or 6 percent with an initial normal left-heart dimension. Thus, both increased left-heart size determined by chest x-ray and pulmonary venous congestion were significant predictors of increased 1-month and 1-year mortality.

Two-dimensional echocardiography has also been shown to predict major cardiac complications after acute myocardial infarction.[58,81,82] Echocardiography was performed within 12 hours of admission to the CCU in 61 consecutive patients in a study at the Mayo Clinic.[82] A left ventricular wall motion index was derived from analysis of regional wall motion; 14 segments were analyzed, each left ventricular wall segment contributing a score as follows: 0 (hyperkinetic), 1 (normal), 2 (hypokinetic), 3 (akinetic), 4 (dyskinetic), 5 (aneurysmal). The sum of these numbers was then divided by the number of visualized segments to define a wall motion index. Thus, a normal ventricle received a wall motion index of 1.0. Patients with a wall motion index greater than or equal to 2.0 had an 89 percent chance of developing congestive heart failure, ventricular arrhythmias, or death compared with 18 percent if the wall motion index was less than 2.0 ($p < 0.0005$). This relationship remained similar among a subset of patients who were in Killip class I on admission, suggesting that early determination of left ventricular function and segmental wall motion may allow prediction of high-risk patients who might otherwise be believed to be at low risk from clinical parameters.

Stamm and colleagues compared the findings of two-dimensional echocardiography in the early hours after acute myocardial infarction with echocardiography and coronary angiography determined prior to hospital discharge.[83] Asynergy of echocardiographic regions remote from the index infarction were found in 77 percent of patients with multivessel coronary artery disease but in none of the patients with single-vessel disease ($p < 0.01$). Compensatory hyperkinesis was found in 50 percent of patients with single-vessel disease compared with 4.5 percent of patients with multivessel disease ($p = 0.005$). Followup echocardiography before discharge revealed improvement in the extent of asynergy in 33 percent of patients with single-vessel disease and in 77 percent of patients with multivessel disease. Thus, early two-dimensional echocardiography can be used to predict multivessel coronary artery disease, but, especially in the multivessel group, will overestimate the extent of left ventricular asynergy present after recovery from myocardial infarction.

Left ventricular dysfunction at hospital discharge after acute myocardial infarction is not always related to the extent of left ventricular dysfunction present on admission. Several studies have shown that the presence of ventricular dysfunction on admission is a predictor of mortality, which is independent of ventricular function determined prior to discharge.[84,85]

The presence of greater than bibasilar rales in patients with acute myocardial infarction was shown to be an independent prognostic factor, which was additive to predischarge radionuclide left ventricular ejection fraction in the Multicenter Postinfarction Research Group trial.[84] Patients with advanced rales but an ejection fraction greater than 0.40 had a 21 percent mortality rate whereas patients with minimal rales and an ejection fraction less than 0.40 had a 15 percent mortality rate. The authors concluded that acute left ventricular dysfunction is an independent risk factor for mortality, which is probably due, in part, to reversible myocardial ischemia.

Warnowicz and associates identified 39 patients who presented with acute myocardial infarction and pulmonary edema.[85] When patients were stratified according to radionuclide left ventricular ejection fraction determined a mean of 10 days after infarction, 16 patients had normal ejection fractions (0.55 ± 0.06) whereas 23 patients had depressed ejection fractions (0.32 ± 0.06). During a mean followup of 9 months, mortality was similar in both groups. Thus, patients presenting with severe left ventricular dysfunction during acute myocardial infarction form a high-risk group, independent of their ultimate left ventricular function at hospital discharge.

Hemodynamic Factors

Continuous hemodynamic monitoring of patients with acute myocardial infarction was made practical by the development of the balloon-tipped, flow-directed pulmonary artery catheter in 1970.[86] In addition to measuring pulmonary capillary wedge, pulmonary artery and right atrial pressures, cardiac output may be calculated by the Fick method or measured directly by thermodilution techniques.[87] Patients with acute myocardial infarction may be divided into hemodynamic subgroups based on the presence or absence of pulmonary congestion (pulmonary capillary wedge pressure greater than 18 mmHg) and peripheral hypoperfusion (cardiac index less than 2.2 liters/min/m^2).[88] When neither pulmonary congestion nor peripheral hypoperfusion was present, the hospital mortality was 3 percent. The presence of pulmonary congestion alone raised mortality to 9 percent; the mortality with a low cardiac index alone was 23 percent. When both pulmonary congestion and a low cardiac index were present, mortality was synergistically increased to 51 percent. The presence of a cardiac index less than 2.2 L/min/m^2 carries a worse prognosis than the presence of a pulmonary capillary wedge pressure greater than 18 mmHg. Similar results have been reported by other investigators.[89–91] Patients may be divided into clinical subgroups comparable to the hemodynamic subgroups described above. The presence of rales or chest X-ray evidence of congestion defines pulmonary congestion, whereas the presence of hypotension, sinus tachycardia, oliguria, and cool skin defines peripheral hypoperfusion. As expected, patients with neither of these findings have a low mortality (less than 1 percent) whereas patients with both have a hospital mortality of 60 percent.[88] Clinical subset determination accurately predicted hemodynamic subset classification in 68 percent of cases.[88]

Residual Ischemia

Residual ischemia after myocardial infarction may present as angina pectoris, electrocardiographically determined ST segment shifts without clinical angina, exercise-induced ischemia, or recurrent myocardial infarction. The risk factors for and the prognosis of patients with recurrent myocardial infarction have already been discussed. Spontaneous electrocardiographic ST segment shifts without angina and exercise-induced ischemia will be discussed subsequently.

The Multicenter Postinfarction Research Group evaluated many demographic, clinical and laboratory parameters in an attempt to determine parameters of postinfarction risk stratification.[44] The presence of an ejection fraction less than 40 percent, ventricular ectopy greater than 10 beats per hour, and the presence of rales heard in the upper two-thirds of the lung fields were independent risk factors predictive of 2-year mortality. Surprisingly, the presence of angina pectoris after infarction was not associated with increased mortality in this study. Failure to give nitrates after myocardial infarction was independently associated with total mortality in a study from the San Francisco General Hospital,[11] suggesting that residual ischemia may be prognostically important.

Objective evidence of myocardial ischemia after acute myocardial infarction, defined as angina with transient ST-T changes, was observed by Bosch and associates in 18 percent of 449 consecutive patients who survived acute myocardial infarction and underwent cardiac catheterization a mean of 10 days after admission.[92] The presence of angina prior to the infarction and the presence of a non-Q-wave infarction were independent predictors of postinfarction ischemia. Patients with postinfarction ischemia had a greater number of epicardial coronary arteries with >70 percent stenosis ($p = 0.008$). Extension of infarction was predicted only by the presence of early ischemia, occurring in 28 percent of patients with early ischemia versus 2.4 percent without ($p < 0.0001$). Mortality was also increased in those patients with early ischemia. With a mean followup of 14 months, cumulative survival was 83 percent in patients with early ischemia versus 92 percent in those patients without ($p = 0.01$).

The prognostic significance of early postinfarction angina with ST segment changes was studied in a group of 70 patients by Schuster and Bulkley.[93] Forty-three patients had electrocardiographic evidence of ischemia remote from the prior infarct zone, whereas 27 patients had ischemia within the infarct zone. Overall mortality during an average followup of 6 months was 56 percent. Patients with remote ischemia had a mortality of 72 percent compared with 33 percent of patients with ischemia within the infarct zone ($p < 0.005$).

PREDISCHARGE CONSIDERATIONS

Left Ventricular Function

Noninvasive evaluation of left ventricular function may be accomplished by various techniques. Radionuclide ventriculography, echocardiography, and electrocardiographic QRS scoring systems have all been employed in an attempt to refine prognosis after acute myocardial infarction.

In a population of 81 patients studied after acute myocardial infarction, Schulze and colleagues found high correlation between a radionuclide left ventricular ejection fraction and high-grade ventricular arrhythmias in the late phase of hospitalization.[94] In addition, patients who died during a 6-month followup were all found to have left ventricular ejection fractions less than 0.40 and high-grade ventricular arrhythmias prior to discharge.

Subsequently, many studies have demonstrated the independent role of left ventricular function on mortality.[11,44,61,95–100] During 1979–1980, the Multicenter Postinfarction Research Group studied 866 patients after acute myocardial infarction with followup from 1 to 3 years.[44] Ninety-four percent of these patients underwent radionuclide ventriculography prior to hospital discharge. A progressive increase in 1-year mortality with decreasing left ventricular ejection fraction was demonstrated by univariate analysis. Multivariate analysis confirmed that the presence of an ejection fraction less than 0.40 was a strong independent predictor of mortality. Ventricular premature beats greater than 10 per hour and the presence of rales in the upper lung fields were also independent prognostic factors. Reanalysis of the data from this study showed that a left ventricular ejection fraction of less than 0.30 was a more optimal breakpoint for predicting mortality.[36] A left ventricular ejection fraction less than 0.30 was a better predictor of early mortality (less than 6 months) whereas the presence of ventricular arrhythmias was a better predictor of late mortality. However, both left ventricular ejection fraction and ventricular premature depolarizations were independent predictors of mortality.

Sanz and coworkers employed cardiac catheterization and coronary arteriography to study 259 consecutive men survivors of acute myocardial infarction.[98] Left ventricular ejection fraction ($p < 0.001$), the number of diseased vessels ($p < 0.005$), and congestive heart failure in the intensive care unit ($p < 0.01$) were the only independent predictors of survival during a mean followup of 34 months. Patients with normal ejection fractions (greater than or equal to 50 percent) had a 4-year survival of from 96 percent to 100 percent depending on the number of diseased vessels, whereas patients with ejection fractions less than 0.20 had a survival of from 30 percent to 75 percent. In the group of patients with an ejection fraction between 21 percent and 49 percent, only patients with three-vessel disease had significantly lower survival (78 percent) than patients with a normal ejection fraction ($p < 0.01$).

An ejection fraction of less than 0.40 was also found to be predictive of sudden cardiac death over a 2-year followup period in the MILIS study.[97] The presence of a radionuclide ejection fraction less than 0.40 after acute myocardial infarction was found to be predictive of subsequent rehospitalization for cardiac events (angina, heart failure, arrhythmia and coronary heart surgery) ($p < 0.001$).[101]

End-systolic left ventricular volume as measured by contrast angiography was found to be a better predictor of overall mortality than either ejection fraction or end-diastolic volume in 605 patients less than 60 years of age who survived an acute myocardial infarction.[102] For the group of patients with ejection fractions greater than 0.50, end-systolic volume added little predictive value. In the group of patients with ejection fractions less than 0.50, however, patients with larger end-systolic volumes had significantly increased mortality compared with patients with smaller end-systolic volumes. These data suggest that ventricular dilatation after myocardial infarction rather than left ventricular dysfunction alone may be significantly related to mortality.

Two-dimensional echocardiography performed prior to hospital discharge has also been shown to correlate with infarct size and future cardiac events. Nixon and associates showed that two-dimensional echocardiography correlated with estimates of infarct involvement as measured by thallium-201 scintigraphy ($r = 0.87$) and with infarct size as estimated by ^{99m}technetium pyrophosphate scintigraphy ($r = 0.74$).[103] Echocardiography was performed 1 day prior to hospital discharge in 47 consecutive survivors of acute myocardial infarction.[104] A wall motion score was derived from endocardial motion in 11 left ventricular segments, such that higher scores reflected worse segmental wall motion. Patients who developed angina, reinfarction, or death during a mean followup of 17 months had significantly higher wall motion scores than patients who did not develop cardiac complications ($p < 0.005$). Stepwise logistic regression analysis revealed that wall motion score and Killip class were the most significant predictors of cardiac complications. Eight of 47 patients (17 percent) were excluded from analysis because of technically inadequate two-dimensional echocardiograms, a factor that limits applicability of this technique.

Although it is clear that a depressed resting ejection fraction determined prior to hospital discharge is predictive of mortality, a significant percentage of patients with normal resting ejection fractions will have cardiac events. In these patients, determination of the dynamic *ejection fraction response to exercise* may be of prognostic value. Corbett and coworkers studied submaximal exercise ejection fraction in 61 patients with a resting mean ejection fraction of 0.55 after myocardial infarction.[105] Patients with major cardiac events during 6-month followup had a significant reduction of peak exercise ejection fraction (0.44 rest to 0.37 exercise) compared with no significant change in those patients with minor cardiac events. Patients with no cardiac events showed an increase in ejection fraction with exercise (0.66 rest to 0.76 exercise). Hung and colleagues performed exercise radionuclide ventriculography in 117 men 3 weeks after a clinically uncomplicated acute myocardial infarction.[106] A peak treadmill work load of 4 METs or less or a decrease in ejection fraction of 0.05 or more below the value at rest identified patients at high risk for cardiac death, nonfatal ventricular fibrillation, or recurrent MI during a mean followup of 11.6 months (23 percent versus 2 percent, $p < 0.001$). Most likely, a poor ejection fraction response to exercise is indicative of multivessel coronary artery disease and may explain the poor outcome in this group of patients.[107]

Other investigators have not found the ejection fraction (EF) response to exercise to be prognostically important.[108–110] Iskandrian and associates found the exercise EF, resting EF, history of prior MI, resting or exercise wall motion score, exercise duration, and exercise heart rate to all be univariate predictors of cardiac death and nonfatal myocardial infarction.[109] The ejection fraction response to exercise was not prognostically important. By multivariate analysis, the exercise ejection fraction was the most powerful predictor of mortality or nonfatal reinfarction ($p < 0.0001$ for each). Similarly, in another study, the exercise ejection fraction but not the change in ejection fraction with exercise was predictive of 1-year mortality and multivessel coronary artery disease.[110]

Two-dimensional echocardiography performed during the immediate recovery phase of low-level exercise testing has been shown to predict future cardiac events.[111,112] A decrease in recovery ejection fraction units of more than 0.10 and new or worsening wall motion abnormalities was found to be predictive of patients who subsequently required coronary bypass surgery, developed recurrent myocardial infarction, or died.[111] In addition, exercise two-dimensional echocardiography was found to be 80 percent sensitive and 95 percent specific in identifying patients at risk for death, recurrent myocardial infarction, unstable angina, or coronary bypass surgery in a study by Ryan and colleagues.[112]

Additional methods for approximation of left ventricular function include Q-wave[113] and R-wave[114] analysis from multiple lead electrocardiographic recordings. Awan and associates computed a Q-index by summing the number of pathologic Q-waves (>0.04 sec) from 35 precordial leads in patients after anterior myocardial infarction. Compared with results obtained at cardiac catheterization, the Q-index correlated well with extent of left ventricular dyssynergy ($r = 0.84$), and inversely with ejection fraction ($r = -0.87$), stroke work index ($r = -0.79$), and cardiac index ($r = -0.66$). Patients with larger Q-indices had higher New York Heart Association functional class ratings and increased mortality at 1 year. The sum of R-wave amplitude calculated from standard electrocardiographic leads aVL, aVF, and V1 to V6 has been shown to correlate with angiographic left ventricular ejection fraction ($r = 0.61$).[114]

A different QRS scoring system was devised by Selvester and coworkers,[115] in which scoring criteria were derived from Q-wave and R-wave durations and amplitude ratios from 10 of 12 standard surface electrocardiographic leads (I, II, aVL, aVF, and V1 to V6). Patients with bundle branch block or left ventricular hypertrophy are excluded in this method. Palmeri and associates[116] used this approach to correlate left ventricular function with QRS score in 55 patients 3 weeks after acute myocardial infarction. The derived QRS score correlated inversely with ejection fraction ($r = -0.88$). Using the same QRS scoring system, moderate correlations between QRS score and infarct size ($r = 0.72$) and multigated radionuclide ejection fraction ($r = -0.72$) have been demonstrated.[117]

Roubin and colleagues studied 181 patients after myocardial infarction and demonstrated a strong inverse correlation between the Palmeri QRS score and angiographic ejection fraction ($r = -0.81$).[118] Linear regression analysis showed ejection fraction to be related to the QRS score as follows: EF (percent) = 66 − 3.3 (QRS score). A QRS score of greater than or equal to 7 had a sensitivity of 59 percent and a specificity of 97 percent for predicting an ejection fraction of less than 45 percent. Jones and coworkers, however, found only moderate correlations between QRS score and radionuclide ejection fraction ($r = -0.70$) or angiographic ejection fraction ($r = -0.66$).[119]

Recent studies[120–122] have shown weak or absent correlations between QRS score and ejection fraction. In addition, QRS score was inferior to ejection fraction for predicting mortality.[120] Although QRS score is a readily available modality, its usefulness in estimating ventricular function as well as in risk stratification after myocardial infarction has not been consistently demonstrated. Further studies are required to resolve the present inconsistencies.

Other parameters obtained from the predischarge 12-lead electrocardiogram have been used to predict mortality after myocardial infarction.[123] The presence of ST segment depression and a prolonged corrected QT interval were univariate predictors of mortality in a study by Fioretti and associates.[123] However, electrocardiographic parameters did not add independent prognostic value compared with clinical and routine laboratory parameters by multivariate analysis.

Another index of left ventricular function shown to predict survival after acute myocardial infarction is the *systolic time interval,* or, more specifically, the pre-ejection period to left ventricular ejection time ratio (PEP/LVET).[124,125] In one study, patients with a PEP/LVET ratio less than 0.42 (i.e., normal) had significantly less mortality than patients with elevated PEP/LVET ratios (12.2 percent versus 39.5 percent, $p < 0.0005$).[125]

ARRHYTHMIAS

ECG or Holter Monitoring

Epidemiologic studies have shown that the presence of *ventricular premature depolarizations* (VPD) detected on a routine 12-lead electrocardiogram after myocardial infarction are associated with an increased risk of sudden death during a followup period of from 2 to 5 years.[126,127] Early studies suggested that the presence and severity of ventricular arrhythmias were correlated with left ventricular ejection fraction but did not independently influence prognosis.[94] Subsequently, ventricular premature depolarizations detected on extended ambulatory (Holter) monitoring approximately 10 days after acute myocardial infarction were determined to be significantly and independently related to prognosis.[36,96,97,128–131] The Multicenter Postinfarction Research Group studied 866 patients less than age 70 after acute myocardial infarction.[44] Of the 806 patients with adequate 24-hour Holter recordings, 475 (59 percent) had fewer than one VPD per hour. The one year cardiac mortality in this group was less than 5 percent. In contrast, patients with greater than 10 VPDs per hour had a 1-year cardiac mortality of more than 14 percent. When mortality is plotted against VPD frequency, the shape of the curve is sigmoidal, with mortality rising rapidly in the region between 1 and 10 VPDs per hour. Higher rates of ventricular ectopy are associated with little increase in cardiac mortality. Further analysis of the data demonstrated that VPDs were independent of left ventricular function in their ability to predict mortality.[36] A VPD frequency of three VPDs per hour was associated with a twofold increase in mortality during 2 years of followup. A left ventricular ejection fraction less than 0.30 was the best predictor of early mortality (less than 6 months) whereas the presence of ventricular arrhythmias was a better predictor of late mortality (after 6 months).

In the MILIS study, frequent VPDs (greater than or equal to 10 per hour) and an ejection fraction less than 0.40 were independent risk factors of sudden death.[97] Patients with both frequent VPDs and left ventricular dysfunction had eleven times the risk of sudden death during a mean followup of 18 months. Seventy-nine percent of all sudden deaths occurred within 7 months of the index myocardial infarction.

Twenty-four-hour ambulatory electrocardiography was performed on patients after myocardial infarction as part of the Beta Blocker Heart Attack Trial—a clinical trial primarily designed to test the effect of long-term adminstration of propranolol after myocardial infarction.[131] The effect of ventricular ectopy on total mortality and sudden death was assessed in the 1640 patients randomized to placebo therapy. During an average followup of 25 months, 163 patients (10 percent) in the placebo group died; 76 died suddenly. Eighty-four percent of patients had at least 1 VPD/24 hours; approximately 13 percent had an average of greater than or equal to 10 VPDs/hour; approximately 33 percent had multiform VPDs; and approximately 20 percent had repetitive VPDs. Using multivariate logistic regression analysis, ventricular ectopic activity was a significant predictor of total mortality, independent of other variables. Patients were also stratified into four clinical subgroups based on the presence or absence of three clinical criteria (ST depression, cardiomegaly, and prior infarction). Mortality rates ranged from 4.7 percent (no criteria present) to 35.5 percent (three criteria present). Ventricular ectopic activity, defined as greater than or equal to 10 VPDs/hour, ventricular tachycardia, or multiform complexes, was independently predictive of mortality in all four subgroups.

Complex ventricular premature beats (bigeminal, multiform, repetitive or R-on-T) were associated with an increased likelihood of both sudden and nonsudden death in a study of 960 patients who survived an acute myocardial infarction.[130] Cardiac death and sudden cardiac death rates for patients with simple (noncomplex) VPDs were intermediate between those with complex VPDs and those patients with no VPDs detected on 6-hour predischarge Holter monitoring. Patients with complex VPDs were significantly more likely to have nonsudden cardiac death than patients with either simple VPDs or no VPDs.

Electrophysiologic Study

Electrophysiologic testing using programmed ventricular stimulation has become an increasingly important tool in the evaluation and treatment of patients with sustained ventricular tachycardia or sudden cardiac death. Recently, programmed ventricular stimulation has been applied to patients in the early postinfarction period in an attempt to predict future arrhythmic events and cardiac mortality.[132–138]

The prevalence of inducible sustained ventricular tachycardia or ventricular fibrillation after myocardial infarction will vary depending on the population of patients selected for study, the timing of the study,[139] the nature of programmed stimulation,[133] and the endpoints of the study. Hamer and associates studied 70 patients from 7 to 20 days after acute myocardial infarction complicated by heart failure or arrhythmias.[137] Up to double ventricular extrastimuli were introduced during sinus rhythm, atrial pacing, and ventricular pacing using two drive cycle lengths. Up to two right ventricular sites were used (apex and outflow tract), and occasionally higher stimulation currents were used in an attempt to induce ventricular tachycardia. Thirty-seven patients underwent the complete protocol; of these, eight had sustained ventricular tachycardia (22 percent) and four had nonsustained ventricular tachycardia (11 percent). Five of the 12 patients with ventricular tachycardia (42 percent) died during a 12-month followup period; four deaths were sudden. In contrast, only 1 of 25 patients without inducible ventricular tachycardia died suddenly ($p < 0.05$).

Richards and colleagues studied 165 hemodynamically stable patients 6 to 28 days after acute myocardial infarction.[138] Ventricular pacing at a rate of 100 beats per minute with up to double extrastimuli was performed at twice diastolic threshold and at 20 milliamperes at the right ventricular apex and outflow tract. At least 10 seconds of ventricular tachycardia or ventricular fibrillation was induced in 38 (23 percent) patients. During a mean followup of 8 months, 26 percent of patients with inducible VT/VF died, compared with 5.5 percent without ($p < 0.001$). The sensitivity and specificity of programmed stimulation as a predictor of instantaneous death or spontaneous ventricular tachycardia were 86 percent and 83 percent, respectively. The predictive accuracy of "noninducibility" as an indicator of the absence of instantaneous death or spontaneous VT was 98 percent, whereas the predictive accuracy of inducibility was only 32 percent.

The prevalence and relative prognostic importance of ventricular tachycardia or ventricular fibrillation induced during programmed stimulation was studied in 403 survivors of transmural myocardial infarction who were 65 years old or younger.[132] Using a protocol similar to Richards and associates, 14 percent of patients had inducible ventricular fibrillation, 20 percent had inducible ventricular tachycardia, and 66 percent had no inducible arrhythmias. At 2 years, the probability of remaining free of cardiac death or nonfatal ventricular tachycardia of fibrillation was 0.92 for those with no inducible arrhythmias, 0.93 for those with inducible VF, and 0.73 for those with inducible VT.

Breithardt and coworkers performed programmed ventricular stimulation on 132 patients not older than 70 years of age who had survived a recent myocardial infarction.[135] Programmed ventricular stimulation was performed using drive cycle rates of 120, 140, 160, and 180 beats per minute with up to double extrastimuli delivered at twice diastolic threshold. Stimulation was stopped if four or more ventricular beats or ventricular fibrillation was induced. It was found that 53.8 percent of patients had fewer than 4 ventricular beats induced, 20.5 percent had 4 to 9 consecutive beats, 4.5 percent had 10 to 18 beats, and 21.2 percent had sustained ventricular tachycardia or ventricular fibrillation induced. Sudden cardiac death and total mortality were not predicted by results of programmed stimulation, but overall mortality was small. In contrast, the development of spontaneous sustained ventricular tachycardia was strongly related to results of programmed stimulation. None of 71 patients with fewer than four ventricular beats induced developed spontaneous VT whereas 9 of 61 (15 percent) patients with greater than or equal to four induced ventricular beats developed sustained ventricular tachycardia. If sustained ventricular tachycardia was induced during programmed stimulation, 25 percent of patients developed a spontaneous episode of ventricular tachycardia.

Several studies have not found an association between results of programmed ventricular stimulation and mortality or the development of spontaneous ventricular arrhythmias.[134,136,140] Roy and associates performed programmed ventricular stimulation on 150 survivors of acute myocardial infarction using a protocol that included up to double extrastimuli at two right ventricular sites.[134] Patients were studied a mean of 12 days after acute myocardial infarction. Twenty-three percent of patients had six or more beats of ventricular tachyarrhythmias induced. There was no significant difference in the rates of death, sudden death, or the development of sustained ventricular tachycardia between patients with and those without inducible ventricular tachyarrhythmias. In this study, only two patients died suddenly, three died nonsuddenly, and another two developed sustained tachycardia. Such small numbers limit the significance of these results. Prognostic variables for sudden death and spontaneous ventricular tachycardia included a lower ejection fraction ($p < 0.01$), presence of a ventricular aneurysm ($p < 0.05$), and exercise-induced ventricular premature contractions ($p < 0.05$). Similar results were obtained by Marchlinski and colleagues in a study of 46 patients.[136] Results of programmed ventricular stimulation did not predict sudden cardiac death during a mean followup of 18 months. An ejection fraction less than 0.40 and the presence of a ventricular aneurysm provided the best prognostic information for sudden cardiac death.

More aggressive stimulation protocols have been used during electrophysiologic testing in an attempt to increase sensitivity for subsequent arrhythmic events and sudden death. Waspe and coworkers used up to triple extrastimuli in 50 survivors of acute myocardial infarction complicated by major new conduction disturbances, congestive heart failure, or sustained ventricular tachyarrhythmias.[133] Seventeen patients had inducible ventricular tachycardia (greater than seven beats), whereas 33 patients did not. Induction of ventricular tachycardia identified all seven patients with subsequent sudden death or those with spontaneous ventricular tachycardia (sensitivity 100 percent). Triple extrastimuli were required to induce prognostically important arrhythmias in five of the seven patients. The specificity of the protocol was 57 percent. Thus, more aggressive stimulation protocols may increase sensitivity of programmed ventricular stimulation at the expense of reduced specificity.

Approximately 15 percent to 25 percent of patients studied after acute myocardial infarction will have inducible ventricular tachyarrhythmias. The prevalence of inducible arrhythmias does not appear to vary substantially among patients with complicated or uncomplicated infarcts. Most studies to date have indicated patients with inducible ventricular arrhythmias are at increased risk for the development of spontaneous ventricular tachycardia and/or sudden cardiac death. Patients without inducible ventricular arrhythmias are at very low risk for sudden death or spontaneous sustained ventricular tachycardia.

Signal-Averaged Electrocardiography

Signal-averaged electrocardiography has been used to assess a patients risk for sustained ventricular tachyarrhythmias and sudden death after myocardial infarction. The technique of signal averaging allows small-amplitude high-frequency signals to be detected in the terminal portion of the QRS and the early portion of the ST segment of the electrocardiographic signals of many patients with sustained ventricular tachycardia.[141] These signals are believed to be the surface electrocardiographic manifestation of delayed depolarizations occurring in areas of myocardium responsible for reentrant ventricular arrhythmias.[142] An abnormal signal-averaged electrocardiogram had a sensitivity of 92 percent and a specificity of 62 percent in identifying patients at risk for sudden death or ventricular tachyarrhythmias with a median followup of 11 months.[143] The signal-averaged electrocardiogram was also shown to contribute prognostic information independent of 24-hour Holter monitoring and radionuclide-determined left ventricular ejection fraction. Results of signal-averaged electrocardiography are independent of infarct size or location.[144]

Denniss and associates performed programmed ventricular stimulation on 403 clinically well survivors of transmural myocardial infarction less than 66 years old.[132] Signal-averaged electrocardiography was performed in a subset of 306 patients without bundle branch block, of which 26 percent had detectable late potentials. At 2 years, the probability of remaining free from cardiac death, ventricular tachycardia, or ventricular fibrillation was 73 percent in patients with late potentials compared with 95 percent in patients without late potentials. In addition, the presence of late potentials correlated significantly with the ability to induce sustained ventricular tachycardia by programmed stimulation.

Several noninvasive indexes have been developed to allow more accurate prediction of patients at risk for ventricular tachycardias.[145–147] These are based mainly on signal-averaged electrocardiography, left ventricular ejection fraction, and 24-hour Holter monitoring. During a mean followup of 12 months, patients with an abnormal signal-averaged electrocardiogram a mean of 10 days after acute myocardial infarction had a significantly increased rate of sustained ventricular tachycardia or sudden death (29 percent versus 3.5 percent, $p = 0.003$).[146] Patients with an abnormal signal-averaged electrocardiogram and an ejection fraction of less than 0.40 had a 36 percent chance of sustained VT or sudden death. If patients with an abnormal signal-averaged electrocardiogram and ejection fraction also had high-grade ectopy on Holter monitoring, their rate of sudden death or sustained ventricular tachycardia rose to 50 percent. Patients with normal findings on all three tests had no recurrent arrhythmic events. Thus, the signal-averaged electrocardiogram appears to be a promising method for risk stratification of patients after myocardial infarction with regard to ventricular tachyarrhythmias and sudden death.

ISCHEMIA

Ischemic ST segment changes detected on continuous electrocardiographic monitoring (Holter) are significant predictors of survival after acute myocardial infarction.[148] Gottlieb and associates detected ischemic ST segment depression greater than 0.1 millivolt in 30 of 103 patients during 24-hour electrocardiographic monitoring a mean of 8.6 days after acute myocardial infarction.[148] Among the group with ST segment depressions, ischemia occurred a median of five times per day with a median total duration of 157 minutes per day. Only 30 percent of patients with ECG-documented ischemia developed clinical angina; 93 percent of patients had no angina while having ECG-documented myocardial ischemia ("silent ischemia"). Patients with ischemia were slightly older (64 versus 57 years, $p < 0.01$) and had a higher percentage of non-Q-wave infarction (50 percent versus 38 percent, $p < 0.05$). Mortality among patients with documented ST segment depressions was 30 percent at 1 year compared with 11 percent among patients without ($p = 0.001$). The prognostic value of ischemic ST segment depression also extended to patients who were unable to undergo exercise treadmill testing.

The use of *graded exercise testing* to assess prognosis and functional capacity after acute myocardial infarction was first formally described in 1964 by Torkelson.[149] Several authors have reported using cycle ergometer testing between 6 weeks and 3 months after infarction utilizing symptom-limited or heart rate-limited protocols.[150,151] These tests were mainly used to assess cardiovascular response to exercise for cardiac rehabilitation programs, although one early study showed an important correlation between exercise findings and 6-year mortality.[150] Since 1977, several studies have been published indicating that symptom-limited or heart rate-limited exercise testing performed 3 weeks or less after myocardial infarction was a safe way to assess a patient's response to physical exercise as well as a source of prognostic information.[152] The presence of angina pectoris, ventricular arrhythmias or, sinus tachycardia at low work levels as correlated with increased mortality during a 2- to 5-year followup.

DeBusk and associates investigated the safety and prognostic information of various modes of exercise.[153] Forty patients underwent cycle ergometry, arm ergometry, forearm flexion, and hand-grip contraction approximately 7 weeks after myocardial infarction. Ischemic ST segment changes and ventricular ectopy were infrequent with forearm flexion and arm ergometry as compared with cycle ergometry. Leg ergometry resulted in higher systolic blood pressure, heart rate response, and workloads than arm exercise. The authors concluded that dynamic leg work was superior to arm exercise for assessing the physical capacity of patients.

The prognostic usefulness of low-level versus symptom-limited exercise testing has been investigated by several authors.[154–156] DeBusk and Haskell studied 200 patients surviving acute myocardial infarction: 107 patients completed a symptom-limited exercise test, and 93 patients underwent a low-level (maximum heart rate of 130 beats per minute) exercise test.[156] There were no significant differences in the prevalence of ST segment depression or ventricular ectopy. Patients exercising to a symptom-limited endpoint achieved higher workloads and heart rates compared with those patients in the low-level group. In another study, Davidson and DeBusk studied 195 patients following myocardial infarction: 113 patients completed a symptom-limited test, whereas 82 underwent low-level exercise testing.[155] Symptom-limited exercise testing was found to provide superior prognostic information. Symptom-limited exercise testing was also found to be superior in elucidating unsuspected myocardial ischemia in a study performed by Starling and coworkers.[154] Thus, while both low-level and symptom-limited exercise tests will provide prognostic information, symptom-limited testing (3 weeks postinfarction) may provide additional information beyond that provided by low-level testing.

Contraindications to exercise testing early after myocardial infarction have been summarized by Goldschlager.[157] Contraindications include chest pain 2 to 5 days prior to the test, systolic hypertension greater than 150 to 180 mmHg, a ventricular gallop or pulmonary rales suggestive of congestive heart failure, poorly controlled atrial or ventricular arrhythmias, sinus tachycardia, unstable resting ECG, and advanced age. Approximately 40 percent to 75 percent of myocardial infarction survivors would be candidates for early exercise testing using these criteria. Endpoints for testing in many laboratories include the development of angina pectoris, dyspnea, lightheadedness, three or more consecutive ventricular premature beats, systolic hypertension >200 mmHg, ST segment depression greater than 2 mm, and achieving a heart rate of approximately 130 beats per minute.

Several large studies have helped to define the prognostic importance of various exercise test variables.[158–161] Weld and colleagues studied 250 patients after acute myocardial infarction.[158] Low-level treadmill exercise testing was performed prior to hospital discharge in 236 patients. Angina pectoris, similar to the patients' pain of their index acute myocardial infarction, occurred in 21 percent of patients. Twenty-two percent of patients had 0.1 mV or more of horizontal to downsloping ST segment depression in lead V5 during or after exercise, and the ST changes were significantly more common in those patients with exercise-induced angina. Forty-three percent of patients had at least 1 VPD per hour during exercise or at 10 minutes after exercise; 24 percent had 10 or more VPDs per hour. Logistic regression analysis revealed that exercise duration and VPD frequency were, in order of decreasing strength of association, significantly predictive of total cardiac mortality at 1 year. Exercise-induced ST segment depression did not correlate with 1-year cardiac mortality. A patient who completed the 9-minute exercise test with no VPDs and no ST depression had a 1 percent cardiac mortality at 1 year compared with more than 36 percent for a patient who exercised 1 minute, had an average VPD frequency of 100 per hour, and had 0.2-mV ST depression.

Krone and coworkers reported the results of low-level treadmill exercise testing on 667 of the 866 patients less than 70 years old who were enrolled in the multicenter postinfarction study of prognosis after myocardial infarction.[160] The 1-year cardiac mortality in the 192 patients who did not take the exercise test (150 for medical and 42 for logistic reasons) was 14 percent versus 5 percent in those who did ($p < 0.0001$). Exercise parameters associated with decreased 1-year mortality included the achievement of a systolic blood pressure of at least 110 mmHg (3 percent versus 18 percent, $p < 0.001$), the ability to complete the 9-minute test (3 percent versus 8 percent, $p < 0.01$), and the absence of couplets (4 percent versus 13 percent, $p < 0.05$) or any VPDs (4 percent versus 7 percent, $p < 0.05$). ST segment depression greater than 0.1 mV was associated with increased bypass surgery (19 percent versus 9 percent, $p < 0.001$) but not cardiac mortality or recurrent myocardial infarction. The development of angina was similarly associated with subsequent bypass surgery (20 percent versus 9 percent, $p < 0.01$). Recurrent myocardial infarction within the first year was correlated with supraventricular ectopic depolarizations during or after exercise testing (15 percent versus 7 percent, $p < 0.01$), a finding independent of the use of beta-blocking drugs or digitalis. Patients with no chest X-ray evidence of congestion who achieved a systolic blood pressure of at least 110 mmHg identified a group of patients (70 percent of those who took the test) with a 1-year cardiac mortality of 1 percent compared with 13 percent in the remaining patients ($p < 0.0001$). Thus, in this study, low-level exercise testing was shown to provide prognostic information for cardiac mortality, reinfarction, and bypass surgery independent of clinical parameters.

A maximal, symptom-limited treadmill exercise test was performed 6 months after index acute myocardial infarction in 473 patients enrolled in the Multicenter Investigation of the Limitation of Infarct Size (MILIS) and was related to the development of death, nonfatal recurrent myocardial infarction, and bypass surgery.[161] Mortality was increased significantly with any of the following exercise variables: inability to perform the test due to cardiac limitations, ST segment elevation of 1 mm or more during exercise, an inadequate blood pressure response to exercise, the development of any VPDs during or after exercise, and inability to exercise beyond stage 1 of the modified Bruce protocol. Mortality in the 12 months after exercise testing ranged from 1 percent if none of these features were present to 17 percent if at least three were present. Recurrent myocardial infarction was predicted by an inability to perform the exercise test but not by any other exercise test variables. The development of at least 1 mm of ST segment depression with exercise was associated with subsequent bypass surgery. Clinically determined parameters, such as the presence of angina or congestive heart failure, were not predictive of mortality in the group of patients who underwent treadmill testing (N = 473). In contrast, in the group of 246 patients who did not undergo exercise testing because of lack of consent, or cardiac or noncardiac reasons, clinical parameters were predictive of subsequent mortality. The authors conlcuded that, among the low-risk group of patients without severely limiting cardiac disease 6 months after acute myocardial infarction (i.e., those able to perform a symptom-limited treadmill test), maximal exercise testing is a valuable tool that provides information independent of and additive to a clinical evaluation performed at the same time.

Other studies have confirmed that *inability to perform a predischarge exercise test* because of cardiac limitations is associated with a poor prognosis.[161–166] Similarly, functional capacity measured as workload achieved, ability to complete a low-level test, or exercise time has consistently been linked to prognosis.[161,167–170] These results are expected inasmuch as functional capacity should closely parallel the overall extent of left ventricular function.

Many, but not all, studies have concluded that *ST segment depression* occurring during exercise testing after myocardial infarction is predictive of future cardiac events.[150,155,160–163,167,171–176] Thirty percent of 62 postinfarction patients who exercised according to a low-level protocol a mean of 18 days after acute myocardial infarction and developed ST segment depression died or had reinfarction compared with 5 percent for patients without ST segment depression.[174] Similarly, Theroux and associates studied 210 patients by low-level exercise testing a mean of 11 days after acute myocardial infarction.[175] The 1-year mortality rate in patients with ST segment depression was 27 percent compared with 2.1 percent without. In addition, 85 percent of all deaths and 91 percent of all sudden deaths occurred in the group with ST segment depression. Using a symptom-limited exercise protocol, Sami and coworkers studied 200 men without clinical evidence of heart failure or unstable angina pectoris 3 weeks after acute myocardial infarction.[173] During a 2-year followup, all patients who had a cardiac arrest and 64 percent of patients undergoing bypass surgery had at least 0.2-mV ST segment depression with exercise ($p < 0.05$). DeBusk and colleagues studied 702 consecutive men less than 71 years old who were alive 21 days after acute myocardial infarction.[163] ST segment depression of at least 0.2 mV or a peak heart rate less than or equal to 135 beats per minute was able to predict subsequent cardiac events in a population predicted by clinical parameters to do well.

In contrast, several studies have conluded that ST segment depression during exercise after an acute myocardial infarction is not associated with subsequent cardiac mortality.[158,160,161,168,169,177] Although not associated with increased postinfarction mortality, exercise-induced ischemic ST segment depression was usually associated with angina pectoris,[158] subsequent bypass surgery,[160,161] or reinfarction.[164]

In contrast to ST segment depression, *exercise-induced ST segment elevation* is uniformly associated with an increased risk of cardiac events after acute myocardial infarction.[161,167,178] ST segment elevation on a low-level exercise test was significantly associated with recurrent cardiac events during a 1-year followup after acute myocardial infarction.[167] In addition, the presence of exercise-induced ST segment elevation was correlated with low ejection fraction as measured by radionuclide ventriculography. Patients enrolled in the MILIS study who had exercise-induced ST segment elevation had a fourfold increase in mortality at 1 year after acute myocardial infarction compared with those without ST segment elevation ($p < 0.01$).[161] However, the presence of ST segment elevation during exercise testing did not predict recurrent nonfatal myocardial infarction in the MILIS study.

Multiple studies have demonstrated an association between *exercise-induced angina pectoris* and mortality or morbidity after acute myocardial infarction.[152,155,160,162,169,171,172,175,176,179] The presence of angina during exercise testing shortly after acute myocardial infarction was associated with increased development of both stable angina[169,175] and unstable angina.[176] In addition, Jelinek and associates demonstrated that patients with exercise-induced angina had approximately a threefold increase of recurrent myocardial infarction during a followup of 27 months.[171] However, exercise-induced angina was not associated with prognosis in other studies.[158,161]

The relationship of the *blood pressure response to exercise* after acute myocardial infarction was evaluated by Fioretti and colleagues.[165] Three hundred patients performed bicycle ergometry a mean of 13 days after myocardial infarction. The exercise variable most strongly associated with mortality was the extent of blood pressure increase with exercise: 42 ± 24 mmHg in survivors compared with 21 ± 14 mmHg in nonsurvivors ($p < 0.001$). Mortality was 3 percent in those patients with an increase of 30 mmHg or more versus 16 percent in those whose blood pressure increased less than 30 mmHg. In those patients who also underwent coronary angiography, patients with three-vessel coronary artery disease had a smaller blood pressure increase with exercise compared with those patients with less extensive coronary disease (26 ± 22 mmHg versus 42 ± 23 mmHg, $p < 0.001$). The magnitude of blood pressure response to exercise was found to be unrelated to resting ejection fraction. Patients who continued to receive beta-blocking drugs during exercise testing had a significantly smaller blood pressure increase, and the predictive accuracy for mortality in these patients was reduced. Thus, these results should be applied with caution to patients receiving beta-blocking drugs during exercise testing. Other investigators have likewise shown a poorer prognosis of patients with an abnormal systolic blood pressure response to exercise.[167,176]

The contribution of *exercise-induced ventricular premature depolarizations* (VPDs) after acute myocardial infarction to prognosis is uncertain. Studies have shown that VPDs have both prognostic[152,158,160,161,164,173,175] and no prognostic significance.[164,165,174] for cardiac morbidity or mortality. Exercise-induced ventricular ectopy was mainly found to be predictive of 1-year cardiac mortality;[158,160,161,170] however, in one study VPBs predicted recurrent myocardial infarction.[173]

Radionuclide cardiac imaging using thallium-201 has been used in conjunction with exercise testing after acute myocardial infarction to enhance detection of myocardial ischemia. In addition, thallium scanning has been found useful in patients known to have frequent false-positive exercise ECG results (e.g., patients receiving digitalis, or those with left bundle branch block or left ventricular hypertrophy). Several studies have reported prognostic findings of thallium-201 scanning as well.[180–182] The detection of multiple thallium defects identified 94 percent of patients at high risk for recurrent cardiac events within 1 year compared with 56 percent for abnormal exercise test results.[181] Gibson and associates compared thallium scanning with submaximal exercise testing and coronary angiography in 140 patients.[182] Each modality predicted mortality equally well; however, thallium scintigraphy was superior in its ability to distinguish those patients likely to develop class III or IV angina or reinfarction. The detection of thallium defects in more than one discrete vascular region, redistribution, or increased lung uptake were significant predictors of future cardiac events.

Exercise thallium-201 scintigraphy has been shown to predict left main or three-vessel coronary artery disease in several studies.[181,183–186] In a group of 40 patients referred for cardiac catheterization after acute myocardial infarction, exercise thallium-201 scintigraphy was performed by Patterson and associates.[184] Thallium defects outside the region of the infarct, a decrease in blood pressure with exercise, failure to achieve 85 percent of predicted maximal heart rate, or ST depression at less than 70 percent of predicted maximal heart rate were predictors of left main or triple-vessel coronary artery disease. Of these criteria, the presence of a thallium defect outside the infarct region was the most reliable to distinguish high-risk from low-risk coronary artery disease ($p = 0.00052$).

Exercise thallium scintigraphy was performed in 65 patients after acute myocardial infarction in a study by Dunn and associates.[185] Multivessel coronary artery disease was predicted by exercise-induced angina, perfusion defects on the thallium scan in more than one specific vascular area, or a positive exercise ECG test with angina, but not a positive exercise ECG test alone. Of the 37 patients with thallium defects in more than one vascular area, multivessel coronary artery disease was present in 92 percent compared with 72 percent of the 39 patients with a positive exercise ECG test ($p < 0.05$).

Dipyridamole-thallium-201 scintigraphy was compared with submaximal exercise testing prior to hospital discharge after acute myocardial infarction by Leppo and coworkers.[187] Eleven of 12 patients who died or had reinfarction during a mean followup of 19 months had shown redistribution or predischarge scintigraphy. Likewise, 22 of 24 patients requiring readmission for angina had redistribution on scanning. The presence of redistribution on dipyridamole-thallium scanning was the only predictor of the events. In the 26 patients receiving both low-level exercise testing and dipyridamole scintigraphy before discharge, 13 subsequently had reinfarction or cardiac death. Of these 13, exercise testing was positive in only 6 patients whereas dipyridamole-thallium scanning showed a redistribution pattern in 12 ($p < 0.001$).

SUMMARY

Patients surviving acute myocardial infarction form a large, heterogeneous group at risk for few or many varied complications with widely varied prognoses. By examining fundamental aspects of cardiac function such as left ventricular function, electrical instability, and residual ischemia as well as comorbid factors such as diabetes, a patient's risk for subsequent morbidity and mortality may be predicted. It is hoped that by identifying patients at increased risk, one may be able to alter the natural history of their disease.

REFERENCES

1. Gomez-Marin, O, Folsom, AR, Kottke, TE, et al: Improvement in long-term survival among patients hospitalized with acute myocardial infarction, 1970 to 1980. N Engl J Med 316:1353, 1987.
2. Kannel, WB, Sorlie, P, and McNamara, PM: Prognosis after myocardial infarction: The Framingham Study. Am J Cardiol 44:53, 1979.
3. Puletti, M, Sunseri, L, Curione, M, et al: Acute myocardial infarction: Sex-related differences in prognosis. Am Heart J 108:63, 1984.
4. Tofler, GH, Stone, PH, Muller, JE, et al: Effects of gender and race on prognosis after myocardial infarction: Adverse prognosis for women, particularly black women. J Am Coll Cardiol 9:473, 1987.
5. Smith, JW, Marcus, FI, and Serokman, R: Prognosis of patients with diabetes mellitus after acute myocardial infarction. Am J Cardiol 54:718, 1984.
6. Ulvenstam, G, Aberg, A, Bergstrand, R, et al: Long-term prognosis after myocardial infarction in men with diabetes. Diabetes 34:787, 1985.
7. Martin, AC, Thompson, PL, Armstrong, BK, et al: Long-term prognosis after recovery from myocardial infarction: A nine year follow-up of the Perth Coronary Register. Circulation 68:961, 1983.
8. Norris, RM, Caughey, E, Mercer, CJ, et al: Prognosis after myocardial infarction six-year follow-up. Br Heart J 36:786, 1974.
9. Henning, R and Wedel, H: The long-term prognosis after myocardial infarction: A five year follow-up study. Eur Heart J 2:65, 1981.
10. Berman, ND: The elderly patient in the coronary care unit: Factors affecting long-term prognosis. J Am Geriatr Soc 31:400, 1983.
11. Rapaport, E and Remedios, P: The high risk patient after recovery from myocardial infarction: Recognition and management. J Am Coll Cardiol 1:391, 1983.
12. Latting, CA and Silverman, ME: Acute myocardial infarction in hospitalized patients over age 70. Am Heart J 100:311, 1980.
13. Olmsted, WL, Groden, DL, and Silverman, ME: Prognosis in survivors of acute myocardial infarction occurring at age 75 years or older. Am J Cardiol 60:971, 1987.
14. The Coronary Drug Project Research Group: Blood pressure in survivors of myocardial infarction. J Am Coll Cardiol 4:1135, 1984.
15. Kannel, WB, Sorlie, P, Castelli, WP, et al: Blood pressure and survival after myocardial infarction: The Framingham study. Am J Cardiol 45:326, 1980.
16. Lowe, GDO, Machado, SG, Krol, WF, et al: White blood cell count and haematocrit as predictors of coronary recurrence after myocardial infarction. Thromb Haemost 54:700, 1985.
17. Gram, J and Jespersen, J: A selective depression of tissue plasminogen activator (t-PA) activity in Euglobulins characterizes a risk group among survivors of acute myocardial infarction. Thromb Haemost 57:137, 1987.
18. Hamsten, A, Bjorkholm, M, Norberg, R, et al: Antibodies to cardiolipin in young survivors of myocardial infarction: An association with recurrent cardiovascular events. Lancet 1(8473):113, 1986.
19. Brush, JE, Brand, DA, Acampora, D, et al: Use of the initial electrocardiogram to predict in-hospital complications of acute myocardial infarction. N Engl J Med 312:1137, 1985.
20. Masters, AM, Dack, S, and Jaffe, HL: Bundle branch and intraventricular block in acute coronary occlusion. Am Heart J 16:285, 1938.

21. Klein, RC, Vera, Z, and Mason, DT: Intraventricular conduction defects in acute myocardial infarction: Incidence, prognosis, and therapy. Am Heart J 108:1007, 1984.
22. Norris, RM and Croxson, MS: Bundle branch block in acute myocardial infarction. Am Heart J 79:728, 1970.
23. Col, JJ and Weinberg, SL: Incidence and mortality of intraventricular conduction defects in acute myocardial infarction. Am J Cardiol 29:344, 1972.
24. Atkins, JM, Leshin, SJ, Blomqvist, CG, et al: Ventricular conduction blocks and sudden death in acute myocardial infarction: Potential indications for pacing. N Engl J Med 288:281, 1973.
25. Waugh, RA, Wagner, GS, Hanley, TL, et al: Immediate and remote prognostic significance of fascicular block during acute myocardial infarction. Circulation 47:765, 1973.
26. Nimetz, AA, Shubrooks, SJ, Hutter, AM, et al: The significance of bundle branch block during acute myocardial infarction. Am Heart J 90:439, 1975.
27. Dubois, C, Pierard, LA, Smeets, JP, et al: Short- and long-term prognostic importance of complete bundle-branch block complicating acute myocardial infarction. Clin Cardiol 11:292, 1988.
28. Mullins, CB and Atkins, JM: Prognosis and management of ventricular conduction blocks in acute myocardial infarction. Mod Concepts Cardiovasc Dis 45:129, 1976.
29. Scheinman, M and Brenman, B: Clinical and anatomic implications of intraventricular conduction blocks in acute myocardial infarction. Circulation 46:753, 1972.
30. Scanlon, PJ, Pryor, R, and Blout, SG Jr: Right bundle-branch block associated with left superior or inferior intraventricular block: Associated with acute myocardial infarction. Circulation 42:1135, 1970.
31. Hindman, MC, Wagner, GS, Jaro, M, et al: The clinical significance of bundle branch block complicating acute myocardial infarction. Circulation 58:679, 1978.
32. Godman, MJ, Lassers, BW, and Julian DG: Complete bundle-branch block complicating acute myocardial infarction. N Engl J Med 282:237, 1970.
33. Nordrehaug, JE, Johannessen, K, and Von der Lippe, G: Serum potassium concentration as a risk factor of ventricular arrhythmias early in acute myocardial infarction. Circulation 71:645, 1985.
34. Geltman, EM, Ehsani, AA, Campbell, MK, et al: The influence of location and extent of myocardial infarction on long-term ventricular dysrhythmia and mortality. Circulation 60:805, 1979.
35. Coromilas, J, Bigger, JT Jr, Gang, ES, et al: Relationship between infarct size and ventricular arrhythmias. In Zipes, DP and Jalife, J (eds): Cardiac Electrophysiology and Arrhythmias. Grune & Stratton, Orlando, 1985, pp 523–530.
36. Bigger, JT, Fleiss, JL, Kleiger, R, et al: The relationships among ventricular arrhythmias, left ventricular dysfunction, and mortality in the 2 years after myocardial infarction. Circulation 69:250, 1984.
37. Tofler, GH, Stone, PH, Muller, JE, et al: Prognosis after cardiac arrest due to ventricular tachycardia or ventricular fibrillation associated with acute myocardial infarction (The MILIS study). Am J Cardiol 60:755, 1987.
38. Schwartz, PJ, Zaza, A, Grazi, S, et al: Effect of ventricular fibrillation complicating acute myocardial infarction on long-term prognosis: Importance of the site of infarction. Am J Cardiol 56:384, 1985.
39. Volpi, A, Maggioni, A, Franzosi, MG, et al: In-hospital prognosis of patients with acute myocardial infarction complicated by primary ventricular fibrillation. N Engl J Med 317:257, 1987.
40. Goldberg, RJ, Gore, JM, Haffajee, CI, et al: Outcome after cardiac arrest during acute myocardial infarction. Am J Cardiol 59:251, 1987.
41. Rotman, M, Wagner, GS, and Wallace, AG: Bradyarrhythmias in acute myocardial infarction. Circulation 44:703, 1972.
42. Meltzer, LE and Kitchell, JB: The incidence of arrhythmias associated with acute myocardial infarction. Prog Cardiovasc Dis 9:50, 1966.
43. Zipes, DP: The clinical significance of bradycardic rhythms in acute myocardial infarction. Am J Cardiol 24:814, 1969.
44. The Multicenter Postinfarction Research Group: Risk stratification and survival after myocardial infarction. N Engl J Med 309:331, 1983.
45. DeSanctis, RW, Block, P, and Hutter, AM: Tachyarrhythmias in myocardial infarction. Circulation 45:681, 1972.
46. James, TN: Myocardial infarction and atrial arrhythmias. Circulation 24:761, 1961.
47. Knoecke, LL and Knoebel, SB: Nonparoxysmal junctional tachycardia complicating acute myocardial infarction. Circulation 45:367, 1972.

48. Miller, RR, Olson, HG, Vismara, LA, et al: Pump dysfunction after myocardial infarction: Importance of location, extent and pattern of abnormal left ventricular segmental contraction. Am J Cardiol 37:340, 1976.
49. Feiring, AJ, Johnson, MR, Kioschos, JM, et al: The importance of the determination of the myocardial area at risk in the evaluation of the outcome of acute myocardial infarction. Circulation 75:980, 1987.
50. Shell, WE, Kjekshus, JK, and Sobel, BE: Quantitative assessment of the extent of myocardial infarction in the conscious dog by means of analysis of serial changes in serum creatine phosphokinase activity. J Clin Invest 50:2614, 1971.
51. Roberts, R, Henry, PD, and Sobel, BE: An improved basis for enzymatic estimation of infarct size. Circulation 52:743, 1975.
52. Roberts, R, Sobel, BE, and Parker, CW: Radioimmunoassay for creatine kinase isoenzymes. Science 194:855, 1976.
53. Grande, P, Hansen, BF, Christiansen, C, et al: Estimation of acute myocardial infarct size in man by serum CK-MB measurements. Circulation 65:756, 1982.
54. Rogers, WJ, McDaniel, HG, Smith, LR, et al: Correlation of angiographic estimates of myocardial infarct size and accumulated release of creatine kinase MB isoenzyme in man. Circulation 56:199, 1977.
55. Sobel, BE, Bresnahan, GF, Shell, WE, et al: Estimation of infarct size in man and its relation to prognosis. Circulation 46:640, 1972.
56. Thompson, PL, Fletcher, EE, and Katavatis, V: Enzymatic indices of myocardial necrosis: Influence on short- and long-term prognosis after myocardial infarction. Circulation 59:113, 1979.
57. Yusuf, S, Lopez, R, Maddison, A, et al: Value of electrocardiogram in predicting and estimating infarct size in man. Br Heart J 42:286, 1979.
58. Heger, JJ, Weyman, AE, Wann, LS, et al: Cross sectional echocardiographic analysis of the extent of left ventricular asynergy in acute myocardial infarction. Circulation 61:1113, 1980.
59. Holman, BL, Chisholm, RJ, and Braunwald, E: The prognostic implications of acute myocardial infarct scintigraphy with 99M Tc-pyrophosphate. Circulation 57:320, 1978.
60. Hands, ME, Lloyd, BL, Robinson, JS, et al: Prognostic significance of electrocardiographic site of infarction after correction for enzymatic size of infarction. Circulation 73:885, 1986.
61. Stadius, ML, Davis, K, Maynard, C, et al: Risk stratification for 1 year survival based on characteristics identified in the early hours of acute myocardial infarction. Circulation 74:703, 1986.
62. Lembo, NJ, Starling MR, Dell'Italia, LJ, et al: Clinical and prognostic importance of persistent precordial (V1–V4) electrocardiographic ST segment depression in patients with inferior transmural myocardial infarction. Circulation 74:56, 1986.
63. Goldberg, RJ, Gore, JM, Alpert, JS, et al: Non-Q-wave myocardial infarction: Recent changes in occurrence and prognosis—A community wide perspective. Am Heart J 113:273, 1987.
64. Thanavaro, S, Krone, RJ, Kleiger, RE, et al: In-hospital prognosis of patients with first nontransmural and transmural infarctions. Circulation 61:29, 1980.
65. Rigo, P, Murry, M, Taylor, DR, et al: Hemodynamic and prognostic findings in patients with transmural and nontransmural infarction. Circulation 51:1064, 1975.
66. Madias, JE, Chanine, RA, Gorlin, R, et al: A comparison of transmural and nontransmural acute myocardial infarction. Circulation 44:498, 1974.
67. Krone, RJ, Friedman, E, Thanavaro, S, et al: Long-term prognosis after first Q-wave (transmural) or non-Q-wave (nontransmural) myocardial infarction: Analysis of 593 patients. Am J Cardiol 52:234, 1983.
68. Hollander, G, Ozick, H, Greengart, A, et al: High mortality early reinfarction with first nontransmural myocardial infarction. Am Heart J 108:1412, 1984.
69. Maisel, AS, Ahnve, S, Gilpin, E, et al: Prognosis after extension of myocardial infarct: The role of Q wave or non-Q wave infarction. Circulation 71:211, 1985.
70. Madigan, NP, Rutherford, BD, and Frye, RL: The clinical course, early prognosis and coronary anatomy of subendocardial infarction. Am J Med 60:634, 1976.
71. Fraker, TD, Wagner, GS, and Rosati, RA: Extension of myocardial infarction: Incidence and prognosis. Circulation 60:1126, 1979.
72. Marmor, A, Sobel, BE, and Roberts, R: Factors presaging early recurrent myocardial infarction ("extension"). Am J Cardiol 48:603, 1981.
73. Muller, JE, Rude, RE, Braunwald, E, et al: Myocardial infarct extension: Occurrence, outcome, and risk factors in the multicenter investigation of limitation of infarct size. Ann Intern Med 108:1, 1988.

74. Vatner, SF, Baig, H, Manders, WT, et al: Effects of coronary artery reperfusion on myocardial infarct size calculated from creatine kinase. J Clin Invest 61:1048, 1978.
75. Ganz, W, Buchbinder, N, Marcus, H, et al: Intracoronary thrombolysis in evolving myocardial infarction. Am Heart J 101:4, 1981.
76. Ong, L, Reiser, P, Coromilas, J, et al: Left ventricular function and rapid release of creatine kinase MB in acute myocardial infarction. N Engl J Med 309:1, 1983.
77. Cox, DA, Stone, PH, Muller, JE, et al: Prognostic implications of an early peak in plasma MB creatine kinase in patients with acute myocardial infarction. J Am Coll Cardiol 10:979, 1987.
78. Nidorf, SM, Thompson, PL, DeKlerk, NH, et al: Prognostic significance of an early rise to peak creatine kinase after acute myocardial infarction. Am J Cardiol 61:1178, 1988.
79. Nicod, P, Gilpin, E, Dittrich, H, et al: Influence on prognosis and morbidity of left ventricular ejection fraction with and without signs of left ventricular failure after acute myocardial infarction. Am J Cardiol 61:1165, 1988.
80. Battler, A, Karliner, JS, Higgins, CB, et al: The initial chest x-ray in acute myocardial infarction. Circulation 61:1004, 1980.
81. Gibson, RS, Bishop, HL, Stamm, RB, et al: Value of early two-dimensional echocardiography in patients with acute myocardial infarction. Am J Cardiol 49:1110, 1982.
82. Nishimura, RA, Tajik, AJ, Shub, C, et al: Role of two-dimensional echocardiography in the prediction of in-hospital complications after acute myocardial infarction. J Am Coll Cardiol 4:1080, 1984.
83. Stamm, RB, Gibson, RS, Bishop, HL, et al: Echocardiographic detection of infarct-localized asynergy and remote asynergy during acute myocardial infarction: Correlation with extent of angiographic coronary disease. Circulation 67:233, 1983.
84. Greenberg, H, McMaster, P, and Dwyer, EM: Left ventricular dysfunction after acute myocardial infarction: Results of a prospective multicenter study. J Am Coll Cardiol 4:867, 1984.
85. Warnowicz, MA, Parker, H, and Cheitlin, MD: Prognosis of patients with acute pulmonary edema and normal ejection fraction after acute myocardial infarction. Circulation 67:330, 1983.
86. Swan, HJC, Ganz, W, Forrester, JS, et al: Catheterization of the heart in man with the use of a flow-directed balloon-tipped catheter. N Engl J Med 283:447, 1970.
87. Forrester, JS, Diamond, G, Chatterjee, K, et al: Medical therapy of acute myocardial infarction by application of hemodynamic subsets. N Engl J Med 295:1356–1362, 1404–1413, 1976.
88. Forrester, JS, Diamond, GA, and Swan, HJC: Correlative classification of clinical and hemodynamic function after myocardial infarction. Am J Cardiol 39:137, 1977.
89. Weber, KT, Janicki, JJ, Russell, RO, et al: Identification of high risk subsets of acute myocardial infarction. Am J Cardiol 41:197, 1978.
90. Shell, W, Peter, T, Mickle, D, et al: Prognostic implications of reduction of left ventricular filling pressure in early transmural acute myocardial infarction. Am Heart J 102:335, 1981.
91. Cohn, JA, Franciosa, JA, Francis, GA, et al: Effects of short term infusion of sodium nitroprusside on mortality rate in acute myocardial infarction complicated by left ventricular failure. N Engl J Med 306:1129, 1982.
92. Bosch, X, Theroux, P, Waters, DD, et al: Early postinfarction ischemia: Clinical. Angiographic and prognostic significance. Circulation 75:988, 1987.
93. Schuster, EH and Bulkley BH: Early post-infarction angina: Ischemia at a distance and ischemia in the infarct zone. N Engl J Med 305:1101, 1981.
94. Schulze, RA Jr, Rouleau, J, Rigo, P, et al: Ventricular arrhythmias in the late hospital phase of acute myocardial infarction: Relation to left ventricular function detected by gated cardiac blood pool scanning. Circulation 52:1006, 1975.
95. Taylor, GJ, Humphries, JO, Mellits, ED, et al: Predictors of clinical course, coronary anatomy and left ventricular function after recovery from acute myocardial infarction. Circulation 62:960, 1980.
96. Bigger, JT, Weld, FM, and Rolnitzky, LM: Prevalence, characteristics and significance of ventricular tachycardia (three or more complexes) detected with ambulatory electrocardiographic recording in the late phase of acute myocardial infarction. Am J Cardiol 48:815, 1981.
97. Mukharji, J, Rude, RE, Poole, K, et al: Risk factors for sudden death after acute myocardial infarction: Two-year follow-up. Am J Cardiol 54:31, 1984.
98. Sanz, G, Castaner, A, Betriu, A, et al: Determinants of prognosis in survivors of myocardial infarction. N Engl J Med 306:1065, 1982.
99. Castaner, A, Betriu, A, Roig, E, et al: Clinical course and risk stratification of myocardial infarct survivors with three-vessel disease. Am Heart J 112:1201, 1986.

100. Tibbits, PA, Evaul, JE, Goldstein, RE, et al: Serial acquisition of data to predict one-year mortality rate after acute myocardial infarction. Am J Cardiol 60:451, 1987.
101. Dwyer, EM, McMaster, P, and Greenberg, H: Nonfatal cardiac events and recurrent infarction in the year after acute myocardial infarction. J Am Coll Cardiol 4:695, 1984.
102. White, HD, Norris, RM, Brown, MA, et al: Left ventricular end-systolic volume as the major determinant of survival after recovery from myocardial infarction. Circulation 76:44, 1987.
103. Nixon, JV, Narahara, A, and Smitherman, TC: Estimation of myocardial involvement in patients with acute myocardial infarction by two-dimensional echocardiography. Circulation 62:1248, 1980.
104. Bhatnager, SK, Moussa, MAA, and Al-Yusuf, AR: The role of prehospital discharge two-dimensional echocardiography in determining the prognosis of survivors of first myocardial infarction. Am Heart J 109:472, 1985.
105. Corbett, JR, Dehmer, GJ, Lewis, SI, et al: The prognostic value of submaximal exercise testing with radionuclide ventriculography before hospital discharge in patients with recent myocardial infarction. Circulation 64:535, 1981.
106. Hung, J, Goris, ML, Nasm, E, et al: Comparative value of maximal treadmill testing, exercise thallium perfusion scintigraphy and exercise radionuclide ventriculography for distinguishing high- and low-risk patients soon after acute myocardial infarction. Am J Cardiol 53:1221, 1984.
107. Wasserman, AG, Katz, RJ, Cleary, P, et al: Noninvasive detection of multivessel disease after myocardial infarction by exercise radionuclide ventriculography. Am J Cardiol 50:1242, 1982.
108. Borer, JS, Rosing, DR, Miller, RH, et al: Natural history of left ventricular function during 1 year after acute myocardial infarction: Comparison with clinical, electrocardiographic and biochemical determinations. Am J Cardiol 46:1, 1980.
109. Iskandrian, AS, Hakki, AH, Goel, IP, et al: The use of rest and exercise radionuclide ventriculography in risk stratification in patients with suspected coronary disease. Am Heart J 110:864, 1985.
110. Abraham, RD, Harris, PJ, Roubin, GS, et al: Usefulness of ejection fraction response to exercise one month after acute myocardial infarction in predicting coronary anatomy and prognosis. Am J Cardiol 60:225, 1987.
111. Applegate, RJ, Dell'italia, LJ, and Crawford, MH: Usefulness of two-dimensional echocardiography during low-level exercise testing early after uncomplicated myocardial infarction. Am J Cardiol 60:10, 1987.
112. Ryan, T, Armstrong, WF, O'Donnell, JA, et al: Risk stratification after acute myocardial infarction by means of exercise two-dimensional echocardiography. Am Heart J 114:1305, 1987.
113. Awan, NA, Miller, RR, Vera, Z, et al: Noninvasive assessment of cardiac function and ventricular dysfunction by precordial Q wave mapping in anterior myocardial infarction. Circulation 55:833, 1977.
114. Askenazi, J, Parisi, AF, Cohn, PF, et al: Value of the QRS complex in assessing left ventricular ejection fraction. Am J Cardiol 41:494, 1978.
115. Selvester, RH, Kalaba, R, Collier, CR, et al: A digital computer model of the vectorcardiogram with distance and boundary effects: Simulated myocardial infarction. Am Heart J 74:792, 1967.
116. Palmeri, ST, Harrison, DG, Cobb, FR, et al: A QRS scoring system for assessing left ventricular function after myocardial infarction. N Engl J Med 306:4, 1982.
117. Seino, Y, Staniloff, HM, Shell, WE, et al: Evaluation of a QRS scoring system in acute myocardial infarction: Relation to infarct size, early stage left ventricular ejection fraction, and exercise performance. Am J Cardiol 52:37, 1983.
118. Roubin, GS, Shen, WF, Kelly, DT, et al: The QRS scoring system for estimating myocardial infarct size: Clinical, angiographic and prognostic correlations. J Am Coll Cardiol 2:38, 1983.
119. Jones, MG, Ramo, BW, Raff, GL, et al: Evaluation of methods of measurement and estimation of left ventricular function after acute myocardial infarction. Am J Cardiol 56:753, 1985.
120. Fioretti, P, Brower, RW, Lazzeroni, E, et al: Limitations of a QRS scoring system to assess left ventricular function and prognosis at hospital discharge after myocardial infarction. Br Heart J 53:248, 1985.
121. Handler, CE, Ellam, SV, Maisey, MN, et al: Use of an exercise QRS score and radionuclide left ventricular ejection fraction in assessing prognosis after myocardial infarction. Eur Heart J 8:243, 1987.
122. Moss, AJ, Bigger, JT, and Odoroff, CL: Postinfarct risk stratification. Prog Cardiovasc Dis 29:389, 1987.
123. Fioretti, P, Tijssen, JGP, Azar, AJ, et al: Prognostic value of predischarge 12 lead electrocardiogram after myocardial infarction compared to other routine clinical variables. Br Heart J 57:306, 1987.

124. Weissler, AM, O'Neill, WW, Sohn, YH, et al: The prognostic significance of systolic time intervals after recovery from myocardial infarction. Am J Cardiol 37:787, 1976.
125. Brubakk, O, Pedersen, TR, and Overskeid, K: Noninvasive evaluation of the effect of timolol on left ventricular performance after myocardial infarction and the consequence for prognosis. J Am Coll Cardiol 9:155, 1987.
126. Chiang, B, Perlman, L, Ostrander, L, et al: Relationship of premature systoles to coronary heart disease and sudden death in the Tecumseh epidemiologic study. Ann Intern Med 70:1159, 1969.
127. Coronary Drug Project Research Group: Prognostic importance of premature beats following myocardial infarction. JAMA 223:1116, 1973.
128. Davis, HT, DeCamilla, J, Bayer, LW, et al: Survivorship patterns in the posthospital phase of myocardial infarction. Circulation 60:1252, 1979.
129. Ruberman, W, Weinblatt, E, Goldberg, JD, et al: Ventricular premature complexes and sudden death after myocardial infarction. Circulation 64:297, 1981.
130. Moss, AJ, Davis, HT, DeCamilla, J, et al: Ventricular ectopic beats and their relation to sudden and nonsudden cardiac death after myocardial infarction. Circulation 60:998, 1979.
131. Kostis, JB, Byington, R, Friedman, LM, et al: Prognostic significance of ventricular ectopic activity in survivors of acute myocardial infarction. J Am Coll Cardiol 10:231, 1987.
132. Denniss, AR, Richards, DA, Cody, DV, et al: Prognostic significance of ventricular tachycardia and fibrillation induced at programmed stimulation and delayed potentials detected on the signal-averaged electrocardiograms of survivors of acute myocardial infarction. Circulation 74:731, 1986.
133. Waspe, LE, Seinfeld, D, Ferrick, A, et al: Prediction of sudden death and spontaneous ventricular tachycardia in survivors of complicated myocardial infarction: Value of the response to programmed stimulation using a maximum of three ventricular extrastimuli. J Am Coll Cardiol 5:1292, 1985.
134. Roy, D, Marchand, E, Theroux, P, et al: Programmed ventricular stimulation in survivors of an acute myocardial infarction. Circulation 72:487, 1985.
135. Breithardt, G, Borggrefe, M, and Haerten, K: Role of programmed ventricular stimulation and noninvasive recording of ventricular late potentials for the identification of patients at risk of ventricular tachyarrhythmias after acute myocardial infarction. In Zipes, DP and Jalife, J (eds): Cardiac Electrophysiology and Arrhythmias. Grune & Stratton, Orlando, 1985, pp 553.
136. Marchlinski, FE, Buxton, AE, Waxman HL, et al: Identifying patients at risk of sudden death after myocardial infarction: Value of the response to programmed stimulation, degree of ventricular ectopic activity and severity of left ventricular dysfunction. Am J Cardiol 52:1190, 1983.
137. Hamer, A, Vohra, J, Hunt, D, et al: Prediction of sudden death by electrophysiologic studies in high risk patients surviving acute myocardial infarction. Am J Cardiol 50:223, 1982.
138. Richards, DA, Cody, DV, Denniss, AR, et al: Ventricular electrical instability: A predictor of death after myocardial infarction. Am J Cardiol 51:75, 1983.
139. Kuck, KH, Costard, A, Schluter, M, et al: Significance of timing of programmed electrical stimulation after acute myocardial infarction. J Am Coll Cardiol 8:1279, 1986.
140. Klein, H, Trappe, HJ, Hartwig, CA, et al: Repeated programmed stimulation within the first year after myocardial infarction. Circulation 72:III-477, 1985.
141. Simson, MB: Use of signals in the terminal QRS complex to identify patients with ventricular tachycardia after myocardial infarction. Circulation 64:235, 1981.
142. Simson, MB, Untereker, WJ, Speilman, ST, et al: The relationship between late potentials on the body surface and directly recorded fragmented electrograms in patients with ventricular tachycardia. Am J Cardiol 51:105, 1983.
143. Kuchar, DL, Thorburn, CW, and Sammel, NL: Late potentials detected after myocardial infarction: Natural history and prognostic significance. Circulation 74:1280, 1986.
144. Gomes, JAC, Barreca, P, Horowitz, S, et al: Signal averaging of the QRS complex in myocardial infarction: Relationship between ejection fraction and wall motion abnormalities (abstr). Circulation 72(Suppl III):III-212, 1985.
145. Kuchar, DL, Thorburn, CW, and Sammel, NL: Prediction of serious arrhythmic events after myocardial infarction: Signal-averaged electrocardiogram, Holter monitoring and radionuclide ventriculography. J Am Coll Cardiol 9:531, 1987.
146. Gomes, JA, Winters, SL, Steward, D, et al: A new noninvasive index to predict sustained ventricular tachycardia and sudden death in the first year after myocardial infarction: Based on signal-averaged electrocardiogram, radionuclide ejection fraction and Holter monitoring. J Am Coll Cardiol 10:349, 1987.

147. Kanovsky, MS, Falcone, RA, Dresden, CA, et al: Identification of patients with ventricular tachycardia after myocardial infarction: Signal-averaged electrocardiogram, Holter monitoring, and cardiac catheterization. Circulation 70:264, 1984.
148. Gottlieb, SO, Gottlieb, SH, Achuff, SC, et al: Silent ischemia on Holter monitoring predicts mortality in high-risk postinfarction patients. JAMA 259:1030, 1988.
149. Torkelson, LO: Rehabilitation of the patient with acute myocardial infarction. J Chronic Dis 17:685, 1964.
150. Kentala, E: Discrimination between subsequent sudden and nonsudden death of post infarction exercise testing. Scand J Rehabil Med 8:73, 1976.
151. Atterhog, JH, Ekelund, LG, and Kaijser, L: Electrocardiographic abnormalities during exercise 3 weeks to 18 months after anterior myocardial infarction. Br Heart J 33:871, 1971.
152. Granath, A, Sodermark, T, Winge, T, et al: Early work load tests for evaluation of long-term prognosis of acute myocardial infarction. Br Heart J 39:758, 1977.
153. DeBusk, RF, Valdez, R, Houston, N, et al: Cardiovascular responses to dynamic and static effort soon after myocardial infarction. Circulation 58:368, 1978.
154. Starling, MR, Crawford, MH, and O'Rourke, RA: Superiority of selected treadmill exercise protocols pre-discharge and six weeks post infarction for detecting ischemic abnormalities. Am Heart J 104:1054, 1982.
155. Davidson, DM and DeBusk, RF: Prognostic value of a single exercise test 3 weeks after uncomplicated myocardial infarction. Circulation 61:236, 1980.
156. DeBusk, RF and Haskell, W: Symptom-limited versus heart-rate-limited exercise testing soon after myocardial infarction. Circulation 61:738, 1980.
157. Goldschlager, N: Is an exercise electrocardiographic study useful and safe in the early post myocardial period? Cardiovasc Clin 13:113, 1983.
158. Weld, FM, Chu, K, Bigger, JT, et al: Risk stratification with low-level exercise testing 2 weeks after acute myocardial infarction. Circulation 64:306, 1981.
159. Akhras, F, Upward, J, Keates, J, et al: Early exercise testing and elective coronary artery bypass surgery after uncomplicated myocardial infarction. Effect on morbidity and mortality. Br Heart J 52:413, 1984.
160. Krone, RJ, Gillespie, JA, Weld, FM, et al: Low-level exercise testing after myocardial infarction: Usefulness in enhancing clinical risk stratification. Circulation 71:80, 1985.
161. Stone, PH, Turi, ZG, Muller, JE, et al: Prognostic significance of the treadmill exercise test performance 6 months after myocardial infarction. J Am Coll Cardiol 8:1007, 1986.
162. Koppes, GM, Kruyer, W, Beckmann, CH, et al: Response to exercise early after uncomplicated acute myocardial infarction in patients receiving no medication: Long-term follow-up. Am J Cardiol 46:764, 1980.
163. DeBusk, RF, Kraemer, HC, and Nash, E: Stepwise risk stratification soon after acute myocardial infarction. Am J Cardiol 52:1161, 1983.
164. Madsen, EB and Gilpin, E: How much prognostic information do exercise test data add to clinical data after acute myocardial infarction? Int J Cardiol 4:15, 1983.
165. Fioretti, P, Brower, RW, Simoons, ML, et al: Prediction of mortality during the first year after acute myocardial infarction from clinical variables and stress test at hospital discharge. Am J Cardiol 55:1313, 1985.
166. Murray, DP, Salih, M, Tan, LB, et al: Prognostic stratification of patients after myocardial infarction. Br Heart J 57:313, 1987.
167. Sullivan, ID, Davies, DW, and Sowton, E: Submaximal exercise testing early after myocardial infarction. Prognostic importance of exercise induced ST segment elevation. Br Heart J 52:147, 1984.
168. Jennings, K, Reid, DS, Hawkins, T, et al: Role of exercise testing early after myocardial infarction in identifying candidates for coronary surgery. Br Med J 288:185, 1984.
169. Williams, WL, Nair, RC, Higginson, LA, et al: Comparison of clinical and treadmill variables for the prediction of outcome after myocardial infarction. J Am Coll Cardiol 4:477, 1984.
170. Madsen, EB, Gilpin, E, and Henning, H: Evaluation of prognosis one year after myocardial infarction. J Am Coll Cardiol 1:985, 1983.
171. Jelinek, VM, McDonald, IG, Ryan, WF, et al: Assessment of cardiac risk ten days after uncomplicated myocardial infarction. Br Med J 284:227, 1982.
172. Lindvall, K and Kaijser, L: Early exercise tests after uncomplicated acute myocardial infarction before early discharge from hospital. Acta Med Scand 210:257, 1981.

173. Sami, M, Kraemer, H, and DeBusk, RF: The prognostic significance of serial exercise testing after myocardial infarction. Circulation 60:1238, 1979.
174. Smith, JW, Dennis, CA, Gassman, A, et al: Exercise testing three weeks after myocardial infarction. Chest 75:12, 1979.
175. Theroux, P, Waters, DD, Halphen, C, et al: Prognostic value of exercise testing soon after myocardial infarction. N Engl J Med 301:341, 1979.
176. Starling, MR, Crawford, MH, Kennedy, GT, et al: Exercise testing early after myocardial infarction: Predictive value for subsequent unstable angina and death. Am J Cardiol 46:900, 1980.
177. Handler, CE and Sowton, E: Diurnal variation and reproducibility of pre-discharge submaximal exercise testing after myocardial infarction. Br Heart J 52:299, 1984.
178. Bruce, RA, Fisher, LD, Pettinger, M, et al: ST segment elevation with exercise: A marker for poor ventricular function and poor prognosis. Circulation 77:897, 1988.
179. Velasco, J, Tormo, V, Ferrer, LM, et al: Early exercise test for evaluation of long-term prognosis after uncomplicated myocardial infarction. Eur Heart J 22:401, 1981.
180. Becker, LC, Silverman, KJ, Bulkley, BH, et al: Comparison of early thallium-201 scintigraphy and gated blood pool imaging for predicting mortality in patients with acute myocardial infarction. Circulation 67:1272, 1983.
181. Gibson, RS, Taylor, GJ, Watson, DD, et al: Predicting the extent and location of coronary artery disease during the early postinfarction period by quantitative thallium-201 scintigraphy. Am J Cardiol 47:1010, 1981.
182. Gibson, RS, Watson, DD, Craddock, GB, et al: Prediction of cardiac events after uncomplicated myocardial infarction: A prospective study comparing predischarge exercise thallium-201 scintigraphy and coronary angiography. Circulation 68:321, 1983.
183. Turner, JD, Schwartz, KM, Logic, JR, et al: Detection of residual jeopardized myocardium 3 weeks after myocardial infarction by exercise testing with thallium-201 myocardial scintigraphy. Circulation 61:729, 1980.
184. Patterson, RE, Horowitz, SF, Eng, C, et al: Can noninvasive exercise test criteria identify patients with left main or 3-vessel coronary disease after a first myocardial infarction. Am J Cardiol 51:361, 1983.
185. Dunn, RF, Freedman, B, Bailey, IK, et al: Noninvasive prediction of multivessel disease after myocardial infarction. Circulation 62:726, 1980.
186. Abraham, RD, Freedman, SB, Dunn, RF, et al: Prediction of multivessel coronary artery disease and prognosis early after acute myocardial infarction by exercise electrocardiography and thallium-201 myocardial perfusion scanning. Am J Cardiol 58:423, 1986.
187. Leppo, JA, O'Brien, J, Rothendler, JA, et al: Dipyridamole-thallium-201 scintigraphy in the prediction of future cardiac events after acute myocardial infarction. N Engl J Med 310:1014, 1984.

Index

An "F" following a page number indicates a figure. A "T" following a page number indicates a table.